The Sociology of Healthcare

Second edition

Alan Clarke

Aberystwyth Univers.

Longman
is an imprint of

Harlow, England • London • Nev
Tokyo • Seoul • Taipei • New Del

7.doc   v:18052005   geggro

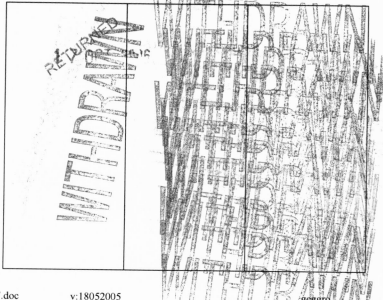

2013 → Truro

Pearson Education Limited
Edinburgh Gate
Harlow
Essex CM20 2JE
England

and Associated Companies throughout the world

Visit us on the World Wide Web at:
www.pearsoned.co.uk

First published 2001
Second edition published 2010

© Pearson Education Limited 2001, 2010

ISBN: 978-1-4058-5849-6

British Library Cataloguing-in-Publication Data
A catalogue record for this book is available from the British Library

Library of Congress Cataloging-in-Publication Data
Clarke, Alan, 1951–
    The sociology of healthcare / Alan Clarke. — 2nd ed.
       p. cm.
    Includes bibliographical references and index.
    ISBN 978-1-4058-5849-6 (pbk.)
1. Social medicine. I. Title.
    RA418.C632 2010
    362.1—dc22

                                        2009049034

10 9 8 7 6 5 4 3 2 1
14 13 12 11 10

Typeset in 10/12.5pt Sabon by 35
Printed in Great Britain by Henry Ling Ltd., at the Dorset Press, Dorchester, Dorset

The publisher's policy is to use paper manufactured from sustainable forests.

Brief contents

Contents

Acknowledgements

I would like to thank Andrew Taylor for his consistent and enthusiastic support throughout the time it took to complete this revised edition of the book. Many thanks are also extended to all those people who have contributed in some way to steering the manuscript through the editorial process, especially Sally Boyles, Philippa Fiszzon and Catherine Morrissey. I am deeply and forever grateful to Sarah for helping to sustain me with her tireless support, insightful comments and cold cups of tea, which she provided in great quantities throughout the preparation of the final manuscript. Equally deserving of mention are Alex (for promptly responding to my requests for help when the 'pooter' crashed), Tom (for his football match reports) and Tom, aka 'Mr Bond', (for making me laugh). Needless to say, none of the above should be blamed for any of the book's deficiencies, for which I take sole responsibility.

Publisher's acknowledgements

We are grateful to the following for permission to reproduce copyright material:

Figures

Figure 3.1 from *Mental Health Matters: A Reader*, Palgrave Macmillan (Tom Heller, Jill Reynolds, Roger Gomm, Rosemary Muston and Stephen Pattison (eds) 2000), reproduced with permission of Palgrave Macmillan; Figure 4.1 from Infant and perinatal mortality 2006: Health areas, England and Wales *Health Statistics Quarterly*, 35, p. ii (2007), Office for National Statistics, web supplement, http://www.statistics.gov.uk/downloads/theme_health/Infant_and_perinatal_report_HSQ35.pdf, Crown Copyright material is reproduced with the permission of the Controller, Office of Public Sector Information (OPSI); Figure 4.2 from *Health Statistics Quarterly*, 34, Summer, p. ii (2007), Web Supplement, http://www.statistics.gov.uk/downloads/theme_health/Death_registration_2006.pdf, Crown Copyright material is reproduced with the permission of the Controller, Office of Public Sector Information (OPSI); Figure 4.3 from http://www.statistics.gov.uk/cci/nugget.asp?id=1899, Crown Copyright material is reproduced with the permission of the Controller, Office of Public Sector Information (OPSI); Figure 4.4 from General Household Survey (2005) Table 7.5, reproduced at http://www.wmpho.org.uk/resources/MPHMM09.pdf as Figure 9.3, Crown Copyright material is reproduced with the permission of the Controller, Office of Public Sector Information (OPSI); Figure 4.5 from The Poverty Site, www.poverty.org.uk (the Figure uses data from the General Household Survey, Office for National Statistics); Figure 4.6 from Office for National Statistics (2006) http://www.statistics.gov.uk/cci/nugget.asp?id=1657, Crown Copyright material is reproduced with the permission of the Controller, Office of Public Sector Information (OPSI); Figure 5.1 from '"Off school sick": mothers' accounts of school sickness', *Sociological Review*, 36, 4, p. 775 (Prout, A. 1988), Wiley-Blackwell; Figure 5.2 from Harris, J. (2001) The effects of computer games on young children: a review of the research, RDS Occasional Paper No. 72, London: Home Office, Figure 4.1, p. 13), http://www.homeoffice.gov.uk/rds/pdfs/occ72-compgames.pdf, Crown Copyright material is reproduced with permission under the terms of the Click-Use Licence; Figure 5.3 from Green, H., McGinnity, A., Meltzer, H., Ford, T. and Goodman, R. (2005) Mental Health of Children and Young People in Great Britain, 2004, Norwich: Palgrave Macmillan/HMSO (Figure 4.1, p. 24), Crown Copyright material is reproduced with permission under the terms of the Click-Use Licence; Figure 5.4 from Green, H., McGinnity, A., Meltzer, H., Ford, T. and Goodman, R. (2005) Mental Health of Children and Young People in Great Britain, 2004, Norwich: Palgrave Macmillan/HMSO, p. 31, Crown Copyright material is reproduced with permission under the terms of the Click-Use Licence; Figure 6.1 from *Social Trends* No. 37, p. 3 (2007), Office for National Statistics/Palgrave Macmillan, Crown Copyright material is reproduced with the permission of the Controller, Office of Public Sector Information (OPSI); Figure 8.1 from *Social Trends* No. 38, p. 20 (2008), Office for National Statistics/Palgrave Macmillan (reproduction of Figure 2.8), Crown Copyright material is reproduced with the permission of the Controller, Office of Public Sector Information (OPSI); Figure 10.1 from Beattie, A. (1991) 'Knowledge and control in health promotion: a test case for social policy and social theory', in J. Gabe, M. Calnan and M. Bury (eds.) *The Sociology of the Health Service*, Routledge (p. 167).

Tables

Table 2.1 from Philo, G., Secker, J., Platt, S., Henderson, L., McLaughlin, G. and Burnside, J., 'Media images of mental distress', p. 165, in Tom Heller, Jill Reynolds, Roger Gomm, Rosemary Muston and Stephen Pattison (eds), *Mental Health Matters: A Reader*, published 1996, Palgrave Macmillan in association with the Open University, reproduced with permission of Palgrave Macmillan; Table 3.1 from Brown, G. W. 'Life events, loss and depressive disorders', p. 37, in Tom Heller, Jill Reynolds, Roger Gomm, Rosemary Muston and Stephen Pattison (eds), *Mental Health Matters: A Reader*, published 1996, Palgrave Macmillan in association with the Open University, reproduced with permission of Palgrave Macmillan; Table 4.1 from Parliamentary Office of Science and Technology (2006) Healthy Life Expectancy, Postnote, February, No. 257, p. 1. Also available at: http://www.parliament.uk/documents/upload/postpn257.pdf., Crown Copyright material is reproduced with permission under the terms of the Click-Use Licence; Table 4.2 compiled using data from News Release, Office for National

Statistics, 24 October 2007, also available at: http://www.statistics.gov.uk/pdfdir/le1007.pdf, Crown Copyright material is reproduced with the permission of the Controller, Office of Public Sector Information (OPSI); Table 4.3 from *Social Trends* No. 37, p. 90 (2007), Office for National Statistics/Palgrave Macmillan, Crown Copyright material is reproduced with the permission of the Controller, Office of Public Sector Information (OPSI); Table 4.4 compiled using data from 'Social inequalities in male mortality for selected causes of death by the National Statistics Socio-economic Classification, England and Wales, 2001–2003' *Health Statistics Quarterly*, 38, p. 19–32 (White, C., Edgar, G. and Siegler, V. 2008), Crown Copyright material is reproduced with the permission of the Controller, Office of Public Sector Information (OPSI); Table 4.5 from National Statistics Online (2008) Standardised Mortality Ratios for Wards in England and Wales, 1999–2003, http://www.statistics.gov.uk/statbase/Product.asp?vlnk=14359., Crown Copyright material is reproduced with the permission of the Controller, Office of Public Sector Information (OPSI); Table 4.6 from Data from Infant Feeding Survey, http://www.statistics.gov.uk/STATBASE/ssdataset.asp?vlnk=5231, Crown Copyright material is reproduced with the permission of the Controller, Office of Public Sector Information (OPSI); Table 4.7 from *Social Trends*, 37, p. 89 (2007), Office for National Statistics/Palgrave Macmillan, Crown Copyright material is reproduced with the permission of the Controller, Office of Public Sector Information (OPSI); Table 4.8 adapted from *Health Statistics Quarterly*, 36, Winter, p. 87 (2007) (Table 4), Crown Copyright material is reproduced with the permission of the Controller, Office of Public Sector Information (OPSI); Table 6.1 adapted from *Social Trends* No. 37, p. 4 (2007) (adapted from Table 1.4) Office for National Statistics/Palgrave Macmillan, Crown Copyright material is reproduced with the permission of the Controller, Office of Public Sector Information (OPSI); Table 8.1 from *Social Trends* No. 39, p. 16 (2009) (Table 2.5) Office for National Statistics/Palgrave Macmillan, Crown Copyright material is reproduced with the permission of the Controller, Office of Public Sector Information (OPSI).

Text

Box 4.3 from 'Social inequalities in male mortality for selected causes of death by the National Statistics Socio-economic Classification, England and Wales, 2001–2003' *Health Statistics Quarterly*, 38, p. 20 (White, C., Edgar, G. and Siegler, V. 2008), Crown Copyright material is reproduced with the permission of the Controller, Office of Public Sector Information (OPSI); Box 5.5 from Layard, R. and Dunn, J. (2009) *A Good Childhood: Searching for Values in a Competitive Age*, © The Children's Society 2009; Box 5.7 from Department for Education and Skills (2001) Promoting Children's Mental Health within Early Years and School Settings, Nottingham: DfES Publications, p. 4, Crown Copyright material is reproduced with permission under the terms of the Click-Use Licence; Box 5.8 from Department for Education and Skills (2001) Promoting Children's Mental Health within Early Years and School Settings, Nottingham: DfES Publications, pp. 5–6, Crown Copyright material is reproduced with permission under the terms of the Click-Use Licence; Box 5.9 adapted from Reproduction of Box 1 in Department for Education and Skills (2004) Every Child Matters: Change for Children, Nottingham: DfES Publications, p. 9, Crown Copyright material is reproduced with permission under the terms of the Click-Use Licence; Box 7.2 from Walter, T. (1996) 'Facing death without tradition', in Glennys Howarth and Peter Jupp (eds), *Contemporary Issues in the Sociology of Death, Dying and Disposal*, p. 195, published 1996, Palgrave Macmillan, reproduced with permission of Palgrave Macmillan; Box 7.9 from 'Dying well: nurses' experiences of "good and bad" deaths', *Journal of Advanced Nursing*, 54, 5, p. 598 (Costello, J. 2006) (Table 1), Wiley-Blackwell; Box 7.10 from 'Dying well: nurses' experiences of "good and bad" deaths', *Journal of Advanced Nursing*, 54, 5, p. 599 (Costello, J. 2006) (Table 2), Wiley-Blackwell; Box 8.6 from Case study, Department of Health (2008) Carers at the heart of 21st-century families and communities, p. 22, Crown Copyright material is reproduced with permission under the terms of the Click-Use Licence; Box 8.7 from Case study, Department of Health (2008) Carers at the heart of 21st-century families and communities, p. 23, Crown Copyright material is reproduced with permission under the terms of the Click-Use Licence; Box 10.3 from Department of Health (2004) Departmental Report 2004, p. 12, Crown Copyright material is reproduced with permission under the terms of the Click-Use Licence; Box 10.4 from Department of Health (2000). The NHS Plan: A Plan for Investment: A Plan for Reform, pp. 3–5, Crown Copyright material is reproduced with permission under the terms of the Click-Use Licence.

In some instances we have been unable to trace the owners of copyright material, and we would appreciate any information that would enable us to do so.

CHAPTER 1

An introduction to the sociology of health and illness

The biomedical model: an introduction and critique

> The dominant disease model is biomedical, with molecular biology as its basic scientific discipline. The biomedical model assumes diseases to be a deviation from the norm of measurable variables, without accounting for the social, psychological and behavioural dimensions of illness.
>
> (Decker, 2005, p. 600)

Health, illness and disease not only are biological and psychological conditions but can also be viewed as *social* states. It is this social dimension that is at the very heart of the sociological study of health and illness. While sociologists acknowledge the importance of biological factors in the aetiology of illness, they are particularly conscious of the pervasive effects of social factors. There is a general perception of health and illness as social products. In other words, people's experiences of health and the incidence of disease are seen as being influenced by the social, economic and cultural characteristics of the society in which they live. As described in Chapter 2, lay definitions of health, illness and disease are embedded in wider socio-cultural contexts and as such are influenced by prevailing social norms and values. These definitions vary across time and place. This also applies in the case of formal medical knowledge, treatment and practice. As will be discussed later in this chapter, some theorists maintain that medical knowledge is subject to the influence of social processes and is not simply the outcome of the objective analysis of scientific 'facts' about the human body and how it works. According to this view, medical knowledge is, in a sense, socially created, the implication being that disease categories are not simply the product of a rigorous scientific analysis of biomedical facts but need to be understood as the creation of a particular set of social, historical and political circumstances.

In order to explore the contention that health, illness and disease are social products, it is perhaps best at the outset to clarify what actually serves to distinguish the Western medical or biomedical model from what has been described as a 'social' (Morgan *et al.*, 1985) or 'sociological' (Turner, 1987) model of medicine. In general, not only has it been observed that the biomedical model forms a contrast to the social model but, as Nettleton notes, 'Many of the central concerns of the sociology of health and illness have emerged as reactions to, and critiques of, this paradigm' (1995, p. 2).

The biomedical model is the dominant model in contemporary medicine and the medical explanations that it provides are based on a number of basic assumptions about the functioning of the human body and the nature of disease. A central distinguishing feature of the model is the way in which it assumes the existence of a dichotomy between mind and body in the conceptualisation of disease. This is referred to as 'mind–body dualism'. The causal agent of illness is identified as being located within the body; hence emphasis is placed on the organic appearances of disease. The body, as the physical site of disease, is the object of treatment and is studied in isolation. Illness itself is perceived as a breakdown in the biochemical or neurophysiological functioning of the body, which essentially means that the relevance of social and psychological factors is overlooked or ignored. It is this expressed belief in the exclusive nature of biomedical explanations of illness and disease that leaves the medical model open to the charge of physical reductionism (Freund and McGuire, 1991, p. 6).

A second assumption characteristic of the medical model, referred to as the 'doctrine of specific aetiology' (Dubos, 1995), is that a specific disease always has a specific cause. As Hart notes, 'This doctrine has been the most influential force in medical research for over a century. It implies that the way to understand disease is to create it in the laboratory and that the ingredients for explanation are found through minute observation of its bio-chemical appearances. In other words, it proposes that the symptoms of disease tell their own story' (1985, pp. 534–5). The idea of specific aetiology emanates from the nineteenth century, when germ theory emerged to account for the causation of infectious diseases. According to this explanation, illness occurs as a result of the human body being invaded by disease-laden micro-organisms, viruses or other causative agents. The different agents produce specific pathological manifestations. The task facing curative medicine is to identify and eradicate the various causal agents and restore the individual body to a healthy, disease-free state.

In portraying disease as the consequence of the malfunctioning of the human body, the medical model adopts a mechanical metaphor as an explanatory device. The body of the sick person is likened to a malfunctioning machine in need of repair. As Freund and McGuire assert, 'Modern medicine has not only retained the metaphor of the machine but also extended it by developing specializations along the lines of machine parts, emphasizing individual systems or organs to the exclusion of the totality of the body' (1991, p. 227). In other words, individual parts of the body can be subjected to treatment without the rest of the body being affected. The doctor is cast in the role of a 'body mechanic' (Hart, 1985, p. 532) working to restore normal functioning to an organism's biochemical system.

The biomedical model is at the heart of modern scientific medicine. Despite having undergone some changes in the light of advances in medical knowledge following the introduction of new medical technologies, many of the fundamental assumptions on which the model is based still find support today. Down the years the medical model, with its emphasis on scientific investigation and explanation, has come to displace or profoundly influence culturally derived belief systems surrounding health, illness and disease. In this regard it has been noted that

> The historical fact we have to face is that in modern Western society biomedicine not only has provided a basis for the scientific study of disease, it has also become our own culturally specific perspective about disease, that is, our folk model. Indeed the biomedical model is now the dominant folk model of disease in the Western world.
>
> (Engel, 1977, p. 130)

For Engel, the medical model has not only become a 'cultural imperative' but also acquired the status of dogma.

The traditional medical model has been the subject of much critical attention. This has come not only from supporters of alternative medical therapies that challenge orthodox biomedical practice, and social scientists engaged in the study of the organisation and delivery of medical care, but also from critiques of the biomedical approach that have emerged from within the medical profession itself. In essence, the stance taken by the various critics can be broadly labelled as essentially either 'pragmatic' or 'fundamental' in nature (Morgan *et al.*, 1985, p. 14). Those who take a pragmatic approach accept in principle the biomedical model of disease but consider that, on the whole, the medical model falls short of providing a full account of the aetiology of disease. In particular, it is claimed that too much emphasis is placed on biochemical processes and insufficient consideration given to the causal significance of social and psychological factors. In marked contrast, critics who adopt a fundamental position challenge the basic assumptions and definitions characteristic of the medical model. For them, medical concepts of disease are not viewed as simply the natural outcome of the application of objective methods of scientific discovery to the study of the human body; there is an important social dimension to the creation of medical knowledge that must not be overlooked. As will be discussed later in this chapter, critics who subscribe to the idea that medical knowledge is socially constructed see medicine as a form of *social* practice and the application of medical labels to physical and mental conditions as the product of social processes.

Despite its dominance the biomedical model does have a number of limitations, particularly when it comes to explaining the role of medicine in improving the health of the population and accounting for the social distribution of health and illness. Firstly, historical research questions the validity of the biomedical model by suggesting that the contribution of medical intervention to the decline in mortality rates from the mid-nineteenth century through to the early decades of the twentieth century has been overstated. For example, McKeown (1976) illustrates how the death rate from respiratory tuberculosis showed a substantial decline well before the introduction of effective medical treatment in the form of antibiotics and the BCG vaccination. Furthermore, with reference to infectious diseases in general, he maintains that improvements in nutrition and hygiene were primarily responsible for the observed decline in mortality from around the middle of the nineteenth century.

Secondly, as a result of its inherent biological determinism, the medical model does not address the relationship between social conditions, such as material deprivation, and poor health. As Nettleton observes, 'The sociology of health and illness has repeatedly demonstrated that health and disease are socially patterned' (1995, pp. 5–6). Variations in mortality and morbidity rates between different socio-economic groups cannot be explained by reference to biological factors alone. As described in Chapter 4, lifestyle and material circumstances are important and these can vary according to non-biological factors such as social class position, ethnic status and gender.

A further shortcoming of the medical model stems from the assumption that there is a clear distinction between the mind and the body. As noted above, this mind–body dualism ensures that an instrumentalist approach is adopted towards the human body. In concentrating on the body as a discrete physical entity the medical model focuses on treating the disease as opposed to the whole person. Adopting an exclusively biomedical framework effectively results in social and psychological factors being ignored. As an alternative to the biomedical model, Engel advocates a 'biopsychosocial model which includes the patient as well as the illness' (1977, p. 133). He stresses the importance of taking the social context in which the patient lives into account. This is not only because psycho-social factors have a role in disease causation but also because, although biochemical abnormalities determine the form a disease takes, it is social and psychological factors that largely determine whether a person suffering from a biochemical dysfunction seeks medical help and adopts the sick role. The importance of structural and cultural elements in the formulation of lay people's definitions of health and illness and the significance of the concept of the sick role in explaining patients' illness behaviour are explored in Chapter 2.

Not only is the body isolated from the person in the medical model but, as described above, it is also depicted as a highly complex biochemical 'machine' whose constituent parts can malfunction or break down. The use of the machine metaphor encourages an interventionist view of medical practice in which doctors are seen to use their expert knowledge and technical skill to diagnose the fault and repair the malfunctioning body part. It is perhaps not difficult to appreciate how a machine metaphor can flourish in the world of modern medicine, especially when the scientific model of medicine extols the virtues of clinical detachment and stresses the importance of the need for medical practitioners to function objectively without emotional involvement. Advances in medical technology and the increasing use of highly sophisticated diagnostic and monitoring equipment and devices also create an atmosphere in which the scientific mode of thinking predominates. It is the application of scientific methods and ideas to the practice of medicine that 'encourages the passivity of the patient, for the scientist knows; the patient, not being a scientist, does not know' (Stacey, 1988, pp. 173–4). How this specialist knowledge produces an imbalance of power in the doctor–patient relationship and subsequently leads to the patient being assigned a passive role in the treatment process is addressed in Chapter 9.

All this is not to deny that biomedical science has had a significant impact on the success of clinical medicine in improving health and relieving suffering. However, as outlined above, the main challenge to the dominance of the medical model is directed at the limitations imposed by its conceptual framework. As summarised by Nettleton, 'The body is isolated from the person, the social and material causes of disease are neglected, and the subjective interpretations and meanings of health and illness are deemed irrelevant' (1995, p. 3).

At a conceptual level, Turner illustrates how 'The sociological model of illness takes a critical and opposed position on the biochemical model of disease' (1987, p. 9). It does this by questioning the very assumptions on which the medical model is founded. Firstly, it rejects the notion of the existence of a clear dichotomy between the mind and the body. Secondly, it challenges the reductionist tendency in the medical model by arguing against the idea that illness can be ultimately reduced to disordered bodily functioning. According to the sociological model of illness it is overly simplistic to think of a disease as having one single cause. Many explanations of specific diseases are multi-causal, describing how physical and biological causes interact with social and environmental factors. Finally, a sociological approach holds that the patient needs to be considered as a 'whole person'. Illness can only be fully understood by taking account of the wider social and cultural context in which physical and mental conditions are observed, diagnosed and treated. As Turner asserts, 'The sociological perspective encourages medical professionals to approach the *person* and not the *patient* as the focus of an enquiry into illness' (1987, p. 9, emphasis added). In order to appreciate the potential contribution a sociological focus can make to our understanding of health, illness and healthcare practice we need to know more about the general nature of sociology and its subject matter.

What is sociology?

. . . sociologists try to understand the world in terms of the relationships between people's choices . . . and the structures that constrain and create the decisions and opportunities available to them. Thus, sociology grounds the study of any particular issue in the empirical world, but moves beyond simple reportage. It examines and explains the regularities and differences that are evident in society . . . [and] offers the potential for a more nuanced and sophisticated understanding of the social world and our own life and others' lives.

(Smith and Natalier, 2004, p. 2)

Sociology is a social science discipline that takes a distinct approach to investigating society. According to Stacey, sociology 'constitutes a body of knowledge about societies and social relations within them and takes as its subject matter all areas of the social' (1991, p. 13). As a consequence of this focus on 'the social' all aspects of human life are open to sociological investigation. It is the study of *social* behaviour that is at the very centre of the sociological enterprise. Explanations of behaviour based solely on individual biological factors or psychological processes often only provide us with a partial understanding of why individuals behave the way they do. From the point of view of the sociologist, human beings are essentially social animals and therefore a full understanding of human behaviour cannot be achieved without taking into account aspects of the social setting in which the behaviour occurs. As Lee and Newby assert, 'Sociologists have . . . repeatedly rejected the possibility of the totally isolated, non-social individual' (1983, p. 17). As a field of enquiry, sociology explores the human processes of social interaction through studying the relationship between individuals, groups and social institutions.

Given its subject matter, one often hears sociology referred to as the 'science of society'. This is a claim that has produced considerable controversy. However, before any such claim to scientific status can be properly evaluated we need to know on what basis the claim is made. In other words, it is important that we understand what it is about a discipline that justifies it being labelled a science. We can begin by considering some of the characteristic features of the natural sciences, such as chemistry and physics. Here systematic observation, sometimes under experimental conditions, produces evidence of general regularities in the natural world. In this way a body of scientific knowledge is constructed, the principal aim being to identify cause and effect relationships in order to explain why particular events occur. This leads to the formulation of scientific theories to describe and explain causal relationships. The whole process is a cumulative one, whereby scientific theories build on one another, with the newer theories amending and extending the older ones.

The fundamental features of the discipline of sociology are such that any claim to scientific status based on the model of the natural sciences is problematic. As Giddens observes, 'Studying human beings . . . is different from observing events in the physical world, and neither the logical framework nor the findings of sociology can adequately be understood simply in terms of comparisons with natural science' (1989, p. 22). A number of specific points are worthy of comment in this context. Firstly, practical considerations and ethical objections prevent sociologists making use of one of the main techniques of investigation used by natural scientists, namely controlled experiments. Secondly, fundamental differences in the nature and character of physical and social phenomena are important when it comes to establishing and maintaining objectivity when carrying out research. In many ways it is easier for natural scientists to adopt a morally neutral and scientifically detached position when studying physical objects than it is for social scientists who have the task of investigating aspects of their own society about which they might have strong personal beliefs or ideological convictions. Finally, not only might sociologists find it difficult to be objective in their approach, but it may prove difficult to obtain truly objective data about human behaviour, since in many cases behaviour is tied up with people's feelings and emotions. Human beings, unlike physical objects, have consciousness and attribute meaning to their own actions. While the natural scientist deals with inanimate objects and can only study physical phenomena from the outside, the sociologist studies conscious beings and therefore needs to understand the meaning the observed behaviour has for the actors concerned.

Whereas the biomedical model is disease oriented and concentrates on biological and physiological criteria, the *social model* takes a much broader view, which involves the consideration of an array of social and environmental factors. Basically these two models represent different, although by and large complementary, approaches to our understanding of health and illness. Sociology as a discipline embraces a wide array of theoretical perspectives; it is to a consideration of some of these perspectives that we now turn.

Sociological perspectives

> To talk in terms of *the* sociological perspective as if it were a unified perspective is, however, quite misleading. In fact nothing could be further from the truth because sociology has always been characterized by its multi-perspective constitution. As well as developing as a series of sub-disciplines, it has also developed as a series of different ways of viewing society, each of which offers only a partial perspective on society, one way of seeing among many potential ways.
>
> (Roslender, 1992, p. 6)

As a discipline sociology accommodates a diverse range of theories and analytic traditions, hence the assertion by Lee and Newby, that sociology has an 'untidy face' in so far as 'there has never been a simple unanimity of view on many of the fundamental questions posed by it and the first experience of this can be perplexing in the extreme' (1983, p. 22). The fact that sociology does not offer a single, monolithic approach to the study of social phenomena can be a cause of considerable consternation to the student approaching the discipline for the first time. However, this lack of uniformity should be viewed in positive rather than negative terms. Given the variety, scope and complexity of human social behaviour it is intellectually naïve to expect that there is only one approach capable of providing a definitive understanding of the social world and how it works. The idea that the social world can be viewed from a number of different theoretical perspectives needs to be grasped by the would-be student at the outset. As stated in one introductory textbook:

> . . . sociology as a discipline or subject is basically best understood by stressing that it is made up of a *number* of separate though more or less interlinked approaches. If students are introduced to sociology in terms of its being a single, monolithic approach, with a single set of terms or concepts, a uniform set of theories and a standard collection of unified findings, we feel that they are either being misled or talked down to . . . we prefer to credit students with both the intelligence and desire to encounter the subject as it currently appears – not rounded off and smoothed for the purpose of easy digestion.
>
> (Cuff *et al.*, 1990, p. 2, emphasis in original)

The separate and sometimes interlinked approaches are commonly referred to as sociological perspectives and represent different ways of looking at and trying to understand the social world. Each perspective gives us a different slant on social behaviour and thereby adds to our knowledge of the nature, structure and content of social relationships and patterns of social interaction.

Cuff *et al.* are keen to point out that the sociological enterprise is not an exercise in discovering ultimate 'truths' about the social world by identifying which perspective or combination of perspectives provides the definitive version of events. As they observe, 'Sociological perspectives merely provide us with *ways* of trying to understand the world; none of them has a built-in assurance that eternal and unshakeable "truth" will or can be provided' (1990, p. 2, emphasis in original). In this sense a perspective represents a way of examining a particular social issue or phenomenon and as such cannot simply be judged as being either right or wrong. A perspective provides a framework for the systematic collection and analysis of empirical data about aspects of contemporary social life.

In any intellectual discipline knowledge is there to be contested. Sociologists use recognised research methods and adopt systematic procedures in their pursuit of knowledge about the social world. Thinking sociologically involves a process of applying 'systematic doubt' to all descriptions and explanations of social phenomena, be they based on common-sense assumptions or sociological theorising (Lee and Newby, 1983, p. 20). Irrespective of the topic under investigation, the kind of issues addressed in a particular study will be largely determined by the research interests and theoretical orientation of the sociologist concerned.

It is beyond the scope of the present chapter to offer an overview of the full range of mainstream sociological perspectives. The intention here is to provide a brief introduction to those perspectives that have had a significant impact on the sociological study of aspects of health, illness and the debates surrounding the provision of healthcare.

Structural functionalism

Basically, as a theoretical perspective structural functionalism focuses on the ways in which social life is organised and social order achieved. This approach played an influential role in sociological thinking and research during the middle decades of the twentieth century. One of the major proponents of this school of thought was the American sociologist Talcott Parsons. His primary interest was in providing a general framework of analysis capable of explaining how it is that societies and social systems manage to function as integrated, cohesive and stable social units. His approach to issues of health and illness is very much influenced by his desire to develop a theoretical understanding of how social systems, despite the existence of potential conflicts over norms and values between constituent social groups, establish a social equilibrium and maintain social order.

The central focus of the functionalist approach is on the societal or macroscopic level of social action. In terms of Parsons' general thesis, securing and maintaining social order is dependent on individuals behaving in accordance with the social norms governing proper conduct, while conforming to what are defined as legitimate social roles. Anything that prevents individuals performing their designated roles and fulfilling their social obligations is seen as a potentially disintegrative force as far as the social system is concerned. Thus the incidence of illness constitutes a threat to the smooth running of society if it prevents individuals from fulfilling what are deemed to be their normal social obligations, such as caring for dependent family members and undertaking paid employment.

According to Parsons' analysis, health is functional not only from the point of view of the individual but also from the perspective of society:

> The problem of health is intimately involved in the functional pre-requisites of the social system . . . Certainly by almost any definition health is included in the functional needs of the individual member of the society so that from the point of view of functioning of the social system, too low a general level of health, too high an incidence of illness is dysfunctional.
>
> (Parsons, 1951, p. 430)

It is the *social* nature of illness that dominates the Parsonian model. Illness is conceived as a social phenomenon rather than a physical property of individuals. Parsons' theoretical interest lay not in illness *per se* but in the implications of illness for the social system. Given the potentially disruptive effects of illness at the societal level, it can be viewed in some contexts as a form of 'motivated deviance' that requires some form of social control (Parsons and Fox, 1953).

For Parsons both the sick role and the medical profession have a prominent part to play in the social control of illness. The idea behind mechanisms of social control is that they function to safeguard the stability and cohesion of the social system by discouraging deviant forms of behaviour and promoting conformity to established norms and social practices. From a structural functionalist perspective it is in the general interests of society that those individuals who experience ill health should feel compelled to seek expert help so as to speed up the process of recovery, thus ensuring that they are able to fulfil their normal social responsibilities both at home and at work. One way in which society attempts to exercise control in the case of illness is through the creation of a socially prescribed role for the sick person. Parsons refers to this as the sick role and it has been described as 'one of the most influential concepts in medical sociology' (Morgan *et al.*, 1985, p. 48). The characteristic features of this role are outlined and discussed in Chapter 2. Basically, the sick role controls the disruptive effects of illness in society by specifying the social rights and obligations enjoyed by those who occupy this role. Members of the medical profession control access to the sick role and in this respect the doctor performs an important social control function.

In summary, the functionalist perspective focuses attention on the functional importance of health and illness for society. For Parsons, health is defined in terms of the ability of the individual to carry out normal daily tasks and perform those social roles that contribute to the maintenance of the social system. From a societal perspective there is a link between health and role performance. In other words, a social definition of health involves the concept of functional fitness. As regards illness, this is defined in terms of the incapacity to perform social roles and fulfil social obligations. Given the potential of a high level of ill health to threaten the stability of a social system, illness presents a problem of social control. Parsons saw doctors as the main agents of social control, acting as official gatekeepers governing access to the sick role. He considered they were best placed to perform this control function on account of the expert biomedical knowledge they possessed. Thus despite focusing on social as opposed to biological processes in the study of health and illness, Parsons did not question the dominance of the biomedical model or the power and influence of the medical profession. As Morgan *et al.* conclude, 'functionalism tends to accept the biomedical model as technical and asocial and focuses on its role in reducing the disruptive effects of illness in society' (1985, p. 33).

As a sociological perspective structural functionalism has been heavily criticised because of its inherent conservatism: as illustrated by its tendency to focus on the existing social structure and the problem of maintaining an orderly society, rather than dealing directly with the dynamics of social change. This approach is sometimes referred to as the consensus perspective on account of the fact that it sees society as being held together largely by the existence of a consensus around a set of basic values. In adopting a consensus-oriented approach to the analysis of the structure of society, functionalism overemphasises the role played by social norms and values in producing cohesion and cooperation in social life. Indeed, many critics are of the opinion that the majority of functionalist theorists fail to recognise and acknowledge the importance of the fact that social structures generate social conflict and that coercion and hostility are characteristic features of social life. One group of critics belongs to what may be loosely termed the conflict perspective.

Conflict perspective

Like structural functionalist or consensus theorists, conflict theorists are also concerned with how society as a whole works and in this respect both approaches may be described as 'structuralist' (Cuff *et al.*, 1990, p. 107). Although these two general perspectives share some common features, they differ significantly when it comes to the assumptions they make about the very nature of society and the kind of relationships that exist between its constituent parts or sub-systems. For example, consensus theorists see society as an integrated system of interdependent parts. Major social, educational and cultural institutions are credited with serving the wider function of social integration. It is by contact with these various institutions that individual members of society, through a process of socialisation, come to identify with a common set of rules governing social behaviour. In theory, the adherence to social norms, coupled with the widespread acceptance of common values and social expectations, produces social cohesion, solidarity and harmony. While consensus theorists see society from the point of view of the maintenance of social order and stability, conflict theorists offer a more radical form of analysis. From a conflict perspective the differential distribution of power and authority in society creates important social divisions which give rise to conflict and hostility between social groups. Thus, as far as conflict theorists are concerned, coercion and not consensus provides the key to understanding the workings of modern society.

When it comes to issues of health and illness, conflict theorists, by and large, take a political economy perspective and focus on how the capitalist system influences the social production of health and illness and determines the social organisation of healthcare. In exploring the complex relationship between the capitalistic organisation of the economy and the practice of scientific medicine in contemporary Western societies, a number of influential theorists make use of Marxist concepts and terminology.

A central theme in Marxist approaches to the sociology of health is the way in which the delivery of healthcare is dominated by the *logic of capitalism*, so much so that the healthcare system is viewed as part of the commodity production process. In a critical analysis of the healthcare industry in the USA, McKinley (1977) claims that the character of modern medicine is determined by the interests of capitalists, as is the case with the production of any consumer product. According to the logic of capital accumulation, manufacturers strive to increase output and sales in order to generate ever-increasing profits. Some of this profit is invested in research and development to produce new products. The 'success' of a particular product is judged not necessarily by its use-value but by its ability to attract new buyers and generate profit. Advertising is used not just to protect existing markets but to open up new ones. This creates a commodity-fetishist culture. McKinley claims that this logic of capitalism applies just as much in the case of the provision of goods and services in healthcare as it does to consumer products and household items in general.

For McKinley, capital is the major factor responsible for determining the very nature of medical treatment and healthcare provision. He maintains that this leaves the consumer or patient open to exploitation as the healthcare industry is concerned first and foremost with maximising its profits. Thus, private healthcare providers may be unwilling to invest in treatments that are costly and have a low profit margin. Furthermore, under certain circumstances, doctors may find themselves restricted to choosing alternative forms of treatment that are less effective but more profitable. According to this analysis the emphasis placed on profitability represents a direct threat to the clinical freedom and occupational autonomy enjoyed by the medical profession.

Critics of McKinley's thesis do not deny that healthcare provision is a highly profitable commercial undertaking in the USA, but they do question his assertion that the relentless search for profit is the major factor responsible for determining the medical treatment patients receive. In comparing the American system of healthcare with that found in Britain, where the bulk of the investment in healthcare comes from public funds, Hart observes that 'the character of medicine is much the same in both societies suggesting that the criterion of profitability is not the major determinant of medical knowledge and technique' (Hart, 1985, p. 639). While this is a valid point it does not undermine the value of taking a political economy perspective towards the study of the relationship between the capitalist organisation of the economy and the nature of healthcare provision.

Conflict theorists following in the Marxist tradition see the healthcare system in capitalist society as performing both economic and ideological functions. With reference to the former, the healthcare sector fulfils four major economic functions: it helps to accumulate capital; it offers opportunities for capital investment (e.g. the pharmaceutical industry); it provides employment opportunities and thus helps to absorb any surplus labour; the services it provides help to maintain the health and productivity of the workforce (Rodberg and Stevenson, 1977).

As regards ideological functions, conflict theorists view medicine as an institution of social control operating at the level of ideology. Navarro (1976) refers to the 'medical bureaucracy' as an 'ideological state mechanism' that helps to maintain the stability of society under capitalism. One way in which it exercises this ideological function is by effectively masking the adverse impact of environmental, occupational and social factors on health by dealing with illness as an individual phenomenon. Navarro (1980) claims that the biomedical model, which emphasises the aetiological significance of individual biological factors over social conditions, came to occupy a dominant place in the explanation of ill health on account of the widespread support it received from powerful and influential social groups in capitalist society. As Doyal and Pennell (1979) argue in their discussion of the conceptual features of modern medicine, focusing on individual characteristics and lifestyle factors obscures the part played by environmental conditions in causing illness. Theorists who subscribe to a conflict perspective maintain that the productive forces of capitalism are instrumental in generating illness and disease, but this is overlooked by the perpetuation of an ideology of health that stresses individual responsibility above all else.

The idea that healthcare needs cannot be understood separately from the capitalist mode of production is a central theme in the conflict perspective. The core features of this approach are neatly summarised by Renaud:

> The view of health and illness is congruent with the larger capitalist environment because it commodifies health needs and legitimates this commodification (Caplan, 1989). It transforms the potentially explosive social problems that are diseases and death into discrete isolable commodities that can be incorporated into the capitalist organisation of the economy in the same way as any other commodity on the economic market. In an

incredible tour de force, it succeeds in providing culturally valued solutions to problems largely created by economic growth and even makes these solutions to a certain extent profitable for capital accumulation and thus for more economic growth. With scientific medicine, health care has grown into an industry which helps maintain the legitimacy of the social order and which in part creates new sectors of production.

(Renaud quoted in White, 1991, p. 24)

According to this view 'medicine in capitalist society is capitalist medicine' (Renaud quoted by White, 1991, p. 24). There is no doubt that healthcare provides many lucrative opportunities for capital investment, especially where the introduction of new medical technologies and the development of pharmaceutical products are concerned. Consequently, conflict theorists ask whether the range of medical treatments on offer is a reflection of the 'real needs' of patients or the unremitting pursuit of profit by private sector organisations.

As is clear from the above brief outline of the consensus and conflict perspectives, the Parsonian brand of structural functionalism and contemporary Marxist interpretations of the political economy of health are based on radically different conceptions of the nature of society. Nevertheless, both perspectives view medicine as an institution of social control that contributes to the production of an orderly and stable society. Despite this similarity, however, there is a major difference between the two approaches when it comes to looking at whose interests are actually served by medicine. According to Parsons, health is defined in terms of the ability to perform social roles and good health is identified as a functional prerequisite for a stable society. Therefore, in their efforts to prevent illness, cure sickness and control access to the sick role, the medical profession is seen to be acting in the interests of society as a whole. The social function performed by medicine is viewed very differently from a Marxist-oriented conflict perspective. Here definitions of health and illness are seen as being shaped by the dominant ideology of capitalism. In helping to maintain a healthy, productive labour force the medical profession acts to protect the interests of capital. In short, viewed from a Marxist perspective, it is not so much the general public interest that is served by medicine but the interests of a particular section of society, namely the ruling capitalist class.

All perspectives have their critics and the political economy perspective is no exception. For example, as Hart (1985) notes, the assumption that medicine has had a major impact on improving human health in the first place is open to question. She holds that contrary to Marxist interpretations there is a case for arguing that medicine has actually helped to *reduce* the productivity of the labour force, when she asserts that 'Since 1948, general practitioners have certified an ever increasing volume of "time off" for sickness, suggesting that the NHS has undermined the health of the workforce rather than improved it' (1985, p. 641). As regards the general state of health in capitalist societies, some critics argue that the political economy perspective largely ignores the fact that marked improvements in living standards and life expectancy have coincided with the growth and development of the capitalist system (Reidy, 1984). However, while this may be so, it is still the case that there are inequalities in health between the social classes in affluent capitalist societies. These inequalities are identified and discussed in Chapter 4.

Interpretive perspectives

As noted above, the two perspectives discussed so far can be described as structuralist, in so far as in seeking to explain social behaviour the focus of analysis is firmly on aspects of the nature, structure and organisation of society. The underlying assumption of this macro-level approach is that the societal environment is largely responsible for determining and shaping patterns of human behaviour. The implication is that in order to understand the actions of individual members of society it is necessary to identify the structural forces at work. As described in Chapter 3, some sociologists have focused on particular aspects of social structure, such as social class, in efforts to explain the incidence and prevalence of various forms of mental illness.

Sociologists working within the interpretivist tradition or social action frame of reference are not interested in exploring the macro-level structures of society; they are more concerned with undertaking a micro-level study of the routine activities of individual social actors engaged in face-to-face social interaction. A particularly influential perspective in this tradition is symbolic interactionism, which has had a major impact on sociological research during the last 50 years. At the heart of this perspective is a belief that social action is *meaningful* action: individual actors not only attribute meaning to their own actions but also interpret the actions of other people. As such, individuals do not passively respond to external stimuli but take an active part in making sense of what happens to them and then react in what they consider to be an appropriate manner. In short, human beings are endowed with the capacity for reflexive communication. Consequently, social life constitutes an amalgam of interconnected interactions based on the perceptions and expectations actors have of each other.

A characteristic feature of the interactionist form of enquiry is the emphasis placed on the importance of obtaining the actor's definition of a social situation or set of circumstances.

> Most often sociology tends to take a holistic point of view, describing situations from the standpoint of the society conceived as a whole. By contrast, symbolic interactionists adopt a 'ground level' perspective, seeking to view situations as they appear to those directly involved in them. In so doing they are less interested in asking whether actors' understandings are 'correct' or 'justified' and much more interested in trying to appreciate *how and why* actors perceive things in the ways they do. The researcher tries to avoid making 'external' judgements about the people he or she studies. Instead, he or she tries to describe their circumstances and actions as *they* see them.
>
> (Cuff *et al.*, 1990, pp. 151–2, emphasis in original)

According to symbolic interactionists, meanings are not seen as being determined by cultural norms or social values that are essentially external to the individual, but are, in fact, viewed as the products of actors' intentions and interactions. As described by Blumer (1969), symbolic interactionism focuses on the subjective or symbolic meanings individuals attach to actions, gestures and words. These meanings are not fixed but are modified during the course of social interaction. Social meaning is not something that is inherent in a particular social context or action. Any behaviour or gesture is open to multiple interpretations. In other words, the same act may be interpreted in a number of different ways; it may hold different meanings for different people. Its meaning may also change from one context to another. Consequently, interactionists endeavour to locate meaningful social action in its social context.

The concept of the *self* has a central place in the symbolic interactionist paradigm. According to the teachings of Mead (1934), during the course of social interaction, by coming to see themselves as others see them, individuals develop a sense of self or a self-consciousness. It is through this process of interaction that the individual ultimately acquires a social identity. Interactionists who adopt a labelling perspective focus on how deviant identities can be produced when individuals with specific physical or mental health problems are assigned to certain social categories. This perspective is covered in some depth in Chapters 2 and 3. In Chapter 2 the implications of the labelling process for the study of illness behaviour are discussed. For example, the role of diagnostic labels in creating deviant or stigmatising social identities is examined, with special reference to epilepsy, AIDS (acquired immunodeficiency syndrome) and mental illness. The contribution of the labelling perspective to the study of mental illness is further explored in Chapter 3.

In general, social research from an interpretive perspective, with its emphasis on human beings as creative social actors, has helped to improve our understanding of what happens to people once they become patients. First of all, as noted in later chapters, there is a wealth of research literature devoted to the study of subjective experiences of illness. This research not only addresses the personal and social problems experienced by chronically sick and disabled people but also describes how they develop coping strategies for managing a spoiled social identity that results from negative public stereotypes and adverse societal reaction. Secondly, by focusing on face-to-face social encounters, research in the interpretive tradition has provided a useful insight into the nature and organisation of social interaction in both formal and informal healthcare settings. Some of the interactional work undertaken by doctors, nurses and patients in a variety of medical and clinical contexts is described in Chapter 8.

Whereas symbolic interactionists concentrate on aspects of people's actions in order to understand human behaviour in different social contexts, functionalist and conflict theorists focus on the wider social structure when constructing theories of society. By focusing on face-to-face interaction and adopting what might be termed a micro-level, as opposed to a macro-level, approach, symbolic interactionism is accused of grossly underestimating or failing to acknowledge the impact of structural forces on behaviour. However, as Cuff *et al.* (1990) observe, interactionist principles have become a part of mainstream sociology and have successfully permeated a number of different theoretical perspectives. Indeed, there are examples of research studies in which macro-level and micro-level approaches are combined in a single analysis. A good example from the sociology of health and illness is Waitzkin's (1989) study of the doctor–patient relationship. In outlining the functional role of medicine in capitalist society he describes how, in terms of the macro-structures of society, medical practice is influenced and shaped by ideological, political and economic factors. For example, he argues that, by associating health with economic productivity, the medical profession effectively reinforces the value system and social relations characteristic of the capitalist class structure. At the level of the micro-politics of social interaction, Waitzkin describes how doctor–patient consultations are conducted in such a way that the health problems patients present are dealt with as discrete scientific or medical issues. 'In medical encounters, technical statements help direct patients' responses to objectified symptoms, signs and treatment. This reification shifts attention away from the totality of social relations and the social issues that are often root causes of personal troubles' (Waitzkin, 1989, p. 223).

Symbolic interactionism is not the only interpretive perspective to take a subjective view of the social world in attempting to discover the meanings and intentions of actors. Ethnomethodology also portrays social reality as the product of a continual process of social interaction during the course of which individuals establish some form of meaningful communication with one another. However, despite this common interest in the study of interpersonal social interaction there are clearly identifiable differences in the way in which symbolic interactionists and ethnomethodologists tackle social phenomena. As Cuff *et al.* observe, one major difference between the two approaches concerns the actual focus of investigation:

> . . . the interactionist is concerned with *actors*, their beliefs, actions and relationships. The ethnomethodologist, in contrast, is concerned with *activities* rather than actors. Ethnomethodological studies inquire not so much into meanings, as into the work which makes meanings possible . . . One could say that ethnomethodological studies *end* at the point where symbolic interactionist studies *begin*.
> (Cuff *et al.*, 1990, pp. 191–2, emphasis in original)

According to Craib, if symbolic interactionism is a theory of persons or social action, ethnomethodology is best described as a theory of 'social cognition', that is '. . . a theory of the way in which we come to agree on what makes up the social world' (Craib, 1984, p. 94).

The development of ethnomethodology as a theoretical perspective owes a great deal to the work of Harold Garfinkel. He defines ethnomethodology as 'the investigation of indexical expressions and other practical actions as contingent on-going accomplishments of organised artful practices of everyday life' (Garfinkel, 1967, p. 11). In simpler terms, ethnomethodology investigates the folk methods people use to make sense of their everyday world and sustain social life. In this respect it differs markedly from those structural sociological perspectives that explain social order as the inevitable outcome of members of society internalising a body of social rules prescribing normative behaviour. For the ethnomethodologist, the norms governing social behaviour are not taken as given in this way; rather, people are seen as having to make order out of the everyday social situations they encounter. This explains how people come to share a commonsense, taken-for-granted knowledge of the social world. The orderliness that characterises many day-to-day social encounters is continually created and sustained by the 'sense-making work' undertaken by social actors. Stable social interaction is therefore something that is achieved or accomplished: to quote Garfinkel, social settings are 'practically accomplished' and social order is 'participant produced'.

Given the significance of verbal communication in everyday social life it is not surprising that conversational interaction has been the subject of much ethnomethodological research. Indeed, '[f]or many ethnomethodologists, the most impressive and powerful body of studies produced under the auspices of ethnomethodology are those of conversation analysis' (Cuff *et al.*, 1990, p. 181). Conversation analysts study the structure and social organisation of talk. One of their key objectives is to describe the procedures speakers adopt to produce or account for their own behaviour and interpret and respond to the behaviour of others. While much attention has been devoted to the analysis of everyday, mundane conversations, there is a growing body of research literature dealing with the study of the organisation of talk in formal settings, such as the classroom (McHoul, 1978), the courtroom (Atkinson and Drew, 1979) and the medical consulting room (Heath, 1981). Using data from medical consultations, Heath (1981) describes how the conversational interaction in doctor–patient encounters follows a pattern of sequential stages. Furthermore, his micro-analysis of interaction in medical settings shows how both speech and non-verbal behaviour are coordinated in face-to-face encounters between doctors and patients (Heath, 1984).

The ideas that interpretive sociologists hold about the nature of social reality, and the creative role they attribute to social actors in the production of shared commonsense knowledge, lead them to question the value of organisationally generated statistics in the study of social behaviour. From their standpoint, when viewing the contents of records of activity produced by formal organisations it is essential to take into account the organisational practices and procedures that give rise to the production of official figures in the first place. Interpretivists challenge the idea that statistics can be regarded as objective measures of social phenomena. From a micro-sociological perspective official statistics are not to be accepted at face value: they are not to be treated as objective social facts but as constructs of practical reasoning.

Consequently, two problems are encountered when attempting to use official records for the purposes of carrying out research. First, there is the problem of inadequate or insufficient data. Garfinkel (1967) describes how patient records can be incomplete and attributes this to the fact that clinic staff may have 'good' organisational reasons for 'bad' record-keeping. Second, where official statistics are used as objective evidence on which to establish theories of social behaviour, interpretivist sociologists have expressed concern about the definitions and procedures used for identifying the behaviour in question. The study of suicide provides a good example in this context. Rather than focusing on official figures and analysing trends and patterns in suicide rates in order to arrive at an explanation of suicide, interpretivists investigate the way suicide rates are socially constructed. This involves looking at the process by which a death comes to be recorded as a suicide. In other words, the social meaning of suicide is treated as problematic.

Studies of the interpretative procedures followed by coroners and other officials involved in investigating cases of sudden death reveal that a verdict of suicide is the outcome of the socially organised practices of the investigators (Garfinkel, 1967; Douglas, 1967; Atkinson, 1978). From this perspective a suicide rate is merely the product of a process whereby commonsense notions are applied to the evidence surrounding a death in order to distinguish accidental deaths from suicides. Coroners examine a wide range of factors surrounding the nature, location and circumstances of a death in search of evidence of intent on the part of the deceased. They select and interpret information obtained from a variety of sources in order to construct a rational account of the course of events leading up to a death. However, studies of the way that evidence is assembled and evaluated by coroners reveal that, while they share a common concern with establishing intent and identifying motives for suicide, opinion varies when it comes to the manner in which an intention to die is inferred from the evidence.

From an interpretivist perspective suicide is not a social phenomenon that can be understood simply by analysing officially produced statistics. 'A suicide rate, in short, is the constituted product of some set of socially organised methods for the "making out" of suicides from a variety of remains' (Heritage, 1984, pp. 174–5). These statistics are socially constructed and the aim is to investigate the procedures by which they are created.

In summary, the interpretivist sociologist aims to gain an insight into the 'actor's point of view' and explore the interactional work undertaken by individuals as they attempt to make sense of everyday social settings in which they find themselves. Dealing as they do with the dynamic aspects of social interaction, these sociologists need to capture social action as it happens in order to generate data for analysis. A method of data collection favoured by interactionists is participant observation; this involves the researcher gathering information by actively participating in the social world he or she is investigating. The researcher records events and participants' reactions in the form of field notes, which are then subjected to qualitative analysis. In studying the methods people use for producing and making sense of everyday social life, ethnomethodologists require a more finely detailed record of behaviour as it occurs in natural settings. Consequently, they prefer to base their analyses on audio-taped and/or video-taped recordings of verbal and non-verbal behaviour.

Feminist perspectives

Feminist sociologists in the 'second-wave feminism' of the 1960s and 1970s criticised conventional sociological theory for being male oriented and ignoring gender divisions in society. As a male-dominated discipline sociology was seen as being biased as its research and theorising offered a predominantly male perspective on the social world. As Abbott and Wallace assert, in mainstream sociology 'sociological knowledge portrayed women as men saw them, not as they saw themselves' (1990a, p. 4). The term 'malestream sociology' was coined to describe this approach, which according to its critics seemed to imply that the sexual division of labour and male domination over women were natural and inevitable consequences of the biological differences between the sexes. Feminist theorists maintain that some sociological theories fail to recognise the significance of the concept of gender in understanding women's life chances and social experiences (Maynard, 1990). With the subsequent emergence of feminist theory much has been done to address the systematic biases found in conventional sociology and develop a 'sociology for women' (Smith, 1987).

According to Abbott and Wallace, '[f]eminism is not a unified intellectual movement' (1990a, p. 212). It is more accurate to refer to *feminisms* rather than feminism (Humm, 1992). However, while it is possible to identify a number of different feminist perspectives, all feminists agree that the economic, social and cultural arrangements in society are such that men exercise power over women in both the public and the private spheres of social life. Feminists aim not only to explain the nature and origins of the subordination and oppression of women but also seek to provide an insight into how the situation might be transformed. While in this respect feminist scholars share a common objective, they do not always agree on the causes of women's oppression or the social reforms and economic policies necessary to secure female emancipation.

It is not possible to review all the feminist perspectives in this brief introduction. In order to illustrate something of the diversity to be found in feminist thought reference will be made to three major feminist perspectives: liberal, radical and socialist.

The values espoused by liberal feminists can be traced to the classical liberal doctrine of those Enlightenment philosophers who advocated the principles of human rights, justice, equality and the sanctity of the individual person. These principles are at the core of contemporary liberal feminism. Feminists in this tradition argue that women should enjoy the same citizenship rights as men. Unfortunately this is not the case as women often find themselves unfairly discriminated against on the basis of their sex. Feminists challenge the view that the differential treatment women receive is a natural consequence of the innate differences between men and women. They argue that the observable differences between the sexes, which are used to justify differential treatment, are a function of the socialisation process by which individuals learn what society considers appropriate behaviour for males and females. In other words, the gender roles allocated to men and women are not determined by biological factors, but are socially constructed. The solution to the problem of women's oppression is through the use of legislation to combat sex discrimination and promote equal rights for women in all sectors of society.

From a radical feminist perspective gender-based inequalities and women's subordination are the products of an autonomous system of patriarchy, through which men dominate and exploit women. The concept of patriarchy is used by radical feminists to account for how and why women are oppressed (Stacey, 1993). Under conditions of patriarchal authority all relations between men and women are power relations. No area of society is free from male domination. As early contemporary radical feminist writers observed, the subordination of women by men is a universal feature of social life. It does not only occur in what might be termed the public sphere of social activity, for example the world of employment, but patriarchal power pervades the private sphere of personal relationships and family life (Millett, 1970; Firestone, 1974). As Annandale notes, the importance attached to the notion of patriarchy is a distinguishing feature of radical feminism: 'One of the limitations of liberal feminism identified by its critics is its willingness to work *within* the patriarchal system. Radical feminism breaks completely with this, arguing that patriarchy is the *root* of women's oppression – there can be no equality on men's terms; patriarchy must be eliminated' (1998, p. 68, emphasis in original).

Although radical feminists share the view that the key to women's emancipation is through the dismantling of patriarchal structures, there are differences when it comes to explaining the significance of biological factors in the production of sexual inequality and female subordination. For writers such as Firestone (1974), inequality between the sexes is rooted in the biological differences between men and women. Firestone claims that as a result of their reproductive function women became dependent on men for their survival. The fact that women gave birth to children, and were then deemed responsible for providing continuous care throughout the early years of life, explained the origins of women's oppression. It is through the forces of reproduction that Firestone identifies women as a 'sex-class'. For her, the sex-class system, in which men exercise power over women, is the primary form of social stratification. Sexual inequality will end only when women are liberated from their biology through advances in reproductive technology. The development of reliable methods of birth control is only the beginning. The biological basis of women's subordination will only be completely overcome when medical science makes it possible for babies to be conceived and developed outside the womb, thus freeing women from their reproductive role.

Not all radical feminists see developments in reproductive technologies as a solution to female oppression. For example, some point out that the biological capacity to give birth only becomes a source of oppression under conditions of patriarchy. They argue that reproductive technologies can be seen as a means by which men can gain some control over women's power to create life (O'Brien, 1981; Corea, 1985).

Many radical feminists do not deny the existence of biological differences but challenge the meanings and significance attached to them. However, there are some radical theorists who reject all biological explanations of female subordination. According to Delphy (1984), biological explanations of gender differences are social constructions. Social norms and cultural mores encourage men and women to behave in ways that are seen as natural. Women are socially conditioned to accept the mothering role as naturally determined and it is argued that biological theories are constructed to justify what are basically socially determined differences.

For radical feminists the systematic exploitation of women by men is a fundamental feature of patriarchal oppression. Although women are exposed to sexual inequality in all spheres of social life, exploitation within marriage is a key issue. As Delphy asserts, '[w]hile the wage labourer sells his labour power, the married woman gives hers away; . . . To supply unpaid labour within the framework of a universal and personal relationship (marriage) constructs primarily a relationship of slavery' (quoted in Abbott and Wallace, 1990a, p. 14). Given the existence of female exploitation, women are seen to share common interests and thus constitute a class in opposition to men. The relations between men and women are therefore political.

Radical feminism has done much to highlight the political and ideological aspects of gender inequality. However, as a perspective it has been criticised for treating women as a homogenous group by ignoring the fact that women from different social, cultural and racial backgrounds do not share the same experiences of oppression and exploitation. For example, patriarchy as a system of oppression has a racial dimension. Black feminist writers have pointed out that the struggle against exploitation is not simply a case of male oppressors versus female victims. Black women can be exploited by white women (hooks, 1984) and black men and black women share common interests in the fight against racism. Thus, interests of racial discrimination and racial disadvantage cut across gender in significant ways.

Socialist feminists have made a major contribution to the debate about female oppression in contemporary societies by arguing that women's subordination is the product of two distinct systems, namely capitalism and patriarchy (Walby, 1990). To understand fully the nature of this subordination it is essential to appreciate how the structure of society under capitalism has led to the exploitation of women in the labour market. From this perspective attention is focused on the sexual division of labour as it occurs both in the world of paid work and in the domestic sphere of life. The fact that women are assigned the role of primary carers in the family unit effectively limits their access to paid employment outside the home. The ideology of marriage and the concept of motherhood, which present the nuclear family and the sexual division of labour as 'natural' arrangements, are used to justify the gender-related nature of women's involvement in the labour market. This masks the fact that the unpaid domestic labour performed by women is of benefit not only to men but also to the capitalist system in general. Thus patriarchal arrangements influence the social relations between men and women in both public and private domains. For socialist feminists, if one is to develop an understanding of how women's oppression is created and maintained in society, it is necessary to examine how the two systems of patriarchy and capitalism work together.

As described above, there are a number of different theoretical perspectives embraced by feminism. What they have in common is the aim of understanding social reality from the point of view of women and the desire to pose questions that are significant to women's lives. When it comes to the study of health and illness, feminist perspectives take the view that health is not simply a straightforward product of women's biological make-up but is socially constructed on account of the gendered nature of women's social experiences.

Social constructionism

As described at the beginning of the chapter, one of the main limitations of the biomedical model of illness is its biological determinism. One of the main contributions of sociology to the study of health and illness has been to draw attention to the fact that health and illness are as much social products as physical entities. For example, Eliot Freidson (1970a) recognises the socially constructed nature of illness when he differentiates between illness as a biophysical condition and illness as a social state:

> While illness as a biophysical state exists independently of human knowledge and evaluation, illness as a social state is *created and shaped by* human knowledge and evaluation.
>
> (Freidson, 1970a, p. 223, emphasis in original)

When a doctor attaches a diagnostic label to a medical condition 'a social state is added to a biophysical state by assigning the meaning of illness to disease' (1970a, p. 223). Thus, at a very basic level, an illness is not simply a physical experience but is also a social experience. The nature of the experience will also depend on how ideas about health and illness are shaped and constructed by society itself. These ideas, because they are social constructions, will be influenced by factors such as cultural beliefs, social context, gender and social class. However, there is more to social constructionism than a belief in the view that knowledge about health and illness is socially created.

In many ways it would be inaccurate to describe social constructionism as constituting a single, unified perspective within sociology. It is essentially multi-disciplinary in nature, drawing as it does from a number of disciplines and a variety of intellectual traditions; these include sociology, philosophy and linguistics. While it is not really possible to identify one all-embracing intellectual or philosophical principle underlying constructionist thought, an attempt can be made to identify the main propositions of contemporary constructionism (Burr, 1995).

The first of these propositions concerns what has been termed the 'problematisation' of taken-for-granted realities (Berger and Berger, 1983). In essence, social constructionism not only entails taking a critical stance towards what we understand to be commonsense knowledge about ourselves and the world around us but also involves treating medical knowledge, or any scientific knowledge for that matter, as problematic. From a constructionist standpoint the ability of scientific methodology to produce objective, unbiased knowledge is brought into question. Scientific facts are viewed as being the product of social processes rather than the outcome of the use of traditional methods of scientific investigation. In the case of the biomedical model, biological determinism dictates that disease and its manifestations are facts waiting to be discovered. However, constructionists see medical knowledge as being socially constructed. For them, 'the objects of medical science are not what they appear to be; the stable realities of the human body and disease are in fact "fabrications", or "inventions" rather than discoveries' (Bury, 1986, p. 139). In other words, diseases are not conceptualised as unchanging natural, biological entities that are simply waiting 'out there' to be discovered but are seen as the products of the social practices involved in the very act of discovery itself. As Bury asserts, 'claims to the discovery of disease are themselves social events and take place in social contexts' (1986, p. 145).

This approach to knowledge is a significant feature of social constructionism. The assumption is that our knowledge of the world, whether based on common ways of understanding or scientific investigation, is sustained by social processes. In a medical context, in order to understand what comes to be regarded as legitimate knowledge it is necessary to explore the social practices that are involved in the production or 'fabrication' of that knowledge. For example, Atkinson (1981) describes how medical students are taught ways of interpreting information in order to assign symptoms to clearly identifiable diagnostic categories.

For constructionists then there is more to medical knowledge than the objective description of illness and disease. Medical diagnostic labels or disease categories play a part in mediating social relations. As Bury notes, '[t]o call an area of experience "medical" is to place it in a significant relationship to other areas of social life, giving it a definite and powerful shape and meaning' (1986, p. 142). Disease categories therefore may be used as a way of justifying certain social arrangements and controlling the behaviour of specific social groups. The disease of hysteria provides a good historical example of this and illustrates how medical thinking can be influenced by wider social, economic and political concerns (Smith-Rosenberg, 1984). In the nineteenth century a strong domestic ideology prevailed, in which it was assumed that the natural and rightful place for women was in the home, caring for their children and husbands. Men were the ones who should be involved in the public sphere of work in order to provide for their families. Although some married women did undertake paid work, men in general saw women's participation in the labour market as constituting a threat to their own paid employment and there was a strong feeling that women should keep to their traditional roles within the household. This division of labour was often justified on the grounds that it was based on the existence of natural biological differences between the sexes. Medical thinking of the day also emphasised the differences between men and women (L'Esperance, 1977). Women were seen as being under the control of their reproductive systems. By denying the biological imperative of reproduction they placed their general physical and mental health in jeopardy. If they neglected the traditional roles of housewife and mother, by seeking paid employment in the public sphere, they ran the risk of developing the disease of hysteria. Furthermore, according to medical opinion education for women beyond the basic level was inadvisable on health grounds, as it was thought to prevent the brain and ovaries developing simultaneously (Smith-Rosenberg, 1984).

What is clear from the constructionist perspective is that 'medical knowledge is not just a description of, nor an attempt to treat, disease and illness, but may also be used to reproduce and reinforce existing social structures and values'

(Nettleton, 1995, p. 26). Whether or not a condition is labelled a disease does not depend on the existence of biological facts alone but is influenced by social and political factors.

Another proposition central to social constructionism concerns the concepts we use to understand and interpret the world in which we live; these are viewed as historically and culturally specific. A good example is provided by the concept of childhood. As described in Chapter 5, social and cultural factors play a major part in the social construction of childhood. In medieval times childhood was not viewed as it is today; from as early as seven years of age children were treated as 'small adults'. Ariès (1962) describes how the creation of childhood as a separate phase of moral and social development emerged as a product of European bourgeois culture in the seventeenth and eighteenth centuries. A social constructionist perspective can also be applied to the study of old age, as described in Chapter 6. Not only is old age a cultural concept that is socially constructed, but, as Bytheway (1995) notes, ageism (that is discrimination against people on the basis of age) can also be seen as a social construct.

Morgan *et al.* neatly summarise the contribution of a constructivist perspective when they note that '[s]ocial constructionism does not imply that disease is imaginery [*sic*] but rather that medicine is a form of social practice, which observes, codifies, and understands these sufferings. Concepts of disease thus have no necessary, transhistorical, universal shape, and reflect a particular way of viewing the world' (1985, p. 29).

The ideas of the French social philosopher Michel Foucault have had a profound impact on the development of constructivist thought in the social sciences in general and in the fields of the sociology of health and illness and the sociology of the body in particular (Foucault, 1965, 1976, 1980a). Indeed, it has been observed that 'Foucault's studies of medical history and his general perspective provide a powerful framework within which to develop medical sociology' (Turner, 1987, p. 14). Consequently, any discussion of social constructionism would be incomplete without reference to some of the key features of Foucault's work.

Two principal themes at the heart of the Foucauldian perspective are the relationship between knowledge and power and the way that the human body is conceptualised. In the case of the former, for Foucault there is no such thing as absolute knowledge. The world in which we live can be understood in a number of different ways and consequently there is more than one interpretation of social reality. All knowledge is equally valid. In essence, individuals and groups make sense of their experiences and surroundings as they communicate with one another. It is through the use of language, in its broadest sense, that we construct a sense of social reality. Foucault uses the term 'discourse' to refer to this phenomenon. In short, a discourse is a way of thinking about the world; it embodies a form of knowledge. By subscribing to a particular discourse we are actively acquiring and applying knowledge and in the process working towards developing a particular view of social reality. In Foucauldian terms, discourses create 'effects of truth' but in themselves cannot be taken as either true or false (Foucault, 1980b).

In *The Birth of the Clinic* Foucault (1976) explores the relationship between knowledge and power in an analysis of the development of medical science and the emergence of hospital-based medicine. As Turner observes, his conception of discourse clearly has important implications as far as the sociological study of medicine is concerned. 'We can no longer regard "diseases" as natural events in the world which occur outside the language with which they are described. A disease entity is the product of medical discourses which in turn reflect the dominant mode of thinking . . . within a society' (Turner, 1987, p. 11). Focusing on changes in medical theory and practice in France in the late eighteenth and early nineteenth centuries, Foucault describes what he sees as a major shift in the medical perception of disease. In essence, disease 'is no longer a pathological species inserting itself into the body . . . it is the body itself that has become ill' (Foucault, 1976, p. 136). The introduction of new techniques of clinical observation and the emphasis placed on physical examinations determined how doctors saw the human body. In this way the body became subject to what Foucault calls the 'clinical gaze' of medical experts.

As a result of this new conceptualisation of disease, 'the core task of medicine became not the elucidation of what the patient said but what the doctor saw in the depths of the body' (Armstrong, 1984, p. 738). The doctor emerged as a passive observer responsible for identifying and charting the nature and course of disease in the human body. This called for the exercise of personal detachment and clinical objectivity. Correspondingly, the patient came to be viewed as a passive, objectified body to whom diseases happen. What is more, the newly emergent clinical discourse viewed the body as a compilation of parts each having their own independent existence for the purposes of medical examination and treatment. As Armstrong (1983a) notes, this clinical gaze gave rise to a new 'anatomical atlas' that provided a set of rules for reading the body and understanding its internal workings. This access to, and control over, a body of medical knowledge was a source of considerable social power. Foucault maintains that the knowledge the medical profession began to accumulate about the human body and the prevalence of illness and disease in the population formed the basis for medical dominance. Thus towards the end of the nineteenth century medicine was playing a significant role in the social and moral regulation of populations by defining what was to be considered 'normal' and promoting a particular image of the body.

The above discussion is testimony to the fact that social constructionism has an important contribution to make to our thinking about health and illness. However, the constructionist perspective attracts its share of critics. A fundamental criticism is levelled at the inherent logic of the social constructionist position, which assumes that *all* knowledge, not just medical knowledge, is socially relative. In this context Bury asks 'if all forms of knowledge are part of "discourses" where does that leave constructionism?' (1986, p. 151). In the absence of a concept of absolute knowledge or truth, what claims can social constructionists make that their accounts or discourses are any more relevant or valid than those they are engaged in criticising? Bury observes that this 'problem of relativism' is either ignored or not taken seriously by some proponents of constructionism.

Clearly, the value of the constructionist approach is that it draws attention to the problematic nature of medical scientific knowledge. However, this does not necessarily constitute a denial of the value of this knowledge in the treatment of illness and disease. As Nettleton asserts, 'the argument that all knowledge is socially contingent is not the same as the statement that all knowledge is worthless' (1995, p. 30). Similarly, Bury takes the view that 'demonstrating the problematic character of medicine is not the same as demonstrating its dispensibility [*sic*]' (1986, p. 165). The constructionist perspective provides us with an alternative account as to how knowledge is created, which stresses how social interests and social contexts can influence the modes of knowledge that are produced.

Summary

- Health and illness can be perceived as social products. Our experiences of health, illness and disease are influenced by the social, economic and cultural surroundings in which we live.
- The biomedical model, characterised by a 'mind–body dualism' and the 'doctrine of specific aetiology', is the dominant model of disease in modern scientific medicine.
- The biomedical model has been criticised for overestimating the contribution of medicine to the decline in mortality rates, failing to recognise fully the impact of social conditions on health, focusing on the disease rather than the whole person and ignoring subjective interpretations of health and illness.
- A sociologically oriented or social model of illness challenges the biomedical approach to disease by roundly rejecting the notion of mind–body dualism, dismissing the idea that illness can be reduced to disordered bodily functioning and urging healthcare professionals to take account of the wider social and cultural milieu in which diseases are diagnosed and treated.
- As a discipline sociology embraces a variety of theoretical perspectives and research methodologies. Each perspective provides us with a different way of looking at the social world. There is no one 'correct' perspective to take. Given the complexity of health and illness a broad approach drawing on different theoretical perspectives is clearly called for.

Questions for discussion

1 What are the fundamental features of the biomedical model of disease?

2 What criticisms have been levelled at the biomedical model?

3 How does sociology contribute to our understanding of health and illness?

4 Compare and contrast structural and interpretivist approaches to the study of society.

Further reading

Busfield, J. (2000) *Health and Health Care in Modern Britain*, Oxford: Oxford University Press.

Churton, M. (2000) *Theory and Method*, Basingstoke: Macmillan.

Cuff, E. C., Sharrock, W. W. and Francis, D. W. (1990) *Perspectives in Sociology*, 3rd edn, London: Unwin Hyman.

Lupton, D. (2000) 'The social construction of medicine and the body', in G. L. Albrecht, R. Fitzpatrick and S. C. Scrimshaw (eds), *Handbook of Social Studies in Health and Medicine*, London: Sage.

Macionis, J. J. and Plummer, K. (2008) *Sociology: A Global Introduction*, 3rd edn, Harlow: Pearson Education.

Marsh, I., Keating, M., Punch, S. and Harden, J. (2009) *Sociology: Making Sense of Society*, 4th edn, Harlow: Pearson Education.

Nettleton, S. (2006) *The Sociology of Health and Illness*, 2nd edn, Cambridge: Polity Press.

Taylor, S. and Field, D. (2003) *Sociology of Health and Health Care*, 3rd revised edn, Oxford: Blackwell, Chapters 1 and 2.

White, K. (1991) 'The sociology of health and illness', *Current Sociology*, 39, 2: 1–115.

Experiences of health and illness

An introduction to the concepts of disease, illness and health

Medicine is becoming more and more 'technologically' powerful. To protect patients, doctors and societies from misuse of this power it is necessary, as before, to indicate, as clearly as possible, the very purposes of medicine. Providing precise definitions of the fundamental concepts of medicine such as 'health'/'illness' ('disease', 'sickness') becomes in this context a crucial issue.

(Niebrój, 2006, p. 251)

At the outset careful consideration needs to be given to the use of the terms disease, health and illness. A useful starting point is Eisenberg's distinction between illness and disease:

... patients suffer 'illnesses'; physicians diagnose and treat 'disease' ... illnesses are experiences of disvalued changes in states of being and social function: diseases are abnormalities in the structure and function of body organs and systems.

(Eisenberg, 1977)

In this definition the term disease is endowed with an 'objective' quality; it refers to a malfunctioning in, or maladaption of, biological, physiological or chemical processes in the body. Thus disease is seen as a pathological condition identified on the basis of the appearance of certain signs and symptoms. Consequently each disease acquires an abstract quality, a 'thing-like' status, and in extreme cases is perceived as a condition which is independent of social behaviour (Fabrega, 1975, p. 969). This approach has been labelled the biomedical or medical model of disease. It is a scientific model with its roots in molecular biology and is the dominant model of disease in modern societies. The central concern is with the organic appearances of disease and the underlying assumption is that disease can be fully understood and accounted for in terms of deviation from some measurable biological norm. This disease-oriented approach to medical knowledge has been criticised for paying insufficient attention to psychological, social and behavioural factors (Engel, 1977).

The terms disease and illness are conceptually distinct: 'Disease is something an organ has: illness is something a man [sic] has' (Helman, 1981, p. 544). Illness refers to the experience of disease and as such deals with the subjective experiences of bodily disorder and feelings of pain and discomfort. In short, illness is defined as 'subjective unwellness', thus distinguishing it from the objective aspects of physical disorder. In contrast, the term disease suggests a biologically altered state, whereas illness relates to the diffuse consequences of the disease process. Illness is about how a person feels and has been defined as 'the human experience of sickness' (Kleinman et al., 1978, p. 251). As such it is a term which can only be fully understood within a social context. As noted above, the definition of disease is heavily based on a medical conception of pathological abnormality. In contrast, illness relies on social definitions of normality, which may or may not correspond to biomedical definitions. This is clearly illustrated by Macintyre (1986) when she quotes Ackernecht's (1947) description of the incidence of dichromic spirochetosis, a form of skin disease, among some South American tribes. The disease was so common that not having the condition was regarded as pathological and men without the disease were prevented from marrying.

To say that disease is a pathological condition and illness is the subjective state experienced by the individual does not imply that the two concepts deal with separate and unrelated sets of phenomena. According to Field (1976) the concepts focus on different levels of experience, namely the physical–organic and the psycho-social, and the relationship between them is a complex one involving the interaction of a number of social, cultural and psychological factors.

Distinguishing between the two concepts in this way has a number of advantages. Firstly, it indicates recognition of the social aspects of ill health and is a clear acknowledgement of the fact that physical impairment can have implications for the social life of an individual. Secondly, evidence from historians, medical anthropologists and sociologists shows that illness and disease are not fixed concepts; definitions can vary not only between societies but within any one society over time and between individuals and groups within the same society at any one time (Stacey, 1988). Definitions of illness have a cultural specificity and can be based on conceptions of normality which do not necessarily conform to biomedical definitions. Ackernecht's study of skin disorders among South American tribes quoted above is a good example. From the perspective of theoretical medicine dichromic spirochetosis is a disease and therefore abnormal but in the social and cultural context examined by Ackernecht it was not identified as such and nor was it considered an illness requiring treatment. Thirdly, distinguishing between the two concepts helps to produce a better understanding of individual and societal responses to ill health. Both Field (1976) and Blaxter (1987) have observed how it is possible to experience illness without the presence of disease and have a disease without feeling ill. To quote Blaxter,

> If 'disease' is defined as biological or clinically-identified abnormality, and 'illness' as the subjective experience of symptoms of ill-health, then it is obviously possible to have disease without illness, and to have illness without disease.
>
> (Blaxter, 1987, p. 5)

It is possible that an individual may have an undiagnosed organic disorder and not experience any symptoms or if they do experience symptoms these may not be recognised as such and be explained away. Research also suggests that what lay people experience as illness may go beyond matters with which the biomedical model deals (Cornwell, 1984). The subject of lay conceptions of health and illness will be returned to later in the chapter. Finally, what is particularly important with regard to the definition of illness is that it is this definition, and not the experience of disease, which is the precursor to the individual taking positive action, such as seeking medical advice. This is an aspect that will be covered in more detail when considering illness behaviour below.

So far the emphasis has been on the concepts of disease and illness and little if nothing has been said about the concept of health. As Dingwall has noted, health and illness are a 'contrasting pair' and our recognition of one depends on our knowledge of the other (Dingwall, 1976, p. 62). Broadly speaking four types of definitions of health can be identified in the medical, sociological and psychological literature (Box 2.1).

According to one proponent of the normative approach:

> Health and disease cannot be defined merely in terms of anatomical, physiological, or mental attributes. Their real measure is the ability of the individual to function in a manner acceptable to himself and to the group of which he is a part.
>
> (Dubos, 1995, p. 9)

Functional fitness can be considered from the perspective of either the individual or the society. In the case of the former the emphasis is on the behavioural manifestations of health. Questionnaire rating scales are used to measure health

Box 2.1   Definition

Four definitions of health

1 *Absence of clinically ascertainable disease*. The emphasis in the medical model's definition is on biophysical abnormalities and disorders to the extent that psychological factors and individual experiences are ignored.

2 *Absence of illness*. This definition focuses on subjective perceptions. A weakness of definitions in this category is that they only allow health to be defined after the event.

3 *Complete well-being*. This is the most comprehensive definition of health, which goes beyond the conventional medical model. It is adopted by the World Health Organisation:

> Health is a state of complete physical, mental and social well-being, not merely the absence of disease and infirmity.
>
> (World Health Organisation Constitution)

This is an *idealised definition of health*, best seen as a goal towards which governments, organisations and individuals should be oriented rather than as a potentially attainable target (Twaddle, 1974).

4 *Normative expectations*. This definition emphasises the capacity of the individual to fit in with society's norms and expectations (Twaddle, 1974).

status or the functional incapacity of individuals in major areas of social activity, such as work, family life and social relationships. The aim is to identify the extent to which individuals can perform the social roles expected of them. Two examples of such scales are the Functional State Index (Fanshel and Bush, 1970) and the Sickness Impact Profile (Bergner *et al.*, 1976). In considering health from a normative or functionalist perspective, the sociologist Talcott Parsons defines health as a 'state of optimum capacity for the effective performance of value tasks' or social roles for which the individual has been socialised (Parsons, 1972, p. 110). The ultimate objective is the maintenance of the social system. From the wider perspective of society Parsons sees illness as disruptive to the smooth running of society and therefore potentially dysfunctional (Parsons, 1951).

Lay perspectives

Lay perspectives do not lack awareness of the natural processes and determinants of disease. However, they are more urgently focused on the need to invest meaning, and consequently also a degree of coherence and sense of control, over arbitrary and chaotic events and experiences which threaten not only the body, but also the self.

(Pollock, 2005, p. 23)

Lay beliefs about health, illness and disease

For many years healthcare policy in Britain has been moving away from an emphasis on curative medicine towards a focus on prevention. This preventive approach has been a major feature in numerous policy documents and government reports over the years. A White Paper published by the Labour Government in the mid-1970s, entitled *Prevention and Health*, stated categorically that:

> Much ill-health in Britain today arises from overindulgence and unwise behaviour . . . The individual can do much to help himself, his family and the community by accepting more direct responsibility for his own health and well-being.
>
> (DHSS, 1976)

A White Paper published some 10 years later, under a Conservative government, presented a similar view. In *Promoting Better Health* (DHSS, 1987) the major health problems, such as heart disease and cancer, are described as being 'lifestyle-based'. The message coming from these publications is that individuals should take responsibility for their own health and the health of others. Many health problems are considered to be behavioural in origin and therefore preventable. Individuals have to begin to make the right choices, which involves taking a number of 'simple steps' to protect and improve their own health (DHSS, 1987, p. 3).

Given this policy strategy, with its emphasis on the individual, considerable importance has been attached to health education. However, the effectiveness of programmes designed to promote health depends on a clear understanding of the nature, content and distribution of health beliefs in the population. Such beliefs need to be explored as products of economic, social and cultural environments. If it is lay concepts of health and illness that play a major part in determining health-related behaviour, then it is essential that any health education strategy identifies and responds to people's own perceptions and needs. This is one justification for undertaking research into lay beliefs about health, illness and disease.

There is another reason for studying lay beliefs. According to the traditional medical model disease produces signs and symptoms indicating its presence. The symptoms are what the patient experiences and the signs are what the doctor looks for in order to identify the nature of the disease. In this model it is the patient who is seen as taking the initiative in seeking medical attention. However, research suggests that people do not behave in such a predictable fashion. Two people may have the same clinical symptoms yet behave differently: one may seek medical help, the other may not consider such a course of action (Mechanic and Volkart, 1961). The fact that there are some people who ignore the symptoms of serious disease and do not seek medical advice, or seek help at a late stage, has been noted by Last (1963). The decision to go to the doctor depends, among other things, on how the symptoms are perceived, interpreted and evaluated. This decision-making process will be influenced by the knowledge and beliefs individuals have about health, illness and the cause of disease. Thus an appreciation of the nature and variety of lay beliefs will enhance our understanding of what is termed 'illness behaviour', that is the process by which individuals with symptoms reach the doctor. This will be discussed in more detail later in the chapter.

Lay definitions of health

One of the first studies to explore the way in which people define health and illness was undertaken by Herzlich (1973). The study was based on interviews with a sample of 80 subjects, drawn mainly from middle-class backgrounds and living in Paris or Normandy. Herzlich discovered three distinct dimensions of health embedded in the accounts of the interviewees. Firstly, there was what she termed 'health-in-a-vacuum', that is a view of health as simply the absence of illness. Within the context of this definition health is seen as a state of 'being'. Secondly, there was the 'reserve of health' approach. According to this interpretation health is defined with regard to the capacity of the individual to maintain good health. This capacity consists of two elements, namely physical strength and the individual's potential for resistance to illness. Individual attributes, such as heredity and temperament, are considered to play a major part in determining the 'reserve of health'. In this context health may be described as a state of 'having'. Finally, Herzlich labelled the third dimension 'equilibrium'. Respondents described equilibrium in terms of feeling strong and having good relationships with others. The existence of health is interpreted in the form of the realisation of the individual's reserve of health and exemplified as a state of 'doing'.

Similar findings are reported by Pill and Stott (1986) who interviewed a sample of 41 mothers, aged between 30 and 35 years, who lived in South Wales and whose husbands were skilled manual workers. Among the definitions of health identified were health as the absence of illness, health as functional fitness and a positive view of health, which was associated with being enthusiastic and cheerful. A study conducted in Scotland into the way in which elderly people describe health also produced similar results (Williams, 1983). Williams' findings are based on data obtained from both a random sample survey of 619 men and women over 60 years of age and intensive, open-ended interviews with a smaller sample of 70 respondents. The subjects were all living at home and drawn from both middle-class and working-class backgrounds. Analysis of the data revealed three dimensions of health similar to those outlined above. On one level there was a negative conception of health according to which health was the absence of disease. In contrast there was a more positive view in which respondents saw health in terms of strength and finally a notion of functional fitness was identified. The relationship between the three dimensions of health was a complex one. In commenting on the similarity between these findings and those of Herzlich (1973), Williams states that, 'These resemblances, in groups which are divergent in age, class composition and nationality, suggest that cultural conceptions of a relatively fundamental kind are involved here' (Williams, 1983, p. 201).

Social class variations in concepts of health have been commented on by a number of researchers. In studies in France, it has been shown how manual workers conceive of health in negative and instrumental terms, whereas those in non-manual managerial and professional occupations are more likely to have a positive definition of health and think of health more in personal and expressive terms (d'Houtaud and Field, 1984, 1986). Blaxter and Paterson (1982) studied attitudes to health and health-related behaviour among women in 58 three-generation working-class families in Scotland. They found that health was primarily defined in negative terms, that is as the absence of illness, rather than in positive terms of physical fitness or a sense of well-being. By all accounts a functional definition of health predominated. The women considered themselves healthy if they were able to carry out 'normal' daily activities and could go out to work. An example of a functional approach to defining health was expressed by one of the interviewees as follows:

> After I was sterilised I had a lot of cystitis, and backache, because of the fibroids. Then when I had a hysterectomy I had bother wi' my waterworks because my bladder lived a life of its own and I had to have a repair . . . Healthwise I would say I'm OK. I did hurt my shoulder – I mean, this is nothing to do with health but I actually now have a disability, I get a gratuity payment every six months . . . I wear a collar and take Valium . . . then, just the headaches – but I'm not really off work a lot with it.
>
> (Blaxter and Paterson, 1982, p. 29)

As the authors point out, this not only represents a functional definition of health but also illustrates the low expectations of health and physical well-being held by the women. It is also evident that the subject in question does not define health simply as the absence of illness.

In a study of 60 women from different social classes living in Outer London, Calnan (1986, 1987) used a variety of questions to explore how respondents conceptualised health. Questions concentrating on the state of the individual's own health elicited more 'negative' definitions (i.e. absence of illness) than positive ones. No social class differences were identified. However, there was a marked contrast between respondents when they were asked about health in abstract terms. Women from working-class backgrounds tended to consider health as a unitary concept and favoured a functional definition, whereas middle-class women operated with a multi-dimensional view of health which included elements such as being active and feeling strong.

The working-class women interviewed by Blaxter and Paterson (1982) defined health in a functional way in terms of the ability to carry out normal daily routines and fulfil social roles such as continuing to work. Calnan concludes from his data that, on the whole, his respondents did not view health in terms of ability to carry out daily tasks. Only a minority of his interviewees found this concept of health familiar and they all came from working-class backgrounds. Thus, Calnan questions the assertion that it is the experience of material deprivation and adverse social conditions which leads to people subscribing to functional definitions of health. He suggests a possible alternative explanation in which social class differences in concepts of health are products of the social context of the research interview. The more elaborate responses to questions about health elicited from middle-class respondents could be a consequence of the nature of the interaction between interviewer and interviewee. Middle-class interviewers may be more successful at developing a rapport with interviewees from similar social backgrounds (Calnan, 1987, p. 35). However, Calnan does not deny that economic circumstances and social background influence the way health is perceived and notes that '. . . in spite of this denial of the functional definition of health, the state of health in which many carried out their daily tasks was quite low' (Calnan, 1987, p. 39).

The reported tendency for working-class respondents to define health in a negative sense, that is as 'not ill', is not confirmed in the findings of the Health and Lifestyle Survey conducted in England, Scotland and Wales and based on a random sample of 9,003 men and women (Cox et al., 1987; Blaxter, 1990). There is no indication of any significant social differentiation in the use of negative definitions of health. The survey does provide useful data regarding the relevance of gender and age in the definitional process. When comparing men and women, the latter provided more expansive answers to the questions on health. Those women in the higher social class categories, or with higher educational qualifications, frequently expressed multi-dimensional concepts of health. It was also found that women, unlike men, were more likely to define health in terms of their social relationships with other people. For example, young women referred to health in terms of being able to 'cope with the family' (Blaxter, 1990, p. 27).

With regard to age, the survey data illustrate how concepts of health differ through the life course. For young male respondents health was clearly viewed in terms of physical fitness and strength. While physical fitness appeared in the definitions given by young women, they placed emphasis on such aspects as vitality and the ability to cope. With the approach of middle age, concepts of health become broader and more complex with the emphasis shifting to notions of total physical and mental well-being. In old age functional definitions predominate, with men in particular focusing on their ability to perform common tasks and carry out normal daily routines.

A feature of the Health and Lifestyle Survey was that respondents were asked first of all to define health in another person and then in relation to themselves. This revealed that many individuals described health 'in others' differently from health 'in themselves'. Health in another person was described as 'positive fitness', as 'the ability to work or perform . . . normal roles' or as 'not being ill'. In contrast, with reference to oneself, health was seen in psychological terms, '. . . respondents were less likely to emphasise physical fitness or lack of disease, but rather to say that health is defined as being unstressed and unworried, able to cope with life, in tune with the world and happy' (Blaxter, 1987, p. 141).

From this brief review of the literature it can be seen that health is a multi-dimensional concept. Lay definitions of health can be divided into three categories, negative (absence of illness), functional (ability to work or perform normal daily activities) and positive (physical fitness and general well-being). The evidence clearly indicates that lay concepts of health are socially situated and as such are influenced by structural and cultural factors. Lay views vary from one social class to another in ways that appear to relate to socio-economic and socio-cultural differences between groups.

Lay definitions of illness

Attention can now be turned to lay perspectives on illness. As stated earlier, illness refers to the experiential aspects of bodily disorder and socio-cultural factors play an important part in shaping and influencing the way in which these disorders are perceived and explained. In their study of socially disadvantaged families, Blaxter and Paterson (1982) describe how the mothers and adult daughters they interviewed adopted a functional definition of health and drew a distinction between normal illnesses and serious illnesses. There was a tendency for respondents to 'normalise' some health conditions and not view them as illnesses. If the condition in question was seen as due to the 'wear and tear' associated with growing old or 'women's troubles' then it was accepted as normal and something they just had to learn to live with (Blaxter and Paterson, 1982, p. 31). While common ailments were accepted as part of everyday life, respondents reserved the label 'illness' for serious conditions such as cancer and heart disease. This distinction between 'normal' and 'real' illness has been identified in other studies (Cornwell, 1984).

Various studies have highlighted the fact that the concept of illness has moral connotations and there is evidence of illness being conceived of in terms of a state of moral, as opposed to physical, malaise. The working-class women in Blaxter and Paterson's study, when considering illness in others, frequently referred not to the experience of symptoms but to the reaction to those symptoms. They viewed much illness as the result of 'imagination' and were of the opinion that 'people were not ill if they did not "lie down to it", "dwell on it", or "let it get them down" . . .' (Blaxter and Paterson, 1982, p. 33). The importance of adopting the right 'attitude of mind' in order to avoid illness, maintain good health or cope with life has been expressed in other studies (Pollock, 1984; Cornwell, 1984). Cornwell studied working-class men and women living in Bethnal Green in East London and observed how they offered 'public' and 'private' accounts of their illnesses. Public accounts concentrated on moral aspects, while private accounts emphasised the practical difficulties and material concerns associated with illness. Cornwell describes how the attitude respondents adopted to employment was reflected in the attitude taken towards health. Although they had very little control over their working lives, they adopted a positive attitude to hard work and approached it with fortitude. As far as health is concerned:

> They experience themselves as having very little control over whether or not they are healthy, and yet they take seriously the idea that having the 'right attitude' is the passport, if not to good health, at least to a life that is tolerable. The moral prescription for a healthy life is in fact a kind of cheerful stoicism, evident in the refusal to worry, or to complain, or to be morbid.
>
> (Cornwell, 1984, p. 129)

As with the respondents in Blaxter and Paterson's study, the men and women interviewed by Cornwell believed in the power of 'mind over matter', expressing the view that a great deal of illness was due to a lack of strength of character on the part of the individual.

Lay explanations of illness and disease

Individuals do not just define health and illness but also attempt to explain and account for changes in their bodily state. It is important to discuss folk ideas about illness causation as these determine the extent to which individuals are likely to accept responsibility for their own health. Chrisman (1977) has identified four basic modes of thought about the cause of illness and disease. He calls these modes of thought 'logics' and they are described in Box 2.2.

Research shows that most people subscribe to multifactorial 'theories' of causality in their attempts to explain illness. Blaxter (1983) identified twelve categories of cause in her study of middle-aged, working-class women in Scotland. The most frequently cited cause was infection, followed by heredity and then environmental factors, such as working conditions. Pill and Stott (1986) studied the lay explanations of illness among a sample of working-class mothers and found that the reason most frequently advanced followed the medical model of infectious illness with symptoms being seen as the result of viruses, bugs or germs. The authors point out that the respondents concentrated on short-term acute illnesses which may reflect the experiences of the group. The sample consisted of young mothers with dependent children who had little or no personal experience of degenerative or age-related diseases.

Lay theories contain explanations of the perceived origins and nature of specific illnesses and diseases. These explanations are constructed by individuals during the course of their daily lives and therefore reflect their experiences. As such, lay views are informed by the biomedical model which individuals acquire knowledge of through direct contact with members of the medical profession or

---

Box 2.2   Definition

Chrisman's four basic 'logics' of illness and disease

1 A *logic of invasion* cites germ theory and other material intrusions as causal agents in the development of illness and disease.

2 A *logic of degeneration* interprets illness as a consequence of the running down of the body.

3 A *mechanical logic* sees illness as the result of damage to, or blockages in, bodily structures.

4 A *logic of balance* views illness as the outcome of a disruption of harmony between parts of the body or between the individual and the environment.

Source: Chrisman, 1977

from information derived from secondary sources, particularly the mass media. Although influenced by scientific medical knowledge, lay perceptions are also structured out of folk ideas and indigenous healing traditions. A characteristic of lay theories is that they contain ideas about the conditions and circumstances under which certain illnesses and diseases arise. Research shows that when people are asked to talk about health and illness they not only describe the signs and symptoms but attempt to identify the cause. Herzlich and Pierret (1986) describe how the majority of middle-class French men and women they interviewed attributed illness to the living conditions prevalent in modern urban society, commenting on how they expose individuals to a variety of health risks through atmospheric pollution and contact with pathological agents. They illustrate how the concept of 'way of life' is used to encompass a variety of factors which can affect health and constitutes 'the prime paradigm of the causality of illness' (Herzlich and Pierret, 1986, p. 84). Conceived in this way illness is seen as something which comes from outside the individual.

Calnan (1987) has examined lay views on the causes of a number of illnesses including coronary heart disease, arthritis and cancer. In the case of heart disease both working-class and middle-class women identified the stresses and strains of daily life as the primary causal factor, followed by obesity. Middle-class women also cited cigarette smoking and excessive drinking as contributory factors, whereas working-class women mentioned smoking and lack of exercise as being important in this respect. As Calnan remarks, these lay ideas fall within Chrisman's 'logic of balance' category in that the emphasis is on the relationship between the individual and the environment with stresses and strains producing an imbalance.

Whilst Calnan found little difference between the two social class groups with regard to the perceived aetiology of coronary heart disease, he did discover social class differences in lay beliefs about the causes of cancer. Middle-class women cited cigarette smoking as one of the major causes of the disease. They also made reference to hereditary factors and expressed the belief that some people might be biologically predisposed to developing the disease. In contrast, the working-class women, in the main, tended to subscribe to the view that cancer was something that was present in some people and was 'triggered off' in some way. Smoking was only rarely mentioned as providing such a trigger. Indeed a number of women expressed the 'trigger theory' without being able to specify the nature or form such a trigger might take.

Pill and Stott (1986) examined how their respondents employed concepts of individual control and external factors when discussing the causes of illness. They found that just over half of the Welsh mothers they interviewed only mentioned external factors such as stress, environment and germs when explaining the cause of illness, whereas the remainder of the sample also referred to behavioural choices made by individuals when discussing aetiology. These intra-class differences were associated with education and housing tenure. The greater the amount of formal education received, the more likely were the women to accept the views of health professionals regarding health promotion. A comparison of attitudes to health held by owner occupiers and council tenants revealed that the former were more likely to mention individual behaviour and lifestyle as causal factors in diseases such as cancer and heart disease. According to Pill and Stott, 'The decision to buy one's house may be regarded as an indicator of a much broader cluster of attitudes with possible relevance for health behaviour: for example, a willingness to postpone immediate gratification, a belief that one is essentially in control of one's Destiny' (Pill and Stott, 1986, p. 277). Blaxter and Paterson (1982) also report differences in attitudes to health and illness among a sample of working-class women. Those who were economically deprived and socially disadvantaged tended to adopt a fatalistic outlook and be pessimistic about future health prospects.

These studies not only illustrate the multi-causal nature of lay explanations of illness but also describe how responsibility for illness is attributed. In the examples quoted above the causal explanations advanced can be divided into two groups: those that see the cause of illness as external to the individual and those that locate the cause within the individual. For example, in the study by Herzlich, illness was perceived as the product of external factors largely outside the control of the individual. Consequently individuals did not consider themselves blameworthy if they became ill. This question of personal responsibility is addressed by Helman (1986) when he describes lay perspectives on colds or chills and fevers or 'flu' in a middle-class suburban community on the outskirts of London. According to Helman colds and chills '. . . are explained as being due to the penetration of the environment – across the boundary of the skin – into the human organism. They are part of the relationship of man [*sic*] to the natural environment in particular, to the idea of "danger without" and "safety within" the human body' (Helman, 1986, p. 218). Natural environmental conditions are assigned causal significance according to this view. Cold and damp or cold and dry weather conditions can affect the body. Although the individual is not seen as being responsible for producing the conditions in the first place he or she is expected to take the necessary precautionary action and dress according to the prevailing weather conditions.

Fevers fall into a different category from colds or chills. They are not viewed as being caused by the weather but are seen as resulting from the presence of germs and bugs that are airborne and invisible and enter the body, thus causing fever. Whereas colds originate in the natural environment, germs originate in other people. Catching a cold is therefore seen as a different process to that of catching a fever. Whether the cause of illness is located with the individual or explained by reference to external factors will influence the attribution of responsibility. Locker (1979) has argued that if the major cause of illness is believed to be outside the individual's control then they are not held responsible for their actions. Under these circumstances the onset of illness is accounted for in terms of bad luck or misfortune and the individual is seen as being blameless and therefore not morally accountable for becoming ill.

The significance of external factors was stressed in the accounts of illness causation given by Herzlich and Pierret's (1986) sample of French men and women.

As described above, they attributed much ill health to modern living conditions, which exposed individuals to a number of health risks as a result of environmental pollution. In accounting for the occurrence of illness interviewees repeatedly referred to the presence of germs, the quality of the air and the nature of modern lifestyles. Illness was perceived as originating outside the individual and consequently individuals were not considered to be blameworthy should they become ill. However, although their notion of illness was based on external factors, they did have a view of health which emphasised individual responsibility. Individuals were seen as possessing an internal reserve of health; this was determined by factors beyond their control but individuals were considered to have a responsibility to maintain their health. Although not considered blameworthy for catching an illness, respondents expressed the view that people could be regarded as responsible for losing their health.

Illness behaviour

Illness is a natural part of life. The fact of illness requires that the sick adapt to illness. This adaptation is moulded by society through cultural, social, institutional and biomedical mechanisms of interaction.

(Young, 2004, p. 9)

From the numerous health surveys conducted over the past few decades it can be concluded that minor health complaints are a regular occurrence for most people. For example, Wadsworth *et al.* (1971) record that 95 per cent of their sample of over 3,000 respondents had experienced one or more symptoms in the two weeks preceding the interview. Similarly, Dunnell and Cartwright (1972) found 91 per cent of adult interviewees claiming to have suffered illness symptoms in the previous two weeks: adults were found to experience symptoms of illness on about one day in four. In a prospective health study, in which 79 women aged between 16 and 44 years kept health diaries over a six-week period, only one woman recorded no symptoms (Scambler *et al.*, 1981).

What is of particular interest to medical sociologists is the fact that the majority of these symptoms do not lead to medical consultations. As Zola claims:

Virtually every day of our lives we are subject to a vast array of bodily discomforts. Only an infinitesimal amount of these get to a physician. Neither the mere presence nor the obviousness of symptoms seems to differentiate those episodes which do and do not get professional treatment.

(Zola, 1983, p. 111)

The terms 'illness iceberg' (Last, 1963), 'symptom iceberg' (Hannay, 1979) and 'iceberg of morbidity' (Freund and McGuire, 1991) have all been used to refer to this phenomenon. In the Dunnell and Cartwright (1972) study only 16 per cent of those with symptoms had visited a doctor before the interview. The 79 women who kept health diaries recorded a total of 863 symptom episodes and 49 medical consultations, giving a ratio of one consultation for approximately every 18 symptom episodes. In a study of 516 women in the 20–44-year-old age group, Banks *et al.* (1975) recorded that for every 37 symptom episodes there was one patient-initiated consultation.

These findings suggest that medical help is sought in connection with only a small proportion of the complaints experienced. It could be the case that the majority of symptoms relate to minor complaints, many of which soon disappear with or without the aid of self-medication, with medical advice only being sought in serious .cases. However, in a national survey of general practitioners it was found that nearly a quarter of the doctors felt that half of the patients they saw presented trivial complaints which did not warrant medical consultation (Cartwright and Anderson, 1981). There is also research evidence which indicates that serious illnesses can go undetected or patients delay in seeking medical advice. In 1969 the London Borough of Southwark conducted a pilot health survey of residents in the borough between the ages of 16 and 60 years. This consisted of setting up a mobile general health screening clinic which carried out comprehensive medical examinations of 3,160 men and women. Over half of those examined were referred to their family doctor for further investigation or treatment. Of these, a quarter were followed up and it was found that nearly 38 per cent of the health problems had not been previously known to the general practitioner. What is more, nearly 22 per cent of findings made known to the family doctor for the first time were considered sufficiently serious to be referred to the hospital for further investigation (Epsom, 1969).

The study of illness behaviour focuses on how individuals perceive, evaluate and react to symptoms. Some people consult a doctor when they feel unwell, while others with the same symptoms do not. This suggests that the decision to consult a doctor is influenced by socio-cultural factors and not simply related to the severity of the symptoms experienced. As previously indicated there is a lack of uniformity in the definitions of health and illness throughout society, and therefore what some groups may define as conditions requiring medical intervention others may consider normal. Even if the symptoms are defined as abnormal it takes more than the experience of illness to bring about a decision to visit the doctor. We need to understand how illness episodes are interpreted.

Kleinman (1980) maintains that the concept of explanatory models can provide an insight into the process by which illness is perceived and treated. Explanatory models offer explanations of the cause of illness, the timing of symptoms, the natural history and severity of symptoms and appropriate methods of treatment. According to Kleinman, explanatory models are held by both lay people and professional medical practitioners and used to make sense of a particular episode of illness. Lay models are heavily influenced by socio-cultural factors and used by individuals to help them to understand and respond to illness.

The lay referral system

Becoming ill is a social process that involves other people besides the patient. Zola (1973) maintains that the decision to consult a doctor is not simply based on how the patient interprets the symptoms but is also influenced by how relatives, friends and work colleagues perceive the problem. Illness behaviour needs to be viewed within a wider socio-cultural framework. Freidson (1970a) uses the concept of the 'lay referral system' to explain help-seeking behaviour. The lay referral system has two components: a 'lay culture' and a 'lay referral structure'. It is within the context of the former that the term 'illness' acquires a social meaning. As Freidson asserts, 'what the layman recognises as a symptom of illness is in part a function of deviation from the culturally and historically variable standard of normality' (1970a, p. 285).

The lay referral structure refers to the social network of personal contacts that may influence an individual when he or she is deciding what action to take regarding a particular symptom episode. Freidson acknowledges that the lay community plays an important part in influencing the utilisation of professional health services when he states that 'it organises the process of becoming ill by pressing the sufferer into or away from the professional consulting room' (1970a, p. 292). The usual lay consultants are family members, although the network can extend to friends and work colleagues. Research suggests that it is common practice for people to seek advice from non-medical sources. One study of a sample of people undergoing medical care found that nearly three-quarters of them had discussed their symptoms with someone before visiting the doctor (Suchman, 1965). One-third of the interviewees in a study of one general practice population reported a serious medical symptom. The majority had done nothing about their condition apart from 15 per cent who had discussed their symptoms with members of the family (Hannay, 1979). In a study of 79 women by Scambler *et al.* (1981) a total of 547 lay consultations were recorded over a six-week period, giving an average of 11 lay consultations for every one medical consultation.

It has been suggested that the structure and composition of lay referral networks can influence decisions to seek medical help. According to Freidson:

> The organization of lay referrals can enforce a particular orientation toward illness, or it can be so loose as to leave the individual fairly free of others' influence, to make decisions contrary to that of his peers without having to suffer their ridicule or scorn.
>
> (Freidson, 1970a, p. 292)

Some researchers have studied the organisational properties of lay referral systems paying particular attention to the strength of social network ties and the relative importance of kinship and friendship networks. There is some evidence to suggest that where there is a tightly knit, cohesive social network there can be a delay in seeking help from professional practitioners. In a study of the use of maternity services by lower-working-class women in a Scottish city, McKinlay (1973) compared mothers who were early and regular attenders at the antenatal clinic with those mothers who had not attended until after the seventeenth week of pregnancy and were not regular attenders. He found that the poor attenders had large interlocking networks of relatives and friends. In contrast, those mothers who made regular use of the maternity services consulted a narrower range of lay persons. In a study of women's social networks and patterns of lay consultations, Scambler *et al.* (1981) did not find a relationship between the extent of the network and the use of general practitioner services. However, when they distinguished between kinship and friendship networks they discovered that extensive kinship networks were associated with high levels of service use and large friendship networks with low levels of service use. They offer the following tentative explanation:

> . . . discussion of symptoms with kin may be intense and protracted and lead to kin referrals to general practitioners. On the other hand, discussion with friends may be more casual and unfocused and result in symptoms being re-defined as unimportant and not in need of medical attention.
>
> (Scambler and Scambler, 1984, p. 43)

Studies of health in families suggest that women are a major source of advice and support in the lay referral system (Graham, 1985). In many families the domestic division of labour is such that the responsibility for healthcare is assigned to women. It is more often the female members of the household who care for the sick.

Social interaction with family and friends can be more significant in prompting the decision to consult a doctor than the nature and severity of the symptoms themselves. In a study of a small number of families in South Wales, Robinson (1971) found that decisions to seek professional medical advice were made when families were uncertain as to the significance of the symptoms. Zola (1973), in an American study of attenders at an outpatient clinic in Boston, observed how patients had coped with their health problems over a considerable period of time before deciding to seek medical help. He identified five non-physiological factors or incidents that appeared to 'trigger' the decision to consult a doctor. Firstly, some form of interpersonal crisis may occur, such as the death of a member of the family. Secondly, the patient may come to seek medical advice when the symptoms begin to disrupt social relationships. Thirdly, there is what Zola calls 'sanctioning'. This occurs when family members, friends or workmates apply pressure on the individual to do something about their problem. Fourthly, medical attention may be sought when symptoms begin to interfere with physical activity and individuals are forced to make marked adjustments to their daily routine. Finally, there is what Zola refers to as the 'temporising of symptoms': this applies where individuals have views about how long certain symptoms should last before medical attention is sought.

Sociological approaches to the study of illness behaviour have generated theoretical models that emphasise the fact that notions of, and responses to, illness are shaped by social and cultural factors. These models concentrate on how individuals come to define themselves as ill and how they respond to the problematic experience of illness. It is suggested that the significance of symptoms is not always immediately self-evident. The individual does not react to the symptom itself but to the meaning attributed to the symptom. As noted above, for Freidson (1970a) it is the lay culture that creates illness as a social meaning. In attributing meaning to an illness experience 'the individual sufferer does not invent the meanings himself but rather uses the meanings and interpretations that his social life has provided him' (Freidson, 1970a, p. 288).

Similarly, Dingwall's (1976) interpretive approach distinguishes between disturbances in body functioning and the meaning given to such events. Dingwall is primarily interested in the decision-making processes involved in the illness action model. He asserts that illness is problematic for the individual in so far as it can disrupt social interaction and prevent the individual from sustaining an identity as a normal person. When faced with an illness, individuals attempt to make sense of what is happening to them. In so doing they make use of lay knowledge and beliefs absorbed from particular cultural, ethnic and religious backgrounds. What determines illness action, that is the decision whether or not to seek help, is the interpretation of the symptoms by the sufferer and significant lay people.

The sick role

Clearly, from a sociological point of view illness is seen as a social state. This is not to deny that for the individual the experience of illness is intensely personal. The signs and symptoms associated with some health problems can cause physical discomfort, emotional distress and considerable anxiety. However, what is of interest to sociologists is how social expectations and cultural beliefs and practices surrounding sickness influence how the sick person behaves. Parsons (1951) developed the concept of the sick role to draw attention to the fact that illness is not purely a biological state but has a social dimension. The concept does not describe how sick persons actually behave; its primary purpose is to outline the social expectations and sanctions that are applied to the sick.

According to Parsons the sick role consists of four components (see Box 2.3) which highlight the rights and responsibilities attributed to the sick person. Firstly, the sick role *legitimates social withdrawal*. In other words, an individual who is deemed to be sick is exempted from normal obligations, such as attending school or going to work. The extent of the withdrawal from daily activities is variable and will depend on the nature of the illness, the degree of incapacity associated with the condition and whether or not the individual is considered to be a danger to others. Secondly, although the individual's incapacity is a form of deviance from prevailing social norms, this is not seen as a deliberate act and *the sick person is not held responsible for her/his condition*. However, the legitimation of sickness as a basis for social withdrawal is not unconditional, as the third and fourth components of the sick role illustrate. The *sick person is expected to define the state of being sick as undesirable* and there is also *a social obligation to get better* by seeking medical attention and cooperating with medical personnel in the treatment of the illness. At no time should the individual seek to take advantage of the benefits associated with the sick role.

Parsons' formulation of the sick role, and his analysis of sickness in society, is essentially functionalist. His principal concern is to account for the stability of society by describing it as a system of interlocking social roles. He holds that society can only function if individuals are motivated by a sense of inter-personal

Box 2.3   Definition

Parsons' sick role

1 The sick person is exempt from the normal social roles that the person takes for the duration of the illness. This exemption is legitimised by society as represented by the physician. Normal role performance and responsibilities are suspended so that the ill person can 'get well'. The strength of the exemption varies directly with the severity of the illness.

2 Sick persons are not responsible for their illnesses. The illness is beyond personal control. A curative process outside the person is required to restore wellness.

3 The sick person has the duty to try to get well. Sickness is societally undesirable and thus society places the obligation to get well on the patient, with the help of the doctor, of course.

4 The sick person must seek competent technical help and cooperate with the caregiver.

Source: Cockerham, 2000, p. 161

responsibility and can be relied upon to perform essential tasks. Any withdrawal from social activities therefore needs to be regulated in some way to ensure that people do not evade their customary duties and responsibilities. This is why the sick role offers temporary release from role expectations at the same time as placing additional obligations on the sick person. For Parsons there is a need for sickness to be subject to a system of social control to prevent people's sense of duty and social responsibility being undermined. The sick role becomes officially sanctioned and members of the medical profession perform the important function of maintaining social responsibility among the ill.

The concept of the sick role has attracted considerable critical comment on a number of grounds. Firstly, in Parsons' original formulation of the sick role it is assumed that the patient will do everything in order to achieve the goal of 'complete recovery'. Consequently, it has been suggested that the concept applies only to acute illnesses and is inapplicable in the case of chronic health problems, where the individual has to cope with long-term illness. However, in his later writings Parsons (1975) responded to this criticism by claiming that although complete recovery from chronic illness, such as diabetes, is not possible, the patient can, with the aid of medical assistance, 'manage' the problem to such an extent that they can follow a fairly normal pattern of daily living.

Secondly, Parsons appears to have been primarily concerned with the sick role as a legitimate means of temporary social withdrawal: a role readily assumed by the sick as a means of escaping from social expectations and obligations. What Parsons does not consider is that not all sections of the population have equal access to the sick role. Research shows that this is particularly the case as far as women are concerned. Not only does the burden of caring for the ill and the disabled fall primarily on women, but also they carry responsibility for maintaining and promoting the health of others. This frequently results in women placing the health needs of their family above their own (Graham, 1979, 1984, 1985). Studies of working-class mothers illustrate how women see their dual roles of wife and mother as indispensable, effectively placing constraints on their adoption of the sick role. This view was expressed by three-quarters of the mothers interviewed in one study. As one woman stated, '. . . I think with a family you can't afford to be ill, you know what I mean? You think, well you'll be ill after you've cooked the tea' (Pill and Stott, 1986, p. 276).

There is evidence that some women are reluctant to lay claim to the sick role. Blaxter and Paterson (1982) in their study of working-class women in Scotland describe how the reaction to symptoms is important. Illness is viewed as something that should not be allowed to occupy the mind for too long. As one grandmother commented, 'I think if you brood too much on your bitties and piecies, I think you would be ill, you would. Self-analysis every morning – tell yourself, get a move on! Dinna sit an' hang aboot' (Blaxter and Paterson, 1982, p. 33). To give in to illness and accept the sick role is seen as a form of weakness and a negation of the responsibilities of a wife and mother, a view endorsed by many of Pill and Stott's interviewees:

> The responsible mother 'carries on' and it is quite clear that this is seen as her duty. Moral opprobrium was heaped on those women who were deemed to be too ready to think they were ill and to seek the advantages of the sick role when the appropriate behaviour was seen as 'not giving in' and 'fighting it off' or by 'keeping going and working it off'.
>
> (Pill and Stott, 1986, p. 276)

The situation with regard to working-class men is different. Cornwell (1984) describes how although the men in her study did not take time off work when suffering from minor ailments they readily adopted the sick role at home and expected to be looked after. As Miles (1991, p. 84) has remarked, such self-indulgence is rarely an option for wives and mothers given their domestic responsibilities.

The view that the sick person voluntarily assumes the sick role because of the advantages it offers does not apply in all cases. Some health problems are so stigmatising that individuals may go to great lengths to avoid being identified as a sufferer. The benefits they would obtain from occupying the sick role may be far outweighed by the social discrimination they are likely to encounter by disclosing their medical condition. Epilepsy provides a good example (Scambler, 1989).

A third criticism levelled at Parsons' model is that the labelling of a condition as an illness by a doctor does not necessarily ensure that the patient is accorded the sick role by others. Miles (1988) describes how husbands of women who were receiving treatment from psychiatrists for neurotic symptoms refused to accept that their wives were ill, even when they were unable to carry out their normal daily activities.

Fourthly, Parsons' theoretical preoccupation with the functions the medical system performs for the wider society led him to adopt an idealised picture of the doctor–patient relationship. The sick-role model presents an image of the patient as passively accepting the medical diagnosis and acting on the advice given. The relationship between doctor and patient is seen as fundamentally reciprocal in character; patient compliance is taken for granted while the potential for conflict is ignored. Consequently, it has been suggested that 'Parsons has merely draped doctors' assumptions about how patients should behave in a sociological cloak' (Bloor and Horobin, 1975, p. 282). In other words, the sick role represents nothing more than Parsons' interpretation as to what doctors consider constitutes the ideal patient.

Another criticism of Parsons' original model concerns the insistence on the obligation to seek medical help as an essential element of the sick role; this effectively overlooks an important conceptual distinction between the sick role and the patient role. As Bloor and Horobin (1975) point out, an individual may adopt the patient role by actively seeking medical treatment, without taking advantage of the sick role. This could be the case with a sexually transmitted disease that is stigmatising but not incapacitating. On the other hand, an individual may readily adopt a sick role, when for example suffering from a heavy cold, and choose self-medication as opposed to a visit to the doctor, thus not adopting the patient role.

Finally, a number of critics have drawn attention to the fact that Parsons' conceptualisation fails to adequately explain variation in illness behaviour displayed by patients from different social, economic, cultural and ethnic backgrounds who share a common illness. For example, research has found cultural and ethnic differences in how patients describe, respond to and account for pain (Zborowski, 1952) and how they talk about their symptoms, account for the onset and progress of their illness and comply with treatment regimes (Zola, 1966; Nilchaikovit *et al.*, 1993; Prior *et al.*, 2000). The classic sick-role model is also seen as having a Western focus, with a strong emphasis on middle-class values of individual responsibility and orientation to work (Hardey, 1999; Cockerham, 2000).

Notwithstanding the many criticisms directed at Parsons' conception of the sick role it has continued to attract the interest of researchers engaged in the study of illness behaviour. Indeed it has been noted that '[m]any of the criticisms are more accurately modifications of the sick role concept to fit changing social norms and a more probabilistic conception of society' (Young, 2004, p. 5). Thus, rather than discarding the concept we should be looking at ways in which it can be used to inform our understanding of the roles assigned to sick people in society. Despite its obvious limitations the concept has proved to be 'a useful analytical tool in the study of illness behaviour' (Miles, 1991, p. 74) and has generated a great deal of research.

Illness as deviance

It may seem strange to think of illness as deviance, particularly if one usually works from a medical model perspective. From the sociological viewpoint, however, where no assumptions are made about aetiology, an illness is a form of deviance just as crime, disloyalty, and sin are.

(Waxler, 1975, p. 39)

Deviance is a term used to refer to behaviour or conduct that violates those social rules and norms that are supported by a significant section of society. Ways of acting which are considered unacceptable in a particular culture can be labelled as deviant. Societies use sanctions as a means of enforcing normative behaviour. These sanctions can be positive, as is the case when rewards or privileges are offered as inducements to conformity, or negative, when breaches of existing norms are punished.

In a sense illness may be seen as a type of deviance in so far as it constitutes a deviation from culturally established standards of good health and normality. In Parsons' conceptualisation of the sick role the individual is allowed to deviate legitimately on the condition that being ill is recognised as an undesirable state and there is an explicit acceptance of an obligation to seek medical attention in an effort to get better. For Parsons the sick role functions to place the deviant in the hands of the medical profession; it represents a form of social regulation, ensuring that sickness is not seen as a way of permanently evading role obligations and responsibilities. It has been remarked that:

> The sick role is analytically significant because it constitutes a form of deviance that is caught up in a process of social control that at once seals the deviant off from non-deviants and prevents him from becoming permanently alienated. It insulates the sick person from the well, depriving the former of unconditional legitimacy and reinforcing the latter's motivation *not* to fall ill . . .
>
> (Freidson, 1970a, p. 227, emphasis in original)

Withdrawal from normal social activities is temporary and conditional. Failure to comply with the obligations attached to the sick role can result in the individual being placed in a deviant category. For example, those with symptoms considered by a medical practitioner to be imaginary rather than real can find themselves treated as 'malingerers' or 'hypochondriacs'.

As described above, Parsons' functional approach attempts to explain how social systems deal with the disruption caused by ill health and maintain stability and cohesion. This provides only a partial insight into responses to illness. In order to understand how signs and symptoms come to be labelled as illness and how the process of diagnosis and treatment can influence social identity it is necessary to turn to research generated within the interactionist perspective.

While the functionalist stance tends to focus on society as a whole and holds that human behaviour is shaped by the social system, interactionists concentrate on how individuals play an active part in organising and managing social interaction. Consequently, whereas for functional theorists roles are fixed, for the interactionist they are constructed and negotiated in the process of social interaction. It is through interacting with others that individuals define social situations, attach meaning to their own behaviour and the behaviour of others and develop a self-concept, that is a picture of themselves as they believe others see them.

The labelling perspective is one approach in the interactionist tradition that can usefully be applied to the study of illness behaviour. The application of this perspective to the study of mental illness is discussed at some length in the next chapter. Briefly, the labelling perspective was originally introduced by sociologists interested in exploring the links between crime and deviance, a central idea being that the definition of deviance is negotiated in the process of social interaction. This is captured in the following statements:

> deviance is not a quality of the act a person commits but rather a consequence of the application by others of rules and sanctions to an offender. The deviant is one to whom that label has successfully been applied; deviant behaviour is behaviour that people so label.
>
> (Becker, 1963, p. 9)

> Forms of behaviour *per se* do not differentiate deviants from nondeviants; it is the responses of the conventional and conforming members of the society who identify and interpret behaviour as deviant which sociologically transforms persons into deviants.
>
> (Kitsuse, 1962, p. 253)

According to this view the nature and quality of societal reaction plays a major part in identifying what is deviant. Attention is drawn to the public labelling of the deviant and the consequences this has for the individual concerned.

The labelling experience readily applies to those who have had a condition medically diagnosed. Being labelled, for example, as an epileptic or HIV (human immunodeficiency virus) positive can form the basis of a deviant identity and have a profound impact on an individual's self-image and their social relationships with others. Thus in some instances formal diagnosis not only identifies a health problem but also creates a deviant status. A strong, negative societal reaction to a particular type of chronic illness or disability can dominate an individual's self-concept to the extent that they come to see themselves as others see them and behave in such a way as to confirm the deviant status ascribed to them.

In certain cases a medical diagnosis can create a deviant identity which, in the eyes of others, becomes the predominant feature in the individual's personal biography. Consequently, the individual acquires a new 'master status' (Hughes, 1945) which largely determines how they are treated by others. AIDS (acquired immunodeficiency syndrome) provides a good example of the dramatic and devastating effects a diagnostic label can have on patients' lives. When AIDS was first identified in 1981 it was exclusively associated with two groups that were already stigmatised as deviant, that is male homosexuals and intravenous drug users. Given this association and the fact that the disease was fatal and there was no effective treatment, sufferers faced social rejection and discrimination. The disease was seen as a consequence of lifestyle choices and AIDS victims were denied access to the sick role. The assumption was that they could have avoided the disease if they had not chosen a deviant way of life. Deuchar (1984) records how sufferers in the USA found themselves ostracised from their own communities and rejected by family and friends.

With the subsequent identification of AIDS among heterosexuals, the growing number of children with AIDS and cases of patients having being infected as a result of receiving contaminated blood products, sufferers are more likely to be seen as innocent victims and worthy of sympathy. Nevertheless, AIDS patients still experience social difficulties in dealing with the social and physical consequences of their condition. The social stigma surrounding AIDS makes it difficult for them to maintain a normal social identity (Weitz, 1989).

Research shows that stigma is a feature of the lives of people suffering from a variety of conditions, including psoriasis (Jobling, 1977; Ginzburg and Link, 1993), diabetes (Hopper, 1981), epilepsy (Scambler, 1989), deafness (Higgins, 1981) and mental illness (Link *et al.*, 1989). It is to the nature and origins of social stigma that we now turn our attention. To illustrate the potentially damaging and harmful effects stigma can have on people's lives and how they develop mechanisms for coping with a stigmatising social identity, reference will be made to studies of the experiences of epileptics, men and women with HIV infection and AIDS and mental health patients.

Social stigma

> . . . if health professionals want to maximise the well-being of the people they treat, they must address stigma as a separate and important factor in its own right.
>
> (Link *et al.*, 1997, p. 177)

Coping with chronic illness, either physical or mental, or living with a disability for many people not only entails coming to terms with physical or mental impairment but also involves dealing with the social stigma associated with their condition. Goffman (1968) identifies three types of stigma:

- physical deformities;
- 'blemishes of individual character';
- 'tribal stigma of race, nation and religion'.

He maintains that these three types share the same sociological features:

> an individual who might have been received easily in ordinary social intercourse possesses a trait that can obtrude itself upon attention and turn those of us whom he meets away from him, breaking the claim that his other attributes have on us. He possesses a stigma, an undesired differentness from what we had anticipated.
>
> (Goffman, 1968, p. 15)

In certain cases the nature of the 'undesired differentness' can result in the stigmatised individual being 'reduced in our minds from a whole and usual person to a tainted, discounted one' (Goffman, 1968, p. 12). Jones *et al.* (1984) describe stigma as a 'mark' that not only serves to set a person apart from others but also in the process associates them with 'undesirable characteristics'. Social stigma is seen as the 'evocation of negative difference' (Susman, 1994, p. 16). It is all about acquiring a tainted or spoiled social identity. For Goffman, when there is a recognisable discrepancy between an individual's *virtual* social identity and his or her *actual* identity, the marked person is likely to experience negative discrimination in social encounters. This discrimination can be widespread, with stigmatising labels being attached to whole groups of people and not just isolated individuals (Dain, 1994).

For Goffman, the visibility of a stigmatising attribute and the extent to which it interferes with social interaction need to be taken into account when considering the coping strategies that are available to the chronically sick and disabled. What is clearly important in this context is whether or not an individual's condition is known to others. Where this is the case, for example when the stigmatising condition is in the form of a clearly observable physical disfigurement or is less obvious but has previously been disclosed, then Goffman refers to it as a *discrediting* attribute. Attributes that remain hidden and undisclosed are termed *discreditable*.

Discredited persons, whose stigma is known about, find that their common problem is one of 'impression management', that is attempting to influence how they present themselves to others. In everyday social encounters with 'normal' people they can find themselves coping with situations that generate tension and have a potential for producing social embarrassment. It is not uncommon for disabled people to find that they have been ascribed a stereotypical identity which forms the basis of their acceptance by others. Scott (1969) maintains that blind people are portrayed as helpless, dependent and susceptible to depression.

A person who is 'discreditable', as opposed to 'discredited', has the option of keeping his or her stigmatising condition a secret. The problem they face is one of 'information management', that is controlling the release of personal information. As Goffman sees it the individual faces a number of difficult decisions: 'To display or not to display; to tell or not to tell; to let on or not to let on; to lie or not to lie; and in each case, to whom, how, when and where' (1968, p. 57). He describes the main strategies available for concealing discrediting information as 'passing' and 'withdrawal'. A person trying to pass as 'normal' will have to withhold information, or provide false information, to avoid attracting a stigmatising label. Living under the constant threat of exposure can be very stressful. Some individuals may cope by keeping their social contacts to a minimum, avoiding difficult social situations or in extreme cases withdrawing from social life altogether.

While passing is not an option available to those whose stigma is known to others, 'covering' represents an alternative coping strategy. Individuals can take active steps to minimise the impact of a stigmatising condition by reducing its obtrusiveness. Blind people may become aware of the rules governing social interaction and conduct themselves accordingly:

> the blind sometimes learn to look directly at the speaker even though this looking accomplishes no seeing, for it prevents the blind from staring off into space or hanging the head or otherwise unknowingly violating the code regarding attention cues through which spoken interaction is organised.

(Goffman, 1968, p. 128)

Although 'covering' relates to impression management and 'passing' to the management of information the two strategies are very similar in terms of the adaptive techniques employed by individuals. As Goffman asserts, 'what will conceal a stigma from unknowing persons may also ease matters for those in the know' (1968, pp. 125–6).

Epilepsy: a stigmatised condition

Epilepsy provides an interesting case study of a stigmatising disorder. It has been suggested that one reason why epileptics are treated as social deviants is because they are perceived as posing a threat to the social order by causing 'ambiguity in social interaction' (Scambler, 1989, p. 50). Scambler identifies three possible ways in which epilepsy may disrupt social interaction. Firstly, its unpredictability may be a cause of concern to others. Secondly, some people may find the sight of an epileptic seizure distressing. Finally, some may fear having to assume responsibility for someone who is having a seizure.

According to Scambler and Hopkins (1986) epileptics and doctors tend to subscribe to what they have termed the 'orthodox viewpoint': this asserts that because of the level of public ignorance surrounding epilepsy, sufferers encounter discriminatory practices and social rejection. Ignorance breeds intolerance: intolerance fosters negative discrimination. It is assumed that it is this response, as much as anything else, which is responsible for the difficulties epileptics experience in coping with their condition. Research findings cast some doubt on the validity of the orthodox viewpoint. Following a brief review of studies of lay knowledge of, and attitudes to, epilepsy, Scambler concludes that there is evidence to suggest that knowledge is on the increase and attitudes are becoming more tolerant. However, he does assert that 'it does not follow . . . that lay discrimination based on stigma is a thing of the past' (Scambler, 1989, p. 47).

Scambler and Hopkins' (1986) study of the experiences of epileptics casts further doubt on the applicability of the orthodox viewpoint. They found that epileptics were distressed on learning of the diagnosis for two main reasons. Firstly, they felt that the diagnostic label attributed to them by the doctor had transformed them from a 'normal' person into an 'epileptic'. Secondly, because they viewed epilepsy as a stigmatising condition they perceived their new status to be both a personal liability and a considerable social burden. While their immediate response to being labelled reflected the views prevalent in the orthodox position, further analysis resulted in this model being challenged and subsequently replaced by the 'hidden distress model' (Scambler, 1989, p. 57).

In order to understand the hidden distress model it is necessary to appreciate the distinction between *enacted* and *felt* stigma. Enacted stigma refers to the actual discrimination epileptics face in society on account of the perceived social unacceptability of their condition. Felt stigma refers to both the shame associated with being 'epileptic' and 'an oppressive fear of enacted stigma' (Scambler, 1984, p. 215). It is this felt stigma which provides the basis for the epileptic's 'special view of the world'. According to Scambler this 'special view of the world' has a major influence on behaviour: it prompts epileptics to conceal their disorder from others by attempting to pass as 'normal'; if this fails and they are assigned a discredited status they adopt the stratagem of covering.

While the orthodox viewpoint emphasises the significance of enacted or actual stigma the hidden distress model draws attention to the behavioural implications of felt stigma. Scambler asserts that by not disclosing their condition epileptics reduced the possibility of enacted stigma but at the same time they increased their vulnerability as far as felt stigma is concerned. For many of the individuals studied by Scambler 'felt stigma . . . was typically the source of more personal anguish and unhappiness than was enacted stigma' (1984, p. 217). In other words, keeping their deviant identity secret produced more stress and unease than coping with the actual discrimination following their exposure as epileptics.

HIV infection and AIDS

Not all illnesses generate the same level of discrediting social attributions. As briefly described above, HIV infection and AIDS draw a particularly negative societal response, which can result in individual sufferers, and the groups to which they belong, being marginalised. Alonzo and Reynolds (1995) note that the research literature contains six main reasons why individuals with HIV/AIDS are stigmatised; these are summarised in Box 2.4.

Of course, as Alonzo and Reynolds argue, individual sufferers do not all experience the same degree of stigma. For example, some groups are likely to be regarded as innocent victims, such as the children of HIV-positive mothers and patients infected after receiving blood transfusions (Pierret, 1992). However, as Lawless *et al.* (1996) found in their study of the experiences of women living with HIV and AIDS in Australia, there was a tendency for medical practitioners to assume that the women's status as HIV positive was a direct result of their engaging in high-risk activities, such as injecting drugs or being sexually promiscuous.

Box 2.4 Research findings

The stigma of HIV and AIDS

Individuals with HIV and AIDS are stigmatised because their illness is:

1 seen as both a product and producer of deviant behaviour;
2 viewed as the responsibility of the individual;
3 considered to be contracted as a result of engaging in what is morally sanctionable behaviour, thought to represent a character blemish;
4 perceived as contagious and a threat to the community;
5 associated with an undesirable and unaesthetic form of death;
6 not very well understood by the lay community and viewed in a negative light by professional healthcare workers.

Source: Alonzo and Reynolds, 1995, p. 305

This was a cause of concern for a number of the interviewees who felt that, although they did not fall into either of these risk categories, they were still discriminated against by healthcare workers. As one interviewee commented:

> I didn't get it by using dirty needles or sleeping around you know. I got it through blood. I went into hospital and I got a death sentence . . . and it does hurt me a lot if people assume that I got it that way. I do find that, you know especially in bigger hospitals they assume everyone used, you know got it through using drugs or being promiscuous . . . I don't like it. I just say look I don't want to be treated any different but I didn't get it that way!
>
> (An HIV-positive woman quoted in Lawless *et al.*, 1996, p. 1373)

The researchers describe how the stigma of sexual deviance and illegal drug use permeates the whole debate about women and HIV/AIDS. There is a discourse of deviance in which infected women are deemed to have fallen from a state of grace by failing to conform to the socially prescribed role of the 'good woman'. A stereotype is created of a group of women who have a chaotic and disorganised lifestyle and are irresponsible, unreliable and undeserving. Individual patients who are continually exposed to this stereotype in their encounters with health workers can internalise the stigma associated with being HIV positive in a process of self-stigmatisation.

In researching stigma as a social construction, researchers have tended to concentrate on how the nature and degree of stigma varies across different types of illnesses rather than explore how stigma changes during the course of a single illness or disease. In the context of HIV/AIDS, Alonzo and Reynolds (1995) use the concept of the 'stigma trajectory', alongside that of the illness trajectory, to help explain how stigma is affected by changes in the biophysical aspects of the disease. As they assert, 'The shape of the stigma trajectory is intrinsically entwined with the disease course but is uniquely tied to the responses of the broader society, family, peers, strangers, healthcare professionals and the identity of the individual who is potentially stigmatizable' (Alonzo and Reynolds, 1995, pp. 305–6). Thus in order to understand the changing nature of the stigma experienced by individuals with HIV/AIDS and identify the coping strategies developed at different stages in the disease process, Alonzo and Reynolds describe the stigma trajectory as having four clearly distinct 'biopsychosocial phases'. These are labelled as follows: at risk, diagnostic, latent and manifest (see Box 2.5).

The first of these stages does not in fact relate to an actual phase in the disease course characteristic of HIV infection. The 'at-risk' phase is one of uncertainty in the stigma trajectory and occurs before diagnosis takes place. At this juncture individuals are described as the 'worried well' who experience a 'potentially felt stigma' or 'pre-stigmatic fear' of the social consequences likely to ensue if they are identified by others as being at risk of infection (Alonzo and Reynolds, 1995, p. 307). A common coping strategy to emerge in this context is denial: essentially a form of avoidance that can take a number of different forms. For example, some individuals may find ways of rejecting claims that certain activities carry a high risk of infection or express the opinion that they do not share

Box 2.5   Research findings

Biopsychosocial phases of the stigma trajectory

- At risk: prior to diagnosis 'worried well' experience pre-stigmatic fear.
- Diagnostic: information management becomes an issue.
- Latent: felt stigma and attempts at concealment.
- Manifest: signs and symptoms become less easy to conceal.

Source: Alonzo and Reynolds, 1995

many of the characteristics associated with those individuals who are deemed to be highly susceptible to infection.

It is at the diagnostic stage that the problem of 'information management' comes to the fore. Decisions have to be made about disclosure and how this might influence social identity and relationships with relatives and friends. The strategies adopted reflect the social circumstances and personal experiences of the individuals concerned. Where disclosure is the favoured option there is the possibility of acquiring a double stigma to be considered, as in the case of HIV-infected individuals with a previously undisclosed gay identity. At this stage in the trajectory and throughout the following latent phase, felt stigma, in the form of fear of social rejection and subsequent isolation, is very much in evidence. In terms of the illness trajectory, the latent or asymptomatic phase can last for a period of up to four years during which time individuals can conceal their condition from others in an attempt to protect themselves against enacted stigma. However, this strategy has its costs. As Alonzo and Reynolds confirm, concealment is emotionally draining as it involves the individual engaging in acts of subterfuge and deceit to hide their deviant status and present a socially acceptable image to those with whom they interact. Furthermore, by keeping the diagnosis a secret the individual is unable to draw on the social support that family and friends normally provide at times of illness. When the disease enters the manifest phase of its trajectory, signs and symptoms become less easy to conceal. The disease and stigma trajectories begin to converge. The individual acquires the 'master status' of an AIDS patient:

> The 'normal' identity of the individual is essentially worn down and the stigmatic AIDS identity becomes fixed by multiple opportunistic infections, repeated hospitalisations, physical changes, weakness, dependence on others, increased contact with medical practitioners, and sometimes either increased contact with estranged family and friends or essential rejection and increased social isolation.
>
> (Alonzo and Reynolds, 1995, p. 311)

Identifying the disease and stigma trajectories for HIV and AIDS makes it possible to appreciate that there are certain critical points in the course of an illness where social stigma may be differentially experienced. Where this is the case, its successful management may depend on individuals altering and adapting their coping strategy to meet the changing circumstances.

The stigma of mental illness

As described above, stigma is a social construction, which takes the form of a discrediting social label that is applied to individuals who fail to live up to normative expectations. To understand the magnitude of the effects a stigmatising label can have on an individual or group, it is necessary to have an insight into the nature and content of societal attitudes towards the behaviour or condition that is the source of the stigma. Surveys of public attitudes towards mental illness reveal that large numbers of people feel that the mentally ill are a cause of embarrassment to others (Huxley, 1993) and with a perceived predisposition to violence are seen as potentially very dangerous (Link and Cullen, 1983, 1986). Research also shows the existence of prejudicial attitudes towards mental illness. Hall *et al*. (1993) asked adult respondents how they felt they would react if they came into contact with people displaying various types of psychiatric symptoms including schizophrenia, depression and obsessional neurosis. The general pattern of responses was similar for the different symptom categories. Whereas the majority of respondents said that if they encountered any individuals displaying the symptoms described they would speak to them, there was evidence that many would prefer their contacts with such symptom sufferers to be limited. For example, less than a third of respondents claimed that they would choose to live next door to someone with symptoms of paranoid schizophrenia and, on average, just under a quarter reported that they would be happy for their child to attend a party at a house in which a mentally ill person lived.

The stigmatisation of psychiatric patients is based on how people perceive mental illness. These perceptions are the product of the knowledge and information people have at their disposal. Information can be gleaned from primary and secondary sources. Primary information comes about through personal contacts with the mentally ill. The first-hand knowledge relatives and friends acquire can dispel many of the myths and stereotypes surrounding mental illness. Indeed, research confirms that negative attitudes and stigma are reduced when there is evidence of previous contact with people suffering from mental health problems (Penn *et al*., 1994). However, the perceptions of many people are based on secondary source material, as produced by the mass media.

Philo *et al*. (1996) undertook a content analysis of the coverage of mental illness by the Scottish media over a one-month period. They included in their analysis not only sources of factual information, such as newspaper articles, television news broadcasts, current affairs programmes and medical items in popular magazines, but also fictional output, as in cartoon strips and soap operas. Five main categories of coverage were identified: these are listed in Table 2.1.

Clearly, the dominant message contained in the media coverage was that mental illness is associated with violence. Philo and colleagues conducted an audience reception study in which they found that the majority of respondents believed this to be true and many claimed that they had reached this view as a result of the information they had obtained from both factual and fictional sources. Although some respondents, as a result of personal experience, rejected the dominant image of mental illness as portrayed in the media, the researchers observed

Table 2.1 Media coverage of mental health/illness, April 1993

Output category	Number of items	Percentage of total items
Violence to others	373	66
Sympathetic coverage	102	18
Harm to self	71	13
'Comic' images	12	2
Criticism of accepted definition of mental illness	4	1
Total	562	100

Source: Philo, G., Secker, J., Platt, S., Henderson, L., McLaughlin, G. and Burnside, J., 'Media images of mental distress', p.165, in Tom Heller, Jill Reynolds, Roger Gomm, Rosemary Muston and Stephen Pattison (eds), *Mental Health Matters: A Reader*, published 1996, Palgrave Macmillan in association with the Open University, reproduced with permission of Palgrave Macmillan

that, 'in our sample several people appeared to believe media messages in preference to the evidence of their own eyes. Where mental illness is concerned it seems that some media accounts can exert exceptional power over readers and viewers' (Philo *et al.*, 1996, p. 169).

Ex-mental patients share with other socially defined deviant individuals the need to develop forms of information management to counter the stigma associated with psychiatric illness. However, the label of ex-mental patient is a particularly powerful and all-embracing one, which once applied constitutes a 'core identity construct' (Thumma, 1991) that can stay with the individual for the rest of his or her life. According to Barham and Hayward, severe mental illness can lead to a 'devastation of personhood' (1996, p. 232). Not all deviant labels are so powerful and enduring. The negative self-image of the mental patient is indicated in the following:

> Having been diagnosed as a psychiatric patient with psychotic tendencies is the worst thing that has ever happened to me. It's shitty to be mentally ill; it's not something to be proud of. It makes you realise just how different you are from everybody else – they're normal and you're not. Things are easy for them; things are hard for you. Life's a ball for them; life's a bitch for you! I'm like a mental cripple! I'm a failure at life . . .
> (Tom, a 45-year-old ex-psychiatric patient, quoted in Herman, 1993, p. 300)

Herman (1993) describes three major strategies of information management employed by individuals: selective concealment, therapeutic disclosure and preventive disclosure.

Selective concealment is what occurs when ex-mental patients decide to keep their mental health status secret from all but a few highly selected individuals. As noted above, when discussing individualised responses to other stigmatising illnesses, this is a stratagem that can produce emotional turmoil. The individual has got to be constantly on his or her guard to ensure that they do not reveal evidence of their current condition or former patient status to others. Therapeutic and preventive disclosures are types of selective disclosure. The former is said to take place when an individual confides in someone whom they feel they can trust.

Among the patients Herman interviewed the trusted person was normally a close relative, friend or former mental patient. One interviewee described the therapeutic value of this management strategy as follows:

> Finally, letting it out, after so many secrets, lies, it was so therapeutic for me. Keeping something like this all bottled up inside is self-destructive. When I came clean, this great burden was lifted from me!
>
> (Vincent, a 29-year-old ex-psychiatric patient, quoted in Herman, 1993, p. 311)

This illustrates the emotional strain that can be engendered by trying to keep an illness secret. Attempts at concealment can leave patients and former patients increasingly vulnerable to the likelihood of experiencing a relapse or a stress-related illness.

Herman describes preventive disclosure as 'selective disclosure to "normals"' (1993, p. 312). This takes the form of individual patients seeking to influence both how they are perceived by significant others and how these 'normal' others view mental illness. By their efforts patients hope to either avoid or at least reduce the impact of future stigma. Herman found that just over one-third of the ex-patients he interviewed chose to disclose details of their illness to selected people at an early stage in the development of a relationship. This represented their way of reducing the degree of disappointment should they be rejected following their disclosure. Over half of the interviewees admitted to using 'medical disclaimers' as part of their overall information management strategy to influence people's general perception of mental illness. A common device was to describe their mental disorder as being like any other disease, something they acquired through no fault of their own. As one ex-patient claimed, 'I just tell them, "Don't blame me, blame my genes!"' (Herman, 1993, p. 314).

Ex-hospital patients can face many difficulties and dilemmas when they try to re-integrate into the community. They not only have to re-establish social relationships with family and friends but also have to establish relationships with the providers of community-based psychiatric care services. A number of discharged mental patients interviewed in a study by Barham and Hayward (1996) spoke as if they felt they had been conscripted into the community mental patient system. The researchers also identified aspects of the relationship between psychiatric professionals and discharged patients that gave rise to tension:

> In attempting to re-establish themselves in social life, participants not infrequently find themselves in conflict with the definitions and ideologies held by psychiatric professionals as to how ex-mental patients ought to think of themselves, conduct their lives and, in the jargon of psychiatric containment, 'fill their time'.
>
> (Barham and Hayward, 1996, pp. 228–9)

Patients described the services provided as offering nothing more than 'protective containment'. While they acknowledged the benefits of medication, they felt that anti-psychotic drugs should be seen as a short-term solution and expressed concern that over-reliance on this form of treatment might be detrimental in the long run. Indeed, the side-effects of certain forms of medication can contribute to negative labelling, which is a potential source of stigma.

Not all researchers view stigma as having a major, long-lasting impact on the lives of mental patients. Walter Gove (1982) is of the opinion that labelling has its positive aspects, in so far as it leads to treatment. Given the effectiveness of much of the treatment that is now available, the contention is that any stigma is short-lived and does not have serious social consequences. However, recent studies conducted in the USA confirm the pervasive and enduring effects of stigma, even within the context of effective mental health treatment programmes (Link et al., 1997; Rosenfield, 1997). Thus, the positive and negative aspects of labelling can exist side by side.

In summary, as the above examples illustrate, certain illness labels have the potential to create a stigmatising identity for the sufferer. Consequently, the labelled individual can experience a loss of social status and be discriminated against on account of his or her 'spoiled' identity. Not all illnesses are equally stigmatising. The significance of the stigmatising aspects of an illness will vary according to factors such as its perceived aetiology, the visibility of the symptoms and the medical prognosis. Also, the situation is exacerbated for those who, in addition to illness-related stigma, are exposed to negative discrimination on account of their gender, ethnicity or sexual orientation.

While there is a tendency for some labelling theorists to portray the labelled person as a passive recipient of a deviant identity, others, such as Goffman, describe the stigmatised person as an active participant in the management and control of information. However, it has been suggested that Goffman's account of coping strategies misrepresents the real concerns of some labelled individuals, such as those with physical disabilities (Higgins, 1981). Many of the disabled, it is argued, are not primarily concerned with the management of stigma but are preoccupied with the practical problems of daily living encountered as a result of their physical condition. Furthermore, it has been argued that Goffman's analysis of individual modes of adaptation to a disvalued social identity overly concentrates on defensive strategies (Gussow and Tracy, 1968) or defensive manoeuvres (Anspach, 1979).

A collective response to information management has emerged in the form of 'identity politics' (Anspach, 1979). This is a feature of the political activism demonstrated by those groups that have challenged, through various forms of social protest, the social construction of a negative social identity. For instance, physically disabled activists have questioned socially accepted definitions of normality and in so doing have fashioned for themselves a new, positive self-image. Other groups have pursued a similar course of action. This politicised response has been described as a process of 'stigma conversion' (Humphreys, 1972). The emphasis is placed on the way society evaluates difference. Those who have attracted a negative social label seek to redefine their situation. All this has implications for those involved in the provision of healthcare. Firstly, health professionals need to realise that for some patients the stigma can be more difficult to cope with than the illness itself (Torrey, 1994). Secondly, carers need to be aware of the importance of social identity and self-image to the patient and take these into account when constructing individualised care plans.

Summary

- An important conceptual distinction can be made between 'disease' and 'illness'. The concept of disease is based on a medical definition of pathological abnormality. Supposedly objective criteria, such as biophysical abnormalities and bodily disorders, are at the centre of the disease-oriented approach to medical knowledge favoured by the medical model. This model can be challenged for failing to pay sufficient attention to social, psychological and behavioural factors. In contrast, the concept of illness refers to the experience of disease. The emphasis is on the subjective experience of physical symptoms and bodily disorders. Whereas the idea of disease is based on a medical conception of pathological abnormality, the concept of illness relies on social definitions of normality.

- It is important to study lay knowledge and beliefs about health and illness as this helps us to understand decision-making and health-related behaviour in different social groups. Lay beliefs are shaped by social, economic and cultural factors. From a lay perspective health is a multi-dimensional concept and research shows that it can be defined in a number of different ways. Health can be defined in terms of the absence of illness (a negative definition), the ability to work (a functional definition) or general physical well-being (a positive definition). There is some evidence of the existence of variations in the concept of health according to social class, age and gender.

- People acquire knowledge about health and illness issues from a wide variety of sources, such as formal encounters with health workers, contact with the mass media and conversations with family members, friends and work colleagues. It is from information of this kind that they construct their own causal theories of illness and disease. Lay explanations do not only account for the occurrence of illness but also attribute responsibility for its occurrence. Research shows that some illnesses are believed to be caused by factors external to individuals and thus outside of their control; consequently it is viewed that in these circumstances they cannot be held responsible for their poor health. An example would be the involuntary exposure to the health risks associated with atmospheric pollution.

- Becoming ill is a social process. To understand what makes people decide to seek medical advice we need to look at how lay referral networks of family members and friends operate. Illness is not only a biological state but also a social state. The concept of the sick role focuses on the social expectations and sanctions applied to those who are defined as sick. Although the concept has been criticised it still constitutes a useful analytical tool in the study of illness behaviour.

- A medical diagnosis can create a deviant identity for the sufferer. Stigma is a social construction that can have damaging consequences for the individual who is trying to come to terms with a chronic health problem or serious physical or mental impairment. Healthcare workers need to appreciate that coping with the social stigma can in some circumstances be more difficult than coping with the illness. Some illness labels are more stigmatising than others: this may be a result of the visibility of the symptoms, the level of public ignorance surrounding the nature of the illness or the general characteristics of those perceived to be sufferers.

Questions for discussion

1 What is the difference between the concepts of illness and disease? Why is it advantageous to maintain this conceptual distinction?

2 What are the characteristic features of lay definitions of health?

3 Why is an understanding of the nature and content of lay definitions of health and illness important for those involved in the provision and delivery of healthcare?

4 What can sociological research tell us about illness behaviour?

5 How useful is the concept of the sick role for understanding illness behaviour?

6 Why are some illnesses, diseases or conditions more stigmatising than others?

7 Why might knowledge of a stigma trajectory for a specific illness or disease be of relevance to healthcare workers?

Further reading

Bury, M. (2005) *Health and Illness*, Cambridge: Polity, especially Chapter 1.

Calnan, M. (1987) *Health and Illness: the Lay Perspective*, London: Tavistock.

Currer, C. and Stacey, M. (eds) (1986) *Concepts of Health, Illness and Disease: a Comparative Perspective*, Leamington Spa: Berg.

Fitzpatrick, R., Hinton, I., Newman, S., Scambler, G. and Thompson, J. (eds) (1984) *The Experience of Illness*, London: Tavistock.

Gabe, J., Bury, M. and Elston, M. A. (2004) *Key Concepts in Medical Sociology*, London: Sage.

Goffman, E. (1968) *Stigma: Notes on the Management of Spoiled Identity*, Harmondsworth: Penguin.

Nettleton, S. (2006) *The Sociology of Health and Illness*, 2nd edn, Cambridge: Polity Press, especially Chapters 3 and 4.

Scambler, G. (1989) *Epilepsy*, London: Routledge.

Scambler, G. (ed.) (2005) *Medical Sociology: Major Themes in Health and Social Welfare*, London: Routledge, Taylor & Francis Group, especially Volume III, Part 9.

Scambler, G. (ed.) (2008) *Sociology as Applied to Medicine*, 6th edn, Oxford: Elsevier Health Sciences, especially Chapter 3.

CHAPTER 3

Perspectives on mental illness

Concepts of mental illness and mental health

> The very concept of mental illness is of profound sociological interest, because there is considerable sociocultural variation in how mental illness is manifest and understood, both across societies and within the various strata comprising a given society.
>
> (Aneshensel and Phelan, 2006, p. 5)

What is mental illness?

Defining mental illness is no easy task. This is a field of study in which 'terminology is a fraught and emotive issue' (Pilgrim and Rogers, 1993, p. vii). Take, for example, the concept of 'mental illness', which has been described as 'extremely elusive' (Ineichen, 1979, p. 21) and 'invincibly obscure' (Gallagher, 1980, p. 19). It is a slippery concept that is open to a number of different interpretations depending upon the perspective adopted. From a lay perspective, individuals who behave in an odd or bizarre way, such as displaying a rapid change in mood from a state of deep depression to one of high elation, may be understood to be suffering from mental illness. However, although some understanding of the general concept of mental illness may be evident in lay definitions, people who act in ways that are considered to be out of the ordinary may find themselves referred to by any one of a number of derogatory terms including 'nutcase', 'fruitcake' or 'loony'. The negative labels will vary according to the socio-cultural milieu in which the behaviour is observed and evaluated. As individuals we learn the appropriate ways of behaving in different social contexts through primary socialisation and we expect adults to perform as competent social actors. For example, while we tolerate strong emotional outbursts in childhood, such behaviour is deemed to be less appropriate in adulthood. Consequently, in this sense, 'mental illness might be understood sociologically as failed or incomplete socialisation' (Rogers and Pilgrim, 2005, p. 105).

Expert definitions of mental illness vary both between and within the disciplines of psychiatry, clinical psychology and psychoanalysis. A description of the various approaches is beyond the scope of this chapter. The intention here is to establish the fact that mental illness is a contested concept. What the different perspectives have in common is that they attempt to identify what constitutes mental illness and speculate as to its causes. However, the nature and content of the explanations they offer is to a large extent determined by the conceptual framework adopted. In terms of the aetiology of mental illness it is possible to make a broad distinction between the biologically oriented explanations and those that are based on social or psychological factors.

Although there are different schools of thought within psychiatry, a medical or biogenic conceptualisation of mental illness as a predominantly biological condition prevails. According to this view the causes of mental illness lie very much within the individual. Explanations are presented in terms of biochemical imbalances, genetically inherited abnormalities, neurological impairment or organic malfunctioning. One consequence of the medical model is that, in one sense, it encourages us to look at mental illness in the same way that we view physical illness. There is a tendency to see mental illness as resulting from some underlying physical pathology, with the illness revealing itself in the form of mental symptoms. Following a diagnosis of the 'disease' on the basis of the observation of the symptoms, the psychiatrist recommends a treatment to cure the condition or alleviate the symptoms. Such an all-embracing concept of mental disorder as an 'illness' can lead to diagnosis and treatment being viewed as mechanistic procedures, and the individual sufferer being regarded as the passive carrier of a disease.

The adoption of what Rogers and Pilgrim (2005) call an 'illness framework' in psychiatry can be problematic as there are qualitative differences between physical sickness and mental illness.

> A fundamental problem with the illness framework in psychiatry is that it deals in the main with symptoms not signs. That is, the judgements made about whether or not a person is mentally ill or healthy focus mainly (and often singularly) on the person's communications.
>
> (Rogers and Pilgrim, 2005, p. 3)

Diagnostic procedures in general medicine involve the doctor looking for physical changes in bodily states, many of which are amenable to some form of objective measurement. In the case of mental illness, abnormal behaviour cannot be detected and measured with the same level of precision and objectivity. The mind, unlike the body, is not merely a physical entity but is also 'an abstract concept' (Gallagher, 1980, p. 19). Biological medicine has had some success in reducing the incidence, or controlling the development, of certain diseases or medical conditions. Tuberculosis and diabetes are two examples. Advances have been made possible by progress in the ability to identify the nature and cause of various types of physical illness. In contrast, in psychiatry there is considerable ambiguity surrounding the classification of mental problems and the identification of diagnostic criteria. This, coupled with the fact that 'the great bulk of what psychiatrists call "mental illness" has no proven bodily cause' (Rogers and Pilgrim, 2005, p. 3), casts doubt on the universal application of the mechanistic medical model in this context.

Nevertheless, British psychiatry lays great store by biological factors in the generation of aetiological theories; this is despite the existence of social and psychoanalytic models of mental illness. The reliance on biological medicine however, does not prevent clinical psychiatrists from presenting the medical model as a broadly eclectic construction. As one psychiatrist stated in Samson's study:

> I always think of looking at three dimensions of treatment: biological, psychological in the sense of what one does for that individual, and social in terms of looking at the setting in which they begin and the setting to which they'll return and the setting in which they live in hospital.
>
> (a psychiatrist quoted in Samson, 1995, p. 249)

However, Samson maintains that while statements such as these reveal that non-biological factors are taken into account, there is no indication that mental illness is primarily understood in terms of social or psychological processes. To quote Samson, the 'social and psychological "factors" simply gave the disease its individual stamp' (1995, p. 250).

Non-biologically oriented explanations of mental illness offer a radically different conceptual framework about mental abnormality based upon social and psychological factors. The Freudian psychoanalytic perspective is one example. In this approach the idea of mental illness is founded upon the assumption that the normal, stable personality develops through a series of sequential stages. If for any reason normal development is interrupted, or there is regression to an earlier stage, mental abnormality can result. Mental illness is therefore viewed as a pathological condition, whose cause can be traced back to early childhood experiences or problems with familial relationships.

The 'myth of mental illness'

The idea that physical illness and mental illness are conceptually different entities is advanced by the American psychiatrist, Thomas Szasz (1961, 1971), when he asserts that the term mental illness is misleading. For him, mental illness is a 'fake illness'; a 'myth' perpetuated by modern psychiatric practice. He claims that the illnesses to which psychiatrists attach the label 'mental' are qualitatively different from illnesses that are described as 'physical'. When it comes to understanding how the human body works, the disciplines of biology, physiology and anatomy provide objective, independent knowledge, from which it is possible to identify what constitutes a normal, healthy state. Not only are physical deviations observable, but it is also possible to describe the nature and form a particular deviation takes. Illness and disease, for Szasz, are seen primarily in terms of the bio-physical state of the organism. Consequently, he claims that as '[t]he mind (whatever it is) is not an organ or part of the body . . . it cannot be diseased in the same sense as the body can' (Szasz, 1974a, p. 97).

It is Szasz's contention that an 'illness' of the mind cannot be conceived of in the way as an illness of the body. He maintains that knowledge of biology and physiology is of little use in helping us to understand what constitutes 'normal functioning' as far as the mind is concerned. He criticises conventional diagnostic procedures in psychiatry, claiming that there is no such thing as mental illness. Mental problems are not diseases. Patients given a psychiatric label do not have an illness as such, but are considered to be suffering from what Szasz calls 'problems in living', which have nothing to do with medicine. As he states:

> The expression 'mental illness' is a metaphor that we have come to mistake for fact. We call people physically ill when their body functioning violates certain anatomical and physiological norms; similarly, we call people mentally ill when their personal conduct violates certain ethical, political, and social norms.
>
> (Szasz, 1974b, p. 23)

Szasz appears to subscribe to the view that physical illness is an objective, value-free concept, whereas 'mental illness' is a label applied by the psychiatrist to certain types of rule-breaking or socially maladaptive behaviour (see Box 3.1).

Box 3.1   Definition

Bad habits are not diseases

The term 'mental illness' is a metaphor. Bodily illness stands in the same relation to mental illness as a defective television set stands to a bad television programme. Of course, the word 'sick' is often used metaphorically. We call jokes 'sick', economies 'sick', sometimes even the whole world 'sick', but only when we call minds 'sick' do we systematically mistake and strategically misinterpret metaphor for fact – and send for the doctor to 'cure' the 'illness'! It is as if a television viewer were to send for a TV repairman because he dislikes the programme he sees on the screen.

Source: Szasz, 1971

In his critique of 'institutional psychiatry', Szasz condemns what he sees as the repressive and coercive nature of Western psychiatric practice. He maintains that psychiatrists diagnose mental illness largely through the observation of non-conforming behaviour. Unlike the detection of physical illness, this involves making value-laden judgements. As he asserts, the psychiatrist does not stand apart from the patient under observation, in the same way that the physician does when diagnosing a physical illness or disease. According to Szasz, 'The psychiatrist is committed to some picture of what he considers reality, and to what he thinks society considers reality, and he observes and judges the patient's behaviour in the light of these beliefs' (1974b, p. 19). Thus, psychiatrists function as powerful agents of social control; they are empowered by society to deprive certain individuals of their freedom. Szasz is concerned that this power is open to abuse. As a result of what he considers a process of 'psychiatric colonisation', more and more vulnerable people or social misfits will find that they are subjected to psychiatric scrutiny and treatment. At his most invective he refers to psychiatrists as 'jailers' and 'torturers' and compares psychiatric institutions to prisons (1961). Throughout his writings he expresses a passionate concern for protecting the civil liberties and human rights of mental patients.

Szasz is not the only writer to criticise the psychiatric profession from within. Ronald Laing (1967) has also challenged the concept of mental illness as employed in conventional psychiatric practice. Drawing on his own experience as a psychoanalyst treating schizophrenic patients, he rejects the notion of schizophrenia as a pathological condition. According to his interpretation, based on what he calls 'existential psychology', the behaviour labelled as schizophrenic does not seem irrational when account is taken of the socio-psychological dynamics of the patient's family life. Some family situations can be pathogenic and emotionally stultifying, to the extent that an individual is forced to behave in ways which in any other context would be seen as irrational. Thus, what is labelled as schizophrenic behaviour is in fact an individual's way of coping with an intolerable situation. In this conceptualisation, schizophrenia is not perceived as a 'disease' or 'illness' located within the individual, but more as a reaction to a particular set of circumstances characteristic of a system of social relationships.

The views by writers such as Szasz and Laing gave rise to what came to be known as the 'anti-psychiatry' movement, which, among other things, called for an end to coercive forms of treatment and the closure of existing psychiatric institutions.

What are we to make of these criticisms levelled at psychiatry? There is no doubt that Szasz has made an important contribution to the debate about the definition of mental illness and encouraged us to take a critical look at the scope and influence of psychiatric practice. For example, Anthony Clare (1980) commends him for producing evidence of the abuses of civil liberties under the involuntary hospitalisation procedures in the USA. However, Szasz's main thesis, that mental illness is a myth, has attracted opposition on three main counts. Firstly, many psychiatrists maintain that mental illness is not diagnosed solely on the basis of the observation of socially maladaptive behaviour, but account is also taken of manifest disturbances of psychological functioning.

Secondly, and more fundamentally, it has been suggested that his concept of illness emphasises the physical aspects while ignoring illness as a social state. Miles (1981) observes that definitions of physical illness are not simply objective, value-free categories, but are also subject to social and cultural influences. Furthermore, Szasz fails to appreciate the importance of the mind–body link. For example, some physical conditions, such as skin complaints, are psychosomatic or psychophysiologic in origin and appear at times of emotional stress. Also, prolonged physical illness can lead to depression and other psychological problems. As Jones asserts, 'Szasz denies the existence of an emotional component in any kind of illness' (Jones, 1988, p. 87). Clearly, the boundary between physical and mental illness is not as easily defined as Szasz would have us believe.

Finally, there is a view that despite his passionately expressed concern for the plight of mental patients, Szasz actually fails to appreciate the full extent of their suffering. His attack on modern psychiatry is directed at what he sees as the dehumanising impact of contemporary therapeutic techniques and the role of psychiatrists as agents of political control of deviant populations. Consequently, he fails to appreciate that mental patients' 'troubles are desperate [and] their sufferings extreme', and that psychiatrists, far from being 'guilty conspirators', are compassionate professionals endeavouring to relieve individual suffering (Roth, 1976, p. 324).

What is mental health?

Mental health, like mental illness, is a complex concept. It is not possible to provide a universal definition of mental health, because, as with mental illness, there are social and cultural variations in what is regarded as 'normal' behaviour. As Warr acknowledges, the concept is value-laden.

> Processes and outcomes which are designated as healthy are typically those accepted and valued by contemporary society, often by the middle-class members of that society. Even within the middle class itself, there are many differences of opinion about which specific behaviours and experiences should be deemed 'healthy' or 'unhealthy'.
>
> (Warr, 1987, p. 24)

However, if primary healthcare services are to promote mental health and play a part in the prevention of mental illness it is necessary to have some understanding of what constitutes mental health.

There are a number of different definitions of mental health available. In a rudimentary sense, mental health may be defined in terms of the absence of mental disorder. However, the World Health Organisation (WHO) offers a much broader definition when it defines mental health as '. . . a state of well-being in which the individual realises his or her own abilities, can cope with the normal stresses of life, can work productively and fruitfully, and is able to make a contribution to his or her community' (WHO, 2001, p. 1). The reference to 'a state of well-being' takes this definition well beyond a consideration of purely psychopathological criteria. In fact, different groups of people tend to stress different aspects when attempting to determine what constitutes a mentally healthy life. On a simplistic level, the definition of mental health can be approached from any one of three broad perspectives: the *personal*, the *societal* and the *professional*. According to the personal perspective, an individual may reach a subjective judgement as to their own state of mental well-being by reflecting on how they feel. Assessments of a person's mental state are also made from the perspective of the wider society. Here the emphasis is on how well the individual copes with the situational and normative requirements imposed by society. In other words, do they behave in what is considered to be a socially responsible and acceptable fashion? Finally, there is the view from the professionals, such as psychiatrists, psychoanalysts and clinical psychologists. Different practitioners highlight different elements of mental health according to their theoretical orientation and professional training. For example, some psychiatrists define mental health in terms of the absence of any manifestations of mental disorder, whereas psychoanalysts see the healthy personality as one in which the three elements (id, ego and superego) are not in conflict and exist in a state of intrapsychic equilibrium.

There is variation both within and between these three broad ways of looking at the definition of mental health. Consequently, from a subjective point of view, it is possible for an individual to feel that their mental state is low, yet because they maintain a 'normal' level of social functioning, they are seen by others to be in good mental health. What the identification of these broad perspectives serves to illustrate, is that mental health is a complex phenomenon.

Many theorists have attempted to arrive at a comprehensive conceptualisation of good mental health. In so doing, they have adopted a wider and more positive definition of mental health than the one implicit in the medical model of mental illness. A primary aim has been to investigate variations in the nature and distribution of mental health among sections of the population not considered mentally ill in a medical sense. A characteristic feature of these approaches is that they attempt to specify the major components of mental health. The psychologist Peter Warr (1987) provides a good example in his study of work, unemployment and mental health. He describes five such components: affective well-being, competence, autonomy, aspiration and integrated functioning. The idea being that in each of these areas it is possible to place the individual on a continuum ranging from 'extremely healthy' to 'extremely unhealthy'. An important feature of this model is its emphasis on how the individual adjusts to and interacts with the environment in meeting personal needs and achieving valued goals.

In a similar vein, Ustun (1998) comments upon operationalising the concept of mental well-being as contained in the WHO's definition of mental health quoted above. He describes the concept of mental well-being as covering four major dimensions: 'the capacity to live, function and enjoy', 'the optimum development of mental abilities', the 'subjective feeling of well-being' and 'the interaction and equilibrium between the individual and the environment' (Ustun, 1998, p. 72). According to this comprehensive approach, the attainment of mental stability is dependent upon the individual having the psychological processes and mental ability to cope with any problems they encounter. There is also the recognition that as a result of environmental factors opportunities for personal growth might be limited, thereby preventing people from realising their full potential.

Sociological approaches to the study of mental illness

> Not all sociological work on explanations of mental disorder is grounded in social epidemiology. Some sociologists of deviance, especially writers of a symbolic inter-actionist persuasion, . . . have paid particular attention to interpersonal dynamics in the development of disorder.
>
> (Busfield, 2001, p. 8)

There is more than one sociological perspective on mental illness. Two major perspectives are reviewed in this section: the *interactionist* and the *social causation* or *structuralist*. These are founded upon different assumptions about such fundamental issues as the nature and origin of mental disorder.

Interactionist perspective

This perspective has its philosophical roots in a theoretical approach in sociology known as symbolic interactionism, which when applied to the study of deviance in the 1950s and 1960s gave rise to social reaction theory, also commonly referred to as the labelling perspective. Thomas Scheff (1966) is often credited with being the first theorist to produce a coherent sociological theory of mental illness based on the labelling approach. To appreciate his contribution we need to understand something about the basic thinking behind the labelling theorists' interpretation of deviant behaviour in general.

The labelling perspective starts from the premise that deviance is relative. Interactionists hold that behaviour cannot be abstractly and objectively categorised as 'normal' or 'deviant', but is best viewed as subjectively problematic. As Gomm notes, 'Deviant and normal . . . have no fixed meanings; rather they represent ways in which people give moral appraisals of social affairs' (1996, p. 80). Deviance is the product of a process of social interaction in which some individuals or groups succeed in applying the label deviant to the behaviour and actions of others. Consequently, in order to understand deviance it is necessary to consider all those groups involved in the labelling process and not just concentrate on those to whom a deviant label has been attached. The idea of deviant behaviour as a socially constructed entity that is generated through social interaction is captured in the following:

> Deviance is not a property *inherent in* certain forms of behavior; it is a property *conferred upon* these forms by the audiences which directly or indirectly witness them. The critical variable in the study of deviance, then, is the social audience which eventually determines whether or not any episode of behavior or any class of episodes is labelled deviant.
>
> (Erikson, 1962, p. 311)

As Erikson states, an act is not referred to as deviant because it possesses some intrinsic quality, but is categorised as deviant on the basis of the judgements made by those individuals and groups that observe the behaviour.

Sociologists who approach the study of deviance from a labelling perspective are not concerned with identifying the causes of deviant behaviour. What is important for them is how the whole social process of labelling works. Thus, they concentrate on how labelling is socially organised within specific social contexts and how being given a deviant label can have a profound impact on an individual's self-image and future social relationships. There is no preoccupation with studying the individual characteristics of those to whom a deviant label has been applied in order to identify underlying causal factors. Deviance is not viewed as individual pathology requiring aetiological analysis. It is the interaction between the labelled and the labellers that is the focus of study for many interactionists.

Behaviour that violates established codes of conduct or contravenes existing social norms is generally regarded as deviant. The type and level of societal reaction generated by rule-breaking behaviour depends upon a host of factors, including the perceived origins of the deviance, the motives imputed to the deviant, the actual form the behaviour takes, the social status of the norm violator and the level of tolerance within the community. For many labelling theorists the public confirmation of a deviant label marks a significant stage in the development of a deviant identity. The labelled individuals come to occupy a distinctive deviant role, which serves to redefine their position in society. According to Cuff *et al.*, '[t]he individual comes to be treated as a deviant *first and foremost*' (1990, p. 156).

The importance of societal reaction in the shaping of a deviant identity was recognised by Lemert (1967) when he formulated the major conceptual distinction between two types of deviance: *primary* and *secondary*. *Primary deviation* refers to those initial deviant acts or occasional transgressions, which arise from a variety of psychological and socio-cultural sources, and are explained away as a temporary aberration and do not lead to the development of a deviant self-image. Most people, at some time in their lives, commit a deviant act, but do not necessarily think of themselves as deviant. In contrast, *secondary deviation* arises as the labelled individual or group responds to the reaction of others to their initial rule-breaking behaviour. As described by Lemert:

> Secondary deviation is deviant behaviour, or social roles based upon it, which becomes a means of defense, attack or adaptation to the overt and covert problems created by the societal reaction to primary deviation.
>
> (Lemert, 1967, p. 17)

The deviance can become the central feature of a labelled person's identity, which has implications for their future conduct. The labels themselves are generally stigmatising and can set in train a self-fulfilling prophecy. Once labelled and processed as a deviant, individuals may find that they are forced into certain situations and groupings where their behaviour is interpreted as confirming their deviant status. Consequently, they may come to see themselves as others see them and accept the deviant role as part of their 'true' identity and act accordingly.

The labelling perspective can be applied to the study of mental illness. In this context it constitutes a direct challenge to the established clinical model. As Scheff asserts, 'The sensitising function of the labelling theory of mental illness derives precisely from its attempt to contradict the major tenets of the medical model' (1975, p. 22). For example, from a medical point of view, deviant behaviour as exemplified by psychiatric patients is seen in terms of individual pathology: an attribute of the person that requires diagnostic classification followed by treatment. In contrast, from an interactionist stance, the defining of someone as mentally ill is best seen from a 'social system perspective' as an 'interpersonal process' (Mercer, 1968). As far as labelling theorists are concerned, the emphasis is on studying how an individual's behaviour is socially defined and labelled in accordance with established value systems and prevailing socio-cultural norms. Cuff *et al.* refer to this approach as an example of a 'meaning and action perspective' (1990, p. 18). Mental illness is not perceived as a condition lying within the individual, but as a social construct, a status conferred upon an individual by other members of society. The severity of the societal reaction to those who have been labelled is partly a function of the nature of the deviant behaviour and the power and influence of the groups who are responsible for applying and endorsing the labels. Psychiatric diagnostic labels are particularly potent given the popular image of medicine as a profession steeped in a body of specialist knowledge.

According to Scheff (1966), it is a particular kind of rule-breaking behaviour that is prone to attract a label of mental illness. As he asserts, there are some basic social norms and conventions that are deemed to be so natural that any violation is viewed with some alarm.

> A host of such norms surround even the simplest conversation: a person engaged in conversation is expected to face his partner, he is expected to look toward the other's eyes, rather than, say, toward his forehead; to stand at a proper conversational distance, neither one inch away nor across the room . . . A person who regularly violated these expectations probably would not be thought to be merely ill-bred, but as strange, bizarre and frightening, because his behaviour violates the assumptive world of the group, the world that is construed to be the only one that is natural, decent and possible.
>
> (Scheff, 1966, p. 32)

He refers to behaviour of this kind as *'residual rule-breaking'* or *'residual deviance'*, adding that its original cause may be due to a host of different factors including organic, physiological, biochemical, psychological and social. It is not the origins of the behaviour that is of central interest to Scheff. He is primarily concerned with exploring the process whereby mental illness labels are applied and in understanding the way in which cultural stereotypes of insanity are created, learned and reaffirmed as part of ordinary social interaction.

Scheff is particularly critical of the way psychiatrists, as agents of social control, attach psychiatric labels to patients. He maintains that it is often all too easy for an individual who has been brought to the attention of the psychiatric services to be 'launched on a career of "chronic" mental illness' (Scheff, 1975, p. 10). Once labelled as a mental patient they are stigmatised and treated differently. Indeed, psychiatric labels have such an all-pervasive quality that there is a tendency for all aspects of a patient's conduct to be evaluated in terms of their diagnosed mental health status. This is one consequence of labelling that is illustrated in Rosenhan's (1973) classic study of voluntary admission to mental hospitals conducted in the USA.

Rosenhan conducted a field experiment whereby 8 supposedly sane men and women presented themselves as voluntary patients at 12 hospitals in 5 different states. Four of the pseudo-patients were mental health professionals; three were psychologists and one was a psychiatrist. However, they did not reveal their true professional identity when interviewed by hospital personnel. All eight pseudo-patients claimed that they could hear voices and were duly admitted as in-patients. Eleven of the admissions were for schizophrenia and one was for manic-depressive psychosis. Following admission to hospital the pseudo-patients ceased to display the fictive symptoms and behaved normally. However, despite this, they were never detected by hospital staff, although they were identified as impostors by the other patients. Those admitted as suffering from schizophrenia were eventually discharged with a diagnosis of schizophrenia 'in remission'.

Certain forms of societal reaction can lead to what has been termed *deviancy amplification*. This occurs when measures to reduce or control deviant behaviour actually result in an increase in deviance. For example, those people to whom a stigmatising label is successfully applied can find themselves socially marginalised and forced out of 'normal' social interaction. Being deprived of valued social relationships can result in a lack of self-esteem and a poor sense of self-worth. The paradox is that some interventions by healthcare professionals can exacerbate the situation either by producing new types of deviant reactions or amplifying existing deviant characteristics (see Box 3.2). It is known that some drug treatments for psychiatric disorders produce adverse side-effects, such as disturbed thought processes, which make it difficult for the patient to engage in everyday social encounters without being treated as a deviant. Gomm sums up the relevance of the concept of deviancy amplification within the context of mental illness when he asserts that, '. . . perhaps the most important deviancy amplifying effect of psychiatric treatment is the way in which it excludes people from the normal opportunities of life, both at the time of treatment and

---

Box 3.2   Definition

The stickiness of psycho-diagnostic labels

A psychiatric label has a life and an influence of its own. Once the impression has been formed that the patient is schizophrenic, the expectation is that he will continue to be schizophrenic. When a sufficient amount of time has passed, during which the patient has done nothing bizarre, he is considered to be in remission and available for discharge. But the label endures beyond discharge, with the unconfirmed expectation that he will behave as a schizophrenic again. Such labels, conferred by mental health professionals, are as influential on the patient as they are on his relatives and friends, and it should not surprise anyone that the diagnosis acts on all of them as a self-fulfilling prophecy. Eventually, the patient himself accepts the diagnosis, with all of its surplus meanings and expectations, and behaves accordingly.

Source: Rosenhan, 1973

---

thereafter because of the persistently stigmatising effect of having been mentally ill' (1996, p. 84).

In general, it can be seen that the labelling perspective makes an important contribution to the study of mental illness, in so far as it:

- draws our attention to the fact that mental illness can be treated as a social concept;
- acknowledges the problematic nature of societal reaction to mental disorder;
- shows how the public application and confirmation of a label can be stigmatising and
- explains how the labelling process can lead to deviancy amplification.

However, labelling theory has not gone unopposed.

One of the leading critics of the application of the labelling perspective to the study of mental disorder is the American sociologist Walter Gove (1970, 1975, 1980 and 1982). Gove challenges some of the basic assumptions made by the supporters of labelling theory when he asserts that there is more to mental illness than simply being labelled. He claims that 'the labelling theory's critique of the psychiatric perspective is both overstated and largely incorrect' (Gove, 1982, p. 285). The idea expounded by the more extreme proponents of the labelling approach, namely that the very act of labelling someone mentally ill actually *creates* mentally ill behaviour, is vigorously challenged. Gove argues that in the majority of cases, persons who receive psychiatric treatment have a serious mental disorder that predates the application of any label. Consequently, labelling theory does not fully address the cause of mental disorder, nor can it account for why some people and not others develop mental illness despite having similar lifestyles, social attributes and family histories.

Labelling theorists are also criticised for creating an impression that the labelling of mental illness is a relatively straightforward, trouble-free process, involving both lay persons and psychiatrists in the defining of certain types of rule-breaking behaviour as symptomatic of an underlying mental disorder. There appears to be an almost unquestionable assumption that the response of labellers is hostile. Indeed, some writers refer to how once the initial label has been applied and a deviant identity created, there is an attempt to confirm the newly ascribed status by looking for evidence of abnormal episodes in the patient's past (Scheff, 1966). Previous behaviour can thus be re-interpreted in the light of a person's newly acquired social identity. However, according to Gove (1982, p. 285) there is empirical evidence to suggest that the reaction from others is not always hostile and negative. He quotes the findings of a study that looked at the experiences of married women living with their mentally ill husbands. The researchers describe how the wives initially refused to accept their husbands' disturbed behaviour as deviant and found various ways of explaining it away as normal. This entailed stretching the definition of what constituted normal behaviour. It was when wives could no longer make adjustments to the pattern of family life in order to minimise or accommodate the abnormal behaviour that they took steps to have their husbands admitted to hospital. As Gove notes, even at this stage the women did not always label their husbands as mentally ill. This is not an isolated research finding. Miles records that 'there is considerable research evidence to show that family members and other lay associates of prospective patients apply the mental illness label with great reluctance and as a last resort' (1981, p. 20).

Critics have also cast doubt on the ease with which labelling theory assumes that the residual norm violator, once identified, obligingly plays the deviant role prescribed by the social audience. As Pilgrim and Rogers assert, if the reactions of lay people are considered to play an instrumental part in the production of mental illness, 'we would expect everyday stereotypes of mental illness to be consistent with the range of behaviours displayed by psychiatric patients' (1993, p. 18). This, they claim, is not the case. Research into the public perception of schizophrenia suggests that the common stereotype of the schizophrenic held by lay people is only loosely related to the description of the schizophrenic patient adhered to by psychiatrists. Furthermore, given the manifestations of schizophrenia, Wing (1973) maintains that it is difficult to see how labelled persons could be forced to display such behaviour 'since this would need special coaching from an expert'.

Gove (1980) attacks Scheff (1966) for assuming that the major factor distinguishing those people who are labelled mentally ill from those who are not so labelled is the label itself. In other words, labelling theorists are of the opinion that there is nothing intrinsically different about the mentally ill. Gove (1982) contests this view, arguing that within the psychiatric literature there is evidence to suggest that those who suffer from certain types of mental illness may be identifiable from their mentally healthy counterparts on the basis of genetic endowment, biological abnormalities or experience of stressful life events.

There is a view that the labelling perspective is too general and makes no attempt to distinguish between different types of mental illness. It is possible that a sociological approach, based on interactionist principles, may be appropriate for understanding some forms of mental disturbance but not others. As Turner (1987) claims, the concept of labelling is of some explanatory value when considering behavioural disorders but is of little causal significance when trying to explain those mental disturbances characterised by organic malfunctioning. He cites the example of dementia, which is caused by the physical decline associated with growing old. While he acknowledges that it would be unreasonable to suggest that dementia is caused by labelling, he maintains that the condition 'may well be complicated by labelling and stereotyping' (Turner, 1987, p. 75).

Where does all this criticism leave labelling theory? Cockerham provides an appropriate summary when he concludes that '. . . Scheff's version of labelling theory should not be dismissed as wrong. Both Scheff and Gove note that it is not simply a case of one view being entirely false and the other being entirely correct. Both viewpoints contain important contributions' (1981, p. 71).

Social causation or structuralist perspective

The term 'structuralist perspective' is used by Cuff *et al.* (1990, p. 17) to refer to a sociological approach to the study of mental illness that examines the relationship between particular aspects of social structure and the incidence and prevalence of mental disorder. Rogers and Pilgrim (2005, p. 12) use the term 'social causation perspective' to describe those sociological approaches which seek to establish a link between social disadvantage and mental illness. These are simply two different terms to describe the same approach, which emphasises the role of social factors in the production of mental illness. Unlike labelling theorists, sociologists working within this perspective broadly accept the conceptual framework used by psychiatrists to understand the nature and origins of mental disturbance. Mental illness is not perceived as a social construct but as something produced within a person, partly as a result of their exposure to particular environmental stresses, socio-economic circumstances or social pressures. The emphasis structurally oriented sociologists place on investigating the nature and impact of the social environment brings them into contact with social psychiatry (Box 3.3). As Henderson (1988) describes, social psychiatry is one of four specialist areas in the study of mental disorder: the other three are psychopathology, biological psychiatry and clinical psychiatry.

Box 3.3   Definition

Social psychiatry

Social psychiatry is concerned with the relationship between disorders of the mind and the human environment. It studies the forces which act at the interface between individuals and those around them; and which may contribute to the onset, or influence the course of mental disorders. The social environment extends from immediate others, as in the family, to the wider society.

Source: Henderson, 1988

Of the many studies in social psychiatry and sociology that identify links between the prevalence of mental disorder and aspects of social structure, there are a considerable number that focus on social stress or life events as factors capable of contributing to a causal explanation of mental illness. Before considering some of the findings from life-events research three observations need to be made.

Firstly, psychiatric disorders, more so than physical diseases, have multiple causes. Therefore, an explanation of the origins and development of a particular mental illness may require drawing on causal models from a number of different disciplines. For example, although the primary cause of some types of functional psychoses may be rooted in biogenic factors, particular life experiences or a combination of social circumstances may be responsible for triggering the onset of an episode of mental disorder.

Secondly, life-events research does not attempt to ascertain the aetiological significance of a single adverse life event, such as the death of a close family member or the loss of a job, but is concerned with the cumulative impact of several stress-inducing events in a person's life (Dohrenwend, 1975). Not only might some single events have a greater impact than others, but their potential for producing stress might be significantly increased when they occur in particular combinations. Furthermore, it needs to be recognised that a patient may experience both physical ill health and mental illness simultaneously. The relationship between physical illness, psychological stress and socio-economic conditions is fairly complex. As Gomm observes, these three form an 'unholy triangle' (Figure 3.1) in which causality can be traced in all directions (1996, p. 113).

For example, the link between material deprivation and poor physical health is well established (Benzeval *et al.*, 1995). Long-term illness, coupled with limited material resources, can lead to increased levels of anxiety and create conditions conducive to the development of depression. The loss of self-esteem, along with other symptoms of psychological stress, can undermine physical recovery, which has implications as far as employment and economic security are concerned. Thus, social deprivation and economic disadvantage are not only important causal factors in the production of physical ill health and mental disorders, but they can also be seen as possible negative outcomes of mental and physical illnesses.

Thirdly, there is some debate surrounding the conceptualisation, measurement and interpretation of adverse life-events. Currently there are two main methods

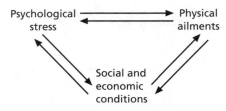

Figure 3.1 Triangle of causality

Source: Gomm, 1996, 2000 p. 112. From *Mental Health Matters: A Reader*, Palgrave Macmillan (Tom Heller, Jill Reynolds, Roger Gomm, Rosemary Muston and Stephen Pattison (eds) 2000), reproduced with permission of Palgrave Macmillan for measuring exposure to stressful events or episodes: the *inventory* method and the *interview* method.

The *inventory method*, also referred to as the 'checklist-dictionary approach' (Brown, 1989, p. 12), was developed by Holmes and Rahe (1967) in the form of the Social Readjustment Rating Scale or Schedule of Recent Experience. Their original rating scale contained a list of 43 life experiences that lead to varying degrees of disruption in a person's life. Each life event is assigned a relative stress value or what the authors call a 'life change' score. Scores for individual life events vary and are based on the extent to which events disrupt the normal pattern of daily living and the amount of adjustment they require a person to make. For example, death of a spouse is ranked the highest with a stress value of 100; divorce is second with a value of 73; birth of a child is ranked 14 with a stress score of 39 and Christmas is the penultimate event in the list with a score of 12. For Holmes and Rahe, life events can be arranged along a continuum of stressfulness and a total life change score obtained by aggregating the values for the various individual events experienced by a person over a specified period of time. It is assumed that the higher the score, the greater the level of stress, hence the greater the likelihood of the individual becoming ill. Inventories or checklists of this kind are quick and easy to administer and have been widely used in research studies. However, care is needed when interpreting the information provided by this method. Two points deserve special mention. First, in trying to quantify life events the qualitative meaning different individuals attach to particular events or experiences can be overlooked. As Brown (1981) maintains, the actual impact a life event has on an individual is partly determined by their personal circumstances and the wider social context surrounding the event. Second, as research shows 'some life events, such as divorce, can be regarded as a *consequence* of stress instead of a *cause*' (Cockerham, 1981, p. 114, emphasis in original).

The *interview method*, developed by Brown and Harris (1978) in their study of the social origins of clinical depression in women, overcomes both these shortcomings. They used specially trained interviewers to collect detailed information so as to be able to locate events accurately in time. This made it possible to eliminate from the analysis any events that were not potential causal factors, but were perceived as being *caused by* the psychiatric condition under study. The interview method, by focusing on the context of events, enables interviewers to obtain a considerable amount of information about the personal circumstances and social conditions prevailing at the time the event occurred. The Life Events and Difficulties Schedule (LEDS) devised by George Brown and his colleagues provides interviewers with a list of 40 types of events grouped into the eight categories described in Box 3.4.

Interviewers are given very detailed instructions as to what events should be included under each heading. For example, when dealing with 'changes in health' they are instructed to record all instances where the interviewee was admitted to hospital, but in the case of close ties or household members they are only required to document admissions to hospital that are classified as urgent or lasting for one week or more. Whereas the checklist or inventory can be either administered

Box 3.4   Definition

The Life Events and Difficulties Schedule

1 Changes in a role for the subject, such as changing a job and losing or gaining an opposite-sex friend for the unmarried.

2 Major changes in a role for close ties or household members, such as a husband's staying off work because of a strike.

3 Major changes in subject's health, including hospital admissions and development of an illness expected to be serious.

4 Major changes in health for close ties or household members.

5 Residence changes or any marked change in amount of contact with close ties or household members.

6 Forecasts of change, such as being told about being rehoused.

7 Fulfillments [sic] or disappointments of a valued goal, such as being offered a house to rent at a reasonable price.

8 Other dramatic events involving either the subject (e.g. witnessing a serious accident or being stopped by the police while driving) or a close tie (e.g. learning of a brother's arrest).

Source: Brown, 1989, p. 22

by an interviewer or completed by the respondent in a relatively short space of time, the interview method takes considerably longer. A single interview can take between two and three hours to complete. Once the information has been obtained it has to be processed. Unlike the inventory method, it is not a case of simply adding together the stress values associated with individual events to produce a total stress score. The information is passed on to a group of specially trained raters who judge the severity of each recorded event according to the amount of threat implied.

Brown and Harris (1978) used the LEDS in their study of women living in Camberwell, an inner-city area in south London. They selected a sample of 114 women, aged between 18 and 65, who were diagnosed as suffering from depression and were receiving either in-patient or out-patient treatment from the local psychiatric services. In addition, they chose a random sample of women from the same district to act as a comparison group. Each member of this group was screened for evidence of psychiatric disturbance. It was found that 17 per cent had an undetected affective disorder and a further 19 per cent displayed symptoms of a less serious nature and were considered 'borderline' cases. The remainder were designated as 'normal' for the purposes of the research study. LEDS was administered to both the patient group and the community sample.

Brown *et al.* draw a conceptual distinction between 'events' and 'long term difficulties'. A severe event is characterised by 'the *experience of a threatened or actual major loss*' (1981, p. 146) of such magnitude that it undermines an

Box 3.5   Case study

Mrs Ferguson: a case history

Mrs Ferguson, a married woman of 51 with two adult children living at home, was one of the seventy-three women admitted as an in-patient. Her husband told her one day 'out of the blue' that he was having an affair. Before this she said she had no reason to think her marriage was not 'fine'. She said she had suspected nothing. Almost at once she said she felt depressed. She began to cry a great deal and did so every day. She felt life was not worth living and she thought carefully about various methods of committing suicide. She began to feel guilty and in some way responsible for the failure of her marriage. She sweated a good deal and generally felt tense. These symptoms came on within a week or so of the event and for the next five to six months she gradually got worse.

Source: Brown and Harris, 1978, p. 111

individual's view of herself and her relationship to others. An example of a severe life event is contained in the brief extract presented in Box 3.5, from the case history of Mrs Ferguson, quoted in Brown and Harris (1978). In contrast, long-term difficulties are defined in Brown and Harris' research not as discrete events, but as problems that the individual interviewee had experienced for at least one month during the twelve-month period prior to interview. Included among ongoing difficulties were housing problems, difficulties with children and short-age of money. The majority of these difficulties were seen as having no causal significance in the onset of affective disorder. However, a small number of problems, which had persisted for at least two years, were labelled major difficulties.

One major aspect of the research was to investigate the relationship between events and difficulties and the onset of depression. Life events rated as 'severe' were nearly four times more likely to be detected among the sample of patients than they were among the symptom-free or 'normal' group of women. Major difficulties were also found to be associated with the onset of depression; these were three times more likely to occur in the patient sample than in the comparison group. In commenting upon the aetiological importance of events and difficulties, Brown *et al.* conclude that, 'Major difficulties . . . although of lesser aetiological importance than events, do appear to play a causal role along with events in the aetiology of affective disturbance' (1981, p. 147). The life-events model or social stress hypothesis is often advanced to account for the preponderance of mental illness in the lower social classes.

> Differences in the rates of mental illness experienced by different social groups and classes are directly associated with the differential prevalence of stressful life events and the vulnerability factors which increase the likelihood of stress. We can argue therefore that the level of adversity, the presence of stressful events, social vulnerability and individual management of stress are important features of this life-events framework.
>
> (Turner, 1987, p. 77)

Social class appears as a salient feature in Brown and Harris' multi-factorial social model of the aaetiology of depressive conditions in women. As already indicated, one of the main aims of their research was to explore the causal links between social structural factors and the onset of depression. Although their research sample was drawn from a predominantly working-class district, it contained a sufficient number of middle-class women to make it possible to investigate class differences in the origins and development of depression.

When the researchers concentrated on those women who had experienced a severely detrimental life event or major difficulty, they discovered that working-class women were five times more likely to develop depression than were their middle-class counterparts (Brown et al., 1981). Interestingly, this class difference in the risk of the onset of psychiatric disturbance was restricted to women with children living at home. In other words, when considering women without children at home there was no observed difference between working-class women and middle-class women in terms of the risk of developing depression or the number of adverse events or difficulties faced. However, what was of particular interest to Brown and Harris was that when they looked at women with children still living at home, and controlled for the number and severity of events and difficulties experienced by both class groups, the working-class women were found to be four times more likely to develop a psychiatric disorder than those in the middle class. In short, life events do not invariably lead to affective disorders. Brown and Harris maintain that it is necessary to take into account what they call 'vulnerability factors' or, as labelled in the simplified causal model in Figure 3.2, 'amplifying factors'.

According to Brown and Harris (1978), adverse life events or major difficulties act as stressors or provoking agents in the onset of depression. This finding was confirmed by a later longitudinal investigation of a sample of working-class women living in Islington, north London (Brown et al., 1986). The women, all of whom had at least one child living at home, were followed up over a twelve-month period. Table 3.1 below illustrates the onset rate for depression for those women who at the time of the first interview were deemed to be at risk of developing depression.

Table 3.1 Onset of depression among 303 women in terms of provoking agent status

Provoking agent status	Number of onsets	Onset rate (%)
A. No provoking agent	2/153	1
B. Provoking agent:		
i. Major difficulty only	1/20	5
ii. Severe event	29/130	22
Total onset rate	32/303	11

Source: Brown, G. W. 'Life events, loss and depressive disorders', p.37, in Tom Heller, Jill Reynolds, Roger Gomm, Rosemary Muston and Stephen Pattison (eds), *Mental Health Matters: A Reader*, published 1996, Palgrave Macmillan in association with the Open University, reproduced with permission of Palgrave Macmillan

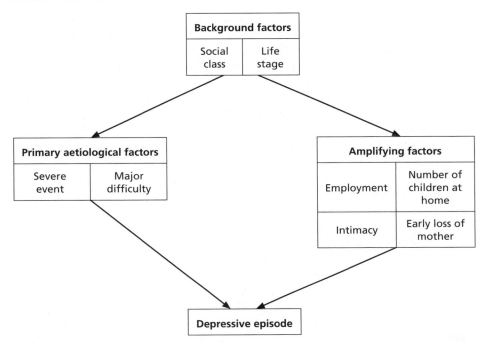

Figure 3.2 A simple causal model of depression
Source: Adapted from Brown *et al.*, 1981, p. 156

As the table shows, of the 32 women who displayed symptoms of depression 29 had experienced a severe life event. However, only 22 per cent of those who experienced severe life events actually developed depression, thus suggesting that there needs to be something more than just provoking life events to produce a depressive condition. Whether or not depression occurs in an individual case depends to a certain extent on how vulnerable a woman is at the time she experiences an event or encounters a difficulty. In the earlier Camberwell study four vulnerability factors were identified:

1 lack of employment, either full-time or part-time, outside the home;

2 having three or more children under 15 years of age living at home;

3 absence of an intimate confiding relationship with a husband or boyfriend;

4 loss of mother before 11 years of age.

The obverse side of these vulnerability factors is that they perform a protective function. For example, those women who had a job outside the home, were in a strong confiding relationship or had not lost their mother in childhood appeared to have a reduced risk of developing psychiatric problems following the occurrence of a severe life event.

The research evidence suggests that the life events and major difficulties experienced by working-class women were closely related to their social situation and economic circumstances. In some instances the duration and intensity of their experiences were such that their situation could be described as chronic. As Brown and Harris comment, 'In interpreting this complex of experiences leading to depression, we outlined a "conveyor belt" of adversities upon which some women were moved inexorably from one crisis to another, starting with lack of care in childhood (often associated with loss of mother) and passing via premarital pregnancy to current working-class status, lack of social support, and high rates of provoking agents' (1989, pp. 371–2).

The availability of social support is of fundamental importance when considering vulnerability factors. Social support refers to the social ties the individual has to other individuals and groups within the community. The term 'social network' is sometimes used to describe the structural and interactional aspects of the personal ties individuals develop with others in their social environment. It is possible to distinguish two broad types of network: informal and formal. The informal network encompasses family members, relatives, friends and neighbours. Contact with individuals and groups outside of these kinship and friendship networks, such as professional healthcare workers and members of welfare organisations, is what constitutes the formal social network.

The range, intensity and duration of social relations available to an individual are key elements when considering the nature of social networks. There is a view, referred to as the 'fund of sociability', that individuals have a need for social interaction with others who share their interests and concerns. According to Weiss (1974), to secure personal and social well-being individuals need to develop and maintain relationships that meet their cognitive and emotional needs. He identifies six types of need that are met through social relationships: these are briefly outlined in Box 3.6.

As Henderson (1988, pp. 98–9) notes, there are three main ways of looking at the relationship between social support and mental illness. Firstly, the lack of social support may be perceived as having a direct impact upon mental health, irrespective of whether or not there is evidence of adversity. Secondly, while it is possible that social support does not have an independent effect on mental health, certain forms of social support may act as a buffer against those stressful life events that have the capacity to push the individual in the direction of mental disorder. Finally, it is possible that social support has a therapeutic effect, for example it may help aid the recovery process for patients suffering from affective disorders. Research has tended to concentrate on the aetiological significance of social support and ignored its therapeutic effects.

There is of course the problem of distinguishing between cause and effect when examining the relationship between some types of mental disorder and the nature and intensity of social networks. Social isolation or exclusion from potentially supportive networks may in fact be seen as a cause of mental disorder or a consequence of having a mental illness. Brown *et al.* (1986), in their Islington study, used a prospective longitudinal research design to explore the role of social support in the onset of depressive illness. They used follow-up interviews to ascertain the type and amount of support received by those women who experienced

Box 3.6   Definition

Provisions of social relationships

1 *Attachment and intimacy.* Both are provided by those relationships that give individuals a sense of personal security and belonging, such as stable sexual partnerships and close friendships. In the absence of such relationships individuals may experience feelings of loneliness and isolation.

2 *Social integration.* This is provided by those relationships that emerge in social networks where individuals share a common purpose, task or objective. This can be a feature of both formal work groups and informal friendship groups.

3 *Nurturance.* Some relationships create opportunities for nurturance, such as when an adult cares for a child. This leads to the development of a sense of being needed.

4 *Reassurance of worth.* This is provided by relationships that necessitate the individual displaying particular skills and competencies. Work roles are an example. In the absence of such reassurance individuals can experience a poor level of self-esteem.

5 *Reliable assistance.* There is an expectation that the relationship with close kin can be depended upon to provide a source of continued assistance in times of need. Feelings of personal vulnerability and anxiety are heightened in relationships where such expectations are absent.

6 *Guidance.* Relationships with 'respected others', such as doctors, nurses and priests can be a source of guidance.

Source: Weiss, 1974

a severe life event. On the basis of the data they obtained they concluded that lack of emotional support from a spouse or close friend was a significant factor in determining vulnerability to depression. Furthermore, they revealed that a particularly high rate of onset of depression was recorded among women who had been 'let down' at a time when they were in greatest need of the help and support a friend or confidant could provide.

A question of perspective: interactionist or social causation/structuralist?

As discussed above, the interactionist and structuralist stances take different approaches to the study of mental illness. In the case of the former, mental illness is not viewed in terms of individual pathology but as a social construct, a socially derived label applied by certain members of society. As such, the interactionist perspective questions the applicability of a disease concept of mental illness and focuses on identifying the process by which individuals are defined and labelled as mentally ill. This is in contrast to the social causation approach, in which there is a general acceptance of the fundamental assumptions underlying diagnostic classification in psychiatry. The primary objective is to identify the role played by social factors in the causation of mental disorder. Busfield (1988) believes that the social stress model offers a *social* analysis, rather than a full-blown structural analysis of the aetiology of mental illness. The emphasis is placed on situational aspects of the lives of individuals, as opposed to aspects of social structure and how they shape social relations at the macro-level of analysis.

Neither the interactionist nor the structuralist or social causation perspective is capable on its own of providing all the answers we need to enable us to appreciate fully the social ramifications of mental illness. Each, in its own way, makes a significant contribution to the sociological understanding of the origins, development and treatment of mental disorder. As Cuff *et al.* (1990) maintain, it is not the case that one perspective is necessarily more correct than the other; they simply constitute markedly different ways of viewing behaviour that is categorised as 'mental illness'.

> ... the kinds of sociological analyses and explanations of mental illness produced by sociologists using meaning and action perspectives differ considerably from those produced by the sociologists using structuralist perspectives. The events and behaviours in the world that both are observing may be 'the same', but because they start from different bedrock assumptions about the nature of the social world and make use of different conceptual frameworks, they produce different sociological analyses.
>
> (Cuff *et al.*, 1990, p. 20)

Explaining the relationship between social class and mental illness

> The inverse relationship between social class and the occurrence of mental disorders is one of the most well established in the field of mental health epidemiology. This relationship was first documented empirically in early mental hygiene studies in the 1930s and such findings continue to be replicated in numerous contemporary studies.
>
> (Perry, 1996, p. 17)

Studies show that mental illness is not randomly distributed across the social classes. In the main, social class patterns in the development and prevalence of diagnosed mental disorder reveal a tendency towards higher rates of mental illness among the lower social classes. This is particularly so with regard to some neurotic disorders (Meltzer *et al.*, 1995) and functional psychoses, such as schizophrenia (Eaton, 1985). Epidemiological analyses indicate that schizophrenia is three times more likely to be found among individuals from working-class backgrounds than among individuals from any of the other social class groupings (Barbigian, 1985). The social class gradient in schizophrenia is well established in the research literature. As Gallagher has stated of a review of 50 studies from a number of countries, 'Almost without exception these studies have found a preponderance of schizophrenia at the lowest social class levels of urban society' (1980, p. 257). Many early ecological studies of mental disorder conducted in the USA report a concentration of high rates of mental disturbance, especially schizophrenia, in the central city districts (Faris and Dunham, 1939; Klee *et al.*, 1967) and among low status socio-economic groups (Hollingshead and Redlich, 1958; Srole *et al.*, 1962). Evidence for a social class gradient for senile dementia of the Alzheimer type is provided by a study of clinically identified cases in Finland, where the highest rate was recorded in the lowest social class (Sulkava *et al.*, 1985).

This social class gradient does not apply to all types of mental disturbance. For example, suicide affects all social groups and the rate tends to be higher for those groups situated at opposite ends of the economic scale (Retterstol, 1993). Eating disorders, such as anorexia nervosa, have their highest incidence in young women from middle-class backgrounds (Cohen and Hart, 1988). Alcohol abuse is found in all social classes but rates are higher in specific occupational categories where there is a culture of heavy drinking and where drinking alcohol is part of the daily routine. Typical high-risk occupations include jobs in the brewing and hotel industries and merchant seamen. High rates of alcohol-related problems are also found among managing directors (Henderson, 1988).

Despite the fact that the lower social classes do not produce the highest rates of mental illness across the whole range of disorders, Gomm concludes that '. . . for nearly every kind of "mental" illness . . . especially those which afflict large numbers of people, poorer people are afflicted more than richer people, more often, more seriously and for longer' (1996, pp. 111–12). To illustrate that there is more mental illness in the lower social classes is not to suggest that being from the working class actually *causes* mental illness but to argue that, in comparison to other social classes, sections of the working class are more susceptible to developing mental-health problems. This raises the question as to how we explain the concentration of mental illness in the lower classes.

Basically, four major explanations or hypotheses have been advanced to account for the fact that, in the main, the lower classes are responsible for producing some of the highest rates of diagnosed mental illness. These four hypotheses are genetic inheritance, social selection, social stress and societal reaction.

Genetic inheritance

According to this hypothesis the pattern of genetic inheritance within the lower social classes ensures that there is a greater predisposition towards mental disturbance within this social category. This explanation has been advanced by some to explain the incidence of schizophrenia. It rests on the basic assumption that there is a direct genetic explanation for schizophrenia. A considerable amount of genetic research has been undertaken to explain the aetiology of schizophrenia. Studies report higher concordance rates for schizophrenia in monozygotic (identical) twins than in dizygotic twins, thus suggesting that genetic factors have some influence. However, genetic transmission alone cannot account for the development of schizophrenia as studies have failed to produce 100 per cent concordance rates for identical twins. Consequently, a view held by many genetic researchers is that both genetic and environmental factors interact to produce schizophrenia. According to some, what is genetically inherited is a *vulnerability* to schizophrenia and not the condition itself (Meehl, 1962). Although genetic mechanisms have a role to play, environmental circumstances and socio-cultural factors also feature in causal explanations (Dunham, 1977).

Social selection

This explanation is also referred to as the *downward drift hypothesis*. It contends that social class is not a cause but a consequence of mental disorder. The reason why there is a preponderance of mental illness in the lower social classes is precisely because mentally disordered persons experience downward social mobility. As a result of their illness they are unable to maintain their position in the class structure and hence 'drift' down into the lower class. For those already in the lower class, their mental condition is such that it prevents them from becoming upwardly socially mobile. Consequently, this process ensures that the lower class contains a residue of mentally disturbed persons.

There is much evidence to support this selection or drift hypothesis. In what is described as a 'methodologically elegant study' (Henderson, 1988, p. 46), Goldberg and Morrison (1963) took a sample of male patients in England and Wales, aged between 25 and 34 years, who were admitted to mental hospital for the first time suffering from schizophrenia. The researchers compared the patients' class of origin (as determined by the occupation of the patients' fathers at the time the patients were born) with their class of destination (that is, their occupational status prior to their admission to hospital). They found that while the social class distribution of the patients' fathers was representative of that appertaining in the general population, a disproportionate number of the sons were located in social class V, that is the unskilled occupational category. Thus it was concluded that downward drift had occurred. Similar findings were also reported by Hare *et al.* (1972) in their study of the social mobility of neurotic and schizophrenic patients in Britain. Downward mobility was a feature of the occupational histories of these patients, particularly the schizophrenics. It is results from studies such as these that lead to the conclusion that 'schizophrenia impairs the functioning of individuals, making it more difficult for them to hold the social class of their origin, particularly where the disorder is chronic or frequently recurrent' (Henderson, 1988, pp. 46–7).

Social stress

This explanation is also referred to as the *social causation hypothesis, environmental stress explanation* (Miles, 1981, p. 171) or the *breeder hypothesis* (Henderson, 1988, p. 45). Basically, psychiatric illness is the result of a combination of factors. The social circumstances, economic conditions and environmental surroundings characteristic of life in the lower social classes are thought to be instrumental in explaining the increased rates of psychiatric illness in the lower reaches of society. Supporters of this approach maintain that certain aspects of lower-class life can be excessively stress-inducing and create a climate in which there is an increased risk of developing mental illness. The role of adverse life events as precipitating factors in the onset of depression has been discussed above. What emerges from this research is the finding that many of the severe life events and ongoing major difficulties experienced by working-class women were of a type that brought a deep sense of insecurity into their lives. Lack of suitable accommodation and unemployment were identified as just two areas of insecurity in working-class life capable of generating stress which in turn provokes psychiatric disorder. However, as Brown and Harris (1989) note, the preponderance of mental illness in the lower social classes is not accounted for solely by the presence of stressful life events, consideration also needs to be given to the existence of specific vulnerability factors.

Miles (1981) maintains that working-class people are generally in a relatively more vulnerable position than their middle-class counterparts when it comes to coping with stressful situations. She suggests that the kinds of stress-inducing events and difficulties experienced by working-class individuals are less responsive to individual action than those encountered by middle-class people.

> Stress in the working-class environment most often arises from structural economic factors over which individuals have little control, and moreover, they have fewer resources, in money and power, to mitigate the consequences of stressful events.
>
> (Miles, 1981, p. 184)

Herein lies a form of double jeopardy: conditions of economic and social deprivation increase the stress-producing potential of the working-class environment and the very lack of material resources makes it difficult to deal with stressful life events and difficulties once they occur.

Societal reaction

This hypothesis accounts for the inverse relationship between social class and the prevalence of mental illness by focusing on the nature and content of the process of psychiatric labelling. The underlying theme is that there are important differences between the social classes in terms of problem-solving activity, behavioural norms and the expression and control of emotions. Members of the mental-health professions are drawn primarily from middle-class backgrounds and their professional socialisation reinforces middle-class attitudes, values and beliefs. Consequently, the normative standards by which they evaluate the behaviour and conduct of patients reflect a middle-class bias. According to some observers, what is interpreted as psychiatric disturbance among patients of working-class origin may in fact be deviation from middle-class norms (Wilkinson, 1975).

Which explanation do we choose?

While the increased incidence of certain types of mental illness in the lower social class is well documented in the research literature, there is much debate surrounding the reasons for this observed distribution. It may be concluded that none of the four hypotheses by themselves provides an adequate explanation. A strong case can be made for all four having some part to play in explaining the complex relationship of psychiatric illness to social class. It is possible that a different combination of elements from more than one explanation will be required to produce a satisfactory account of the origin and development of particular types of psychiatric illness. Mental illness is such a complex phenomenon covering a range of diverse conditions that it makes little sense to search for a single causal explanation.

Gender and mental illness

> Despite the continuing interest in gender and mental health, there is still not a clear sociological account of why women are over-represented in the way they are in psychiatric populations.
>
> (Rogers and Pilgrim, 2005, p. 7)

Evidence from both epidemiological research based on self-report population surveys and official records kept by the psychiatric services suggests that mental illness is more prevalent among women than among men. Statistics show that, in general, the rates of mental illness are higher for women than for men. Closer examination reveals that while there are no consistent differences by sex as far as psychotic disorders are concerned, the rates of minor psychiatric disturbances, particularly depression and anxiety, are consistently higher for women. This difference in prevalence rates between the sexes is generally found to be greatest in adults between 20 and 45 years of age (Henderson, 1988, p. 36). In the case of personality disorders, the rate of hospital admissions is consistently higher among men than among women. More men than women commit suicide but women have a higher rate of attempted suicide (Retterstol, 1993).

There is controversy surrounding the statistical findings, with some observers arguing that they do not reveal the *true* prevalence rates for women and men. The higher reported rates of mental disorder among women is seen as a reflection of differences in the culturally defined roles of men and women in Western societies (Phillips and Segal, 1969; Horwitz, 1977). It is argued that as a consequence of gender socialisation women are more likely than men to discuss their feelings and seek professional help when they experience emotional problems. Men, on the other hand, are expected to display independence and self-reliance and therefore it is less socially acceptable for them to admit to having psychological problems. Thus, social conditioning not only leads to men underreporting psychiatric symptoms in mental health surveys but also to them being reticent when it comes to consulting health professionals. However, there is research that suggests that there are *real* differences between the sexes, particularly in the case of certain psychiatric disturbances, such as depression (Weissman and Klerman, 1977). Furthermore, the observed overrepresentation of women in the reporting of psychiatric symptoms cannot be simply dismissed as a methodological artefact of differential response patterns in self-report studies (Clancy and Gove, 1974).

How do we explain the higher rates of female psychiatric morbidity? Basically, explanations fall into three broad categories:

* biological explanations;
* social causation explanations;
* feminist perspectives.

Biological explanations

It has been suggested that biological factors or hormonal changes, especially those taking place during menstruation, in the postpartum period and at the time of the menopause, might account for the sex differences in mental illness rates. However, the research evidence is far from conclusive. For example, while some people maintain that women are particularly susceptible to developing depressive disorders at the pre-menstrual stage, others claim that there is no strong empirical evidence to link depression with the menstrual cycle (Weissman, 1979). Also, there is no support for the view that women are more vulnerable to mental illness during the menopause (Weissman, 1979). Research has yet to establish the role of endocrine changes in the onset of involutional melancholia, which is experienced by some menopausal women. In general terms, the biological determinism of the medical model is seen as being unable to offer an adequate explanation of women's higher rates of mental illness for two main reasons. Firstly, overrepresentation of women is not found in all societies. Secondly, 'differences in rates of illness according to marital status appear more complex than a simple biological model can explain' (Payne, 1991, p. 165).

Social causation explanations

Explanations that fall into this category focus on how the relative social positions of men and women might account for the differences in mental illness rates. Structural inequalities can be a source of social stress, which can be detrimental mental health and psychological well-being. Levels of material deprivation and poverty are higher for women than for men (Belle, 1990). Many women, who are major full-time carers of children and other dependent kin, have limited opportunities for taking paid employment outside the home. Those who are single parents are particularly vulnerable to poverty (Platt *et al.*, 1990). Providing care also has its emotional costs and women who are confined to the home can experience feelings of social isolation.

Walter Gove and his co-researchers have studied epidemiological data on gender and mental illness over a number of years in the USA and come to the conclusion that the overrepresentation of women in the mental health statistics can be accounted for by differences in sex roles (Gove, 1972, 1984; Gove and Tudor, 1973). Their research shows that there is a higher rate of diagnosed and self-reported psychiatric disturbance among married women than among married men. This applies particularly to anxiety and depression. Bebbington (1987), in a study of national hospital admission statistics for in England, reports a similar relationship between marital status and depression. These findings seem to suggest that for women marriage might not be a protective institution as far as their mental health is concerned.

For Gove et al., the explanation lies in the stress associated with the social or marital role assigned to women in contemporary industrial societies. This role is described as 'more frustrating and less rewarding' than the adult role prescribed for men (Gove and Tudor, 1973, p. 816). They argue that, in the main, women are restricted to a single occupational and social role, namely that of being a housewife. This is an exclusively domestic role that is frustrating because it requires little skill, is low in social prestige and offers few rewards. In contrast, married men have a role outside the home, in the world of paid employment, which gives them a social identity and source of gratification beyond the scope of that provided by their domestic role.

For those married women employed outside the home the situation can be exacerbated. Not only do they have the domestic burden of household tasks still to contend with but also they may face discrimination and prejudice in the workplace, which can also be stressful. If they are pursuing a professional career, it is possible that they may experience role conflict or role strain, as they strive to achieve their occupational goals while simultaneously trying to meet the demands imposed on them in the form of the traditional sex role of the woman. As Cockerham (1981, p. 212) notes, women can find themselves in a 'double bind' in that not only may they find the traditional role of housewife frustrating but also, if they do enter the labour force, they may experience frustration as they try to reconcile their family and work roles.

The marital role explanation of the perceived gender bias in mental illness rates has attracted some criticism. There is a view that the sex differences in prevalence rates for specific psychiatric disorders are not solely a function of marital status. As Pilgrim and Rogers assert, 'there are larger discrepancies in mental ill health between single and married people than between married men and women' (1993, p. 28). Also, Busfield (1988) questions whether marital status provides an adequate measure of role performance in marriage as there are likely to be differences in the actual marital role adopted by persons of the same marital status. Furthermore, she comments that Gove appears to be too eager to interpret the difference in psychiatric morbidity between married women and married men as being primarily due to differences in marital roles. This lends support to the argument that the recorded sex differences in minor psychiatric morbidity may be a statistical artefact of the utilisation of epidemiological methods of inquiry.

Feminist perspectives

Feminist theorists have made a significant contribution to our understanding of the relationship between gender and mental health. On one level they have highlighted the specific social and economic inequalities prevalent in societies structured by gender and described how these inequalities impinge upon women's everyday lives. Women are exploited, subjugated and oppressed: mental illness is a product of their disadvantageous social position. Their powerlessness means that they are not only the victims of social structural forces but also victims of personal violence and abuse. Knowledge of the incidence and impact of emotional, physical and sexual abuse is important when considering the aetiology of mental health difficulties experienced by women. It is estimated that at least half of all the women who use community-based and hospital-centred psychiatric health services have experienced sexual and/or physical abuse as children and as adults (Williams *et al.*, 1993 quoted in Williams and Watson, 1996). There is growing evidence that the physical and sexual abuse of children (Polusny and Follette, 1995) and adults (Goodman *et al.*, 1993) can have a major impact on future mental well-being.

On another level, feminist theorists have drawn our attention to differential labelling as a possible explanation of the overrepresentation of women in mental illness statistics. According to this view, the behaviour and conduct of women is evaluated from a distinctly male-oriented cultural perspective. Such is the influence of male authority that when women are seen to fail to conform to traditional, stereotypical gender roles, they run the risk of attracting a psychiatric label. Any deviation from, or rejection of, conventional female roles may be judged to be pathological and a sign of impending psychiatric impairment or potential mental disorder.

In exploring the gendered views of mental health and mental illness feminist theorists draw on both the labelling perspective and social constructionism. The latter focuses on how psychiatric knowledge is socially constructed. The diagnostic categories and theoretical formulations employed by psychiatrists are not taken for granted but are seen as inherently problematic. Psychiatry is looked at as a social practice and is itself subjected to critical analysis. Some critics argue that, as psychiatry is a male-dominated profession, a general cultural sexism pervades professional practice (Chesler, 1972). Stereotypical sex roles, with their in-built assumptions about male superiority and female inferiority and their sex-specific definitions of normality, shape psychiatric evaluations. This represents the feminisation of mental illness. The labelling of women as mentally ill is interpreted as evidence of the patriarchal power of the medical profession in action.

The existence of sex stereotyping by medical practitioners is a contested issue. While some writers claim that hard evidence to support its occurrence is hard to come by (Miles, 1981), others maintain that such evidence does exist (Rogers and Pilgrim, 2005). Interestingly, there is a suggestion that sexist stereotyping of female roles is not confined to male-dominated professional groups. Pilgrim and Rogers note that in a study of social workers working with women with severe psychiatric problems, Davis *et al.* (1985) found evidence of sexist stereotyping. This suggests that sex role stereotypes can become embedded within the culture or discourse of a professional group. As Rogers and Pilgrim observe, 'It is likely that sexism in psychiatry has its roots in, and can be transmitted in, the type of knowledge, diagnostic categories and practices followed by the professions as well, which can still be called "patriarchal" even when used by women doctors' (2005, p. 71).

Which explanation do we choose?

The sex difference in psychiatric morbidity is well established. The question is how do we explain the observed difference? What needs to be borne in mind is that it is highly unlikely that any single explanation accounts for all the sex difference in mental illness rates. Depending on the type of psychiatric illness, it may be necessary to combine elements from more than one approach to reach a satisfactory level of understanding of the processes and mechanisms at work. For example, as Busfield (1988) describes, despite the contrasting nature of the social causation and differential labelling perspectives they are not necessarily incompatible. One way forward is to work towards identifying the relative contributions of male–female biological and psycho-social differences in those psychiatric disturbances in which gender is an important variable, while recognising the possibility of bias in the construction of notions of mental health and illness.

Mental health of minority ethnic groups

> Understanding differences in health outcomes and the experiences of living in the UK within, as well as between, 'South Asian', 'Black Caribbean' and 'White' groups is vital, and underlines the need to view ethnicity as a complex social, economic and cultural matrix.
>
> (Weich and McManus, 2002, p. 26)

Problems measuring psychiatric morbidity

Estimating the occurrence of mental illness in different ethnic groups is beset with technical problems and methodological difficulties. Many of these problems are not unique to studies that focus on ethnicity but are a feature of the methods employed when researching psychiatric morbidity in general. Basically, there are two major research strategies for investigating the distribution of mental illness. One relies on official statistics on service users collected as a matter of routine, such as hospital admission rates, or information collected by way of sample surveys of general practitioners and hospital doctors. The other method involves screening for evidence of mental illness by surveying samples of individuals taken from the general population. Data from these population surveys are then used to explore the prevalence of mental illness in relation to a variety of social and economic factors. Thus while '[p]sychiatric epidemiology has traditionally been tied closely in to service utilisation . . . [b]y contrast, *social* epidemiology links the genesis of mental health problems with broader social and economic influences' (Rogers and Pilgrim, 2005, p. 84).

Statistics on service use and population surveys both have shortcomings as measures of psychiatric morbidity. Data collected from administrative records and surveys of medical personnel give details of those individuals who have been identified as having a mental disorder and as such provide a measure of treatment, rather than an indication of the prevalence of mental health problems in the community at large. Not all individuals who experience psychiatric symptoms seek treatment; this method has no way of estimating the extent of undiagnosed psychiatric illness. As for community prevalence surveys, these are capable of uncovering undiagnosed mental illness but they can face the problem of low response rates. There is no way of knowing if those who refuse to take part in a survey possess attributes that would significantly influence the findings if they had agreed to be included. Furthermore, there is the possibility that people with psychotic conditions may be less inclined than those with common mental disorders to participate in a survey.

These problems apply irrespective of the cultural and socio-demographic characteristics of the group being investigated. However, when the aim is to compare the prevalence rates of mental illness between ethnic groups, a number of additional problems arise. First, it is very difficult to measure morbidity in different cultural groups, as the questions asked in the course of making a diagnosis may have different meanings for people from different cultural backgrounds. There may be cultural differences in the way in which mental illness is experienced and described (Kleinman, 1987). Consequently, research instruments that employ diagnostic categories and conceptualisations of mental illness characteristic of Western psychiatric medicine may produce misleading findings when applied across a diverse range of ethnic groups. Certain types of psychological symptoms may not be picked up at all, thus leading to an underestimation of some common mental disorders (Bhui, 1999). Furthermore, there is a view that South Asians, particularly women, express mental or psychological distress in the form of physical symptoms and complaints. This idea that bodily symptoms can mask a real mental illness is known as the 'somatisation thesis' (Currer, 1986). However, it has been suggested that acceptance of the core assumption, that the presentation of physical symptoms serves to disguise an underlying mental illness, 'may reflect a form of Western cultural imperialism on the part of the psychiatric profession' (Rogers and Pilgrim, 2005, p. 94).

A second problem encountered when measuring psychiatric morbidity concerns the difficulty in general population surveys of getting a sufficiently large and representative sample of people from the various minority ethnic groups. Small sample sizes make it impossible to conduct any meaningful statistical analysis on which to draw conclusions about comparative prevalence rates. There is a third issue, in that how ethnicity is determined can influence the findings of research studies. As Rogers and Pilgrim (2005) note, some studies of the ethnic composition of psychiatric inpatients use place of birth to determine ethnic background. This concentration on immigrants excludes from the analysis members of minority ethnic groups who were born in Britain. Finally, on a general level, there is the issue of the stigma associated with mental illness, which 'creates the risk that white doctors or researchers may be suspected of racial bias if they find that one minority group or another has a higher (or lower) rate of illness than others' (Berthoud and Nazroo, 1997, p. 309).

Epidemiology of mental health and ethnicity

Treatment statistics and survey findings reveal differences in the distribution of mental disorders by ethnic group. This applies in both the cases of common mental disorders (such as anxiety and depression) and the more serious psychotic illnesses such as schizophrenia and other delusional disorders. However, research findings in this area have not always presented a consistent picture with regard to the prevalence of various types of mental disorder across the different ethnic groups (Iley and Nazroo, 2001). While some studies have found relatively low rates for psychiatric treatment among Asian immigrants living in Britain, others report the opposite (Carpenter and Brockington, 1980). In a study of psychiatric hospital admission rates in England for 1971 and 1981, Cochrane and Bal (1989) found that when compared to the white majority population, migrants from the South Asian subcontinent had a lower rate of depression. As for African-Caribbeans, they also displayed low rates of depression but were overrepresented in the psychotic disorders. Taking psychiatric admissions for all disorders, Cochrane and Bal report that Irish immigrants were more likely to be admitted to hospital than were immigrants from the Caribbean.

Studies of variations in mental disorder across ethnic groups require careful evaluation. Where hospital admission rates provide the main source of data there is a possibility that observed variations are not an accurate reflection of the incidence of psychiatric disorders in the community. Hospital records may reflect biases in the application of diagnostic labels by psychiatrists. Fernando (1988, 1991) maintains that ethnocentrism and racial bias are evident in the theory and practice of Western psychiatry; their presence may account for differential labelling. With reference to the work of Ranger (1989), Rogers and Pilgrim assert that, 'Cannabis psychosis is a label attached selectively to African-Caribbean people when British psychiatrists are perplexed by their behaviour' (2005, p. 93).

Evidence of variations between ethnic groups in the prevalence of mental illness is provided by the results of community and national surveys. In one survey, based on a national sample of members of minority ethnic groups and white people living in Britain, Nazroo (1997) drew the following general conclusions:

- the rate of depression was higher among married, non-migrant Caribbean people than among white British people; there was no difference in rates between white people and Caribbeans who came to Britain after their eleventh birthday;
- contrary to previous research findings Caribbean men were at no greater risk from psychosis than white men; although the rate for Caribbean women was higher this was not statistically significant;
- the prevalence rates for both depression and psychosis were lower for South Asians. For example, Bangladeshi men and women had a risk of depression

that was half that found among the white British sample; these relatively low rates applied only in the case of those who had migrated after the age of eleven.

A later national survey entitled the Study of Ethnic Minority Psychiatric Illness in the Community (EMPIRIC), covering individuals aged between 16 and 74 years of age and living in private households, focused on five main ethnic groups (Bangladeshi, African-Caribbean, Indian, Irish and Pakistani) and used a white group from the general population for purposes of comparison (Sproston and Nazroo, 2002). With regard to psychiatric morbidity it found:

- small but statistically significant differences in the prevalence of common mental disorders across the ethnic groups;
- African-Caribbean people had lower rates of anxiety but higher rates of depression when compared with whites;
- Irish men showed significantly higher rates of common mental disorders than white British men;
- rates of depression were lowest in the Bangladeshi group;
- Pakistani and Indian groups had higher rates of positive screening for psychosis than the white group (although this was not statistically significant);
- among the African-Caribbean group 'non-migrants' had similar rates of psychosis to 'migrants';
- rates of psychotic illness were higher among African-Caribbean and white people who were in a poor economic position.

How do we explain the relative prevalence of mental illness among different ethnic groups?

There is still considerable debate surrounding the reasons for the observed variation in mental illness rates between different ethnic groups. In broad terms, four major types of explanation have been advanced; each has its strengths and weaknesses.

1 There is the argument that differences in prevalence rates may be explained by reference to inherent differences between ethnic groups, particularly in terms of their collective cultural attitudes or genetic profile. Some groups, when compared to others, might have a greater susceptibility to mental illness.

2 The social stress hypothesis suggests that the stresses caused by the material deprivation and social disadvantages experienced by minority ethnic groups, coupled with the burden of racial discrimination, play an important role in the aetiology of mental illness. While on the face of it this might seem a reasonable hypothesis, as Rogers and Pilgrim remark, it is not supported by data relating to *all* minority ethnic groups. As they assert, 'in poor inner-city areas, Asian people as well as African-Caribbean people suffer recurrent racism. And yet, overall, the evidence seems to point to only the latter being

over-represented in psychiatric records, not the former' (Rogers and Pilgrim, 2005, p. 86). More systematic research is needed to measure the impact of racial disadvantage and racism on mental health. It may be the case that some ethnic groups are more discriminated against than others or that some groups are better able to cope with negative discrimination.

3 Ethnocentric attitudes and racial or cultural bias on the part of professionals in the psychiatric services might account for differences between ethnic groups in terms of diagnosis and treatment.

4 Cultural bias in the definition and measurement of psychiatric illness can result in misleading inferences being drawn from the results of comparative studies. Also, the method used to detect psychiatric symptoms in community surveys may underestimate mental illness among some groups. This is recognised by Berthoud and Nazroo when commenting on the relatively low rates of psychiatric illness among the South Asians in their survey: 'the finding that low prevalence rates were observed among the sub-group who are least familiar with white Western social and cultural conventions is also consistent with the idea that the questions may not have been picking up some real mental illness' (1997, p. 323).

This is a complex field of study, not least because of the methodological problems surrounding the interpretation of the evidence. Research findings are not always consistent and are sometimes inconclusive, as illustrated by two findings from the EMPIRIC study. First, while research shows that the rate of psychotic disorders is higher for African-Caribbean people than white people (the illness rate), the differential in rates is far less than that recorded in studies based on service contact figures (the treatment rate). Thus, Nazroo and King (2002) maintain that while this might suggest that African-Caribbeans may be more susceptible to developing a psychotic disorder, it also suggests that they are treated differently. Possible reasons advanced to explain differential treatment include racism (both within the community and the mental health and social welfare services), misdiagnosis due to a misunderstanding of cultural expressions of emotional distress and social exclusion resulting from racial prejudice and discrimination (Nazroo and King, 2002, p. 54).

Second, studies at the individual level and the area level show an association between social disadvantage and mental health status. For example, using data relating to individuals, Lynch *et al.* (1997) found that people living in 'economic hardship' on a long-term basis were much more likely to suffer from clinical depression than those not living in such conditions. At the area level, Boardman *et al.* (1997) found a strong correlation between social indicators of deprivation and psychiatric admissions not only for psychotic illnesses but also for neurotic disorders. However, the link between socio-economic deprivation and mental disorders is not uniform across all ethnic groups. In the EMPIRIC study the rate of morbidity for common mental disorders was comparatively low for the Bangladeshi group, which led to the observation that:

Given the very high levels of socio-economic deprivation among the Bangladeshi group in particular, these findings would appear to run counter to the hypothesis that members of this ethnic minority group should, as a consequence, experience higher rates of severe mental illness than less deprived groups.

(Weich and McManus, 2002, p. 34)

As the authors comment, the variables used in the study to measure deprivation were employment status, housing tenure and education and it is possible that these were not sensitive enough to reflect the most stressful features of life as experienced by different minority ethnic groups in England.

Where minority ethnic populations include recent immigrants, the migratory experience itself may have an influence on mental health. Migration has been described as 'a psycho-social process of loss and change' and likened to a 'grief process' in the psychiatry of migration (Carta et al., 2005). Emigrants are seen to 'lose' any number of the following in leaving their country of birth: family and friends; homeland; culture; language; status. How successfully the individual immigrant adjusts to these experiences is determined by a complex combination of factors including the motivation to migrate, the social, economic and political circumstances surrounding the decision to migrate and how well they are received in their new country. Psychopathological risk and the need for mental healthcare and psychiatric treatment are not easy to determine as migrants do not constitute a homogeneous group. It is important to try and identify those factors which may, in specific circumstances, lead to an increased risk of mental disorder. The constellation of causal factors will vary not only within a single ethnic group but also between ethnic groups. Variations in psychiatric morbidity may also reflect gender and social class differences. For example, in the case of the former, suicide rates among young women immigrants from the Indian subcontinent are higher than those of their male counterparts. Also, the suicide rate for this group of women is higher than that found among women in the country of destination (Patel and Gaw, 1996).

Experiences prior to migration can have a profound impact on mental health. This is particularly the case with asylum seekers and refugees, who are fleeing for their safety and have very little hope of being able to return to their country of origin in the near future. The sense of loss in such circumstances may be quite extreme. Consequently, such migrants may be less emotionally and economically equipped to be able to cope with any racial prejudice or negative discrimination they might encounter in their host country. Indeed, the most common mental health problem presented by asylum seekers and refugees is post-traumatic stress disorder (LeTouze and Watters, 2003). Bhui et al. (2003) found that among Somali refugees living in the UK it was the trauma of their experiences of war prior to migration that featured as a risk factor as far as their psychiatric symptoms were concerned.

As noted by Nazroo and Sproston (2002, p. 9), 'The relative prevalence of mental illness among different ethnic groups in Britain is both a controversial and complex field of inquiry.' Any attempt at providing an explanation needs to take into account a wide range of individual, social and economic factors. It is not possible to isolate the relative impact of any single risk factor, as these will fluctuate over time and combine to produce a cumulative effect. However, as with the study of physical health and illness, we can conclude that material disadvantage and the experience of racism can cause stress and thereby increase susceptibility to illness. Furthermore, these conditions can affect the health outcomes not just of newly migrant groups but of future generations.

Summary

- Mental illness is not an easy concept to define and there is considerable debate surrounding the causes of mental illness. A general distinction can be made between biogenic explanations and those based on social and psychological factors. Biologically oriented explanations are dominant in the medical model.

- Szasz contends that an 'illness' of the mind cannot be understood in the same way that we understand an illness of the body. For him, mental illness is a label psychiatrists apply to certain types of rule-breaking behaviour. Psychiatric patients do not have illness but suffer from 'problems in living'. Critics of this approach claim that Szasz fails to appreciate the mind–body link in health and illness: chronic physical illness can lead to depression.

- Mental health, like mental illness, is also difficult to define. Some definitions focus on the absence of psychopathological symptoms, while others include notions of mental and social well-being.

- The labelling perspective and the social structure approach constitute two contrasting sociological approaches to the study of mental illness. According to the former, mental illness is a form of deviant behaviour and deviant behaviour is a socially constructed phenomenon. Labelling theorists do not attempt to identify what causes mental illness but are concerned with how the whole process of labelling someone as mentally ill works. In this sense the perspective represents a challenge to the medical model. In contrast, the structuralist or social causation perspective explores the relationship between aspects of the social structure (e.g. social class, gender and ethnicity) and the incidence and prevalence of mental illness. Research shows how adverse life events or major difficulties act as stressors or provoking agents in producing depression in women. Both perspectives make an important contribution to the sociological understanding of mental illness.

- Mental illness is not randomly distributed across the social classes. There is much research evidence to support the premise that there is a relationship between socio-economic status and the rates of certain types of mental disorder. Rates of schizophrenia are higher in the lower social classes. The higher social classes have higher rates of anxiety disorders.

- Evidence from both epidemiological studies and self-report surveys suggests that psychiatric morbidity is higher among women than among men. The difference is greatest when comparing men and women in the 20- to 45-year-old age group. This cannot be accounted for by biological differences between the sexes. Gender differences in structural inequalities and differential labelling have been advanced as possible explanations.

- There is much controversy surrounding the existence and explanation of mental disorder in minority ethnic populations. While some commentators claim that the relatively high incidence rates observed among some ethnic groups are not 'real' but are a result of poor quality data, others maintain that the statistics reflect the ethnocentrism or racism endemic in British psychiatry.

Clearly, the relationship between mental illness, ethnicity and socio-economic conditions is a complex one that requires further systematic research before any firm conclusions can be drawn.

Questions for discussion

1 What is the medical model of mental illness?

2 In what sense is mental illness a contested concept?

3 Critically evaluate Szasz's concept of mental health.

4 What contribution does the labelling perspective make to the study of mental illness?

5 Outline the four major explanations advanced to account for the relationship between social class and psychiatric morbidity.

6 Discuss the main reasons given for the overrepresentation of women in mental health statistics?

7 What can research tell us about psychiatric morbidity and ethnicity in Britain?

Further reading

Bentley, K. J. (2005) 'Women, mental health and the psychiatric enterprise: A review', *Health and Social Work*, 30, 1: 56–63.

Busfield, J. (ed.) (2001) *Rethinking the Sociology of Mental Health*, Oxford: Blackwell.

Fernando, S. (ed.) (1995) *Mental Health in a Multi-ethnic Society: A Multi-Disciplinary Handbook*, London: Routledge.

Heller, T., Reynolds, J., Gomm, R., Muston, R. and Pattison, S. (2000) *Mental Health Matters: A Reader*, Basingstoke: Palgrave Macmillan.

McLeod, J. D. and Wright, E. R. (eds) (2009) *The Sociology of Mental Illness: A Comprehensive Reader*, Oxford: Oxford University Press.

Prior, P. M. (1999) *Gender and Mental Health*, Basingstoke: Macmillan.

Rogers, A. and Pilgrim, D. (2005) *A Sociology of Mental Health and Illness*, 3rd edn, Maidenhead: Open University Press.

Tausig, M., Michello, J. and Subedi, S. (2004) *A Sociology of Mental Illness*, Upper Saddle River, NJ: Pearson/Prentice Hall.

Useful websites

Mental Health Foundation: http://www.mentalhealth.org.uk/welcome/
MIND: http://www.mentalhealth.org.uk/welcome/
National BME Mental Health Network: http://bmementalhealth.org.uk/index.php?option
=com_frontpage&Itemid=1
The Royal College of Psychiatrists: http://www.rcpsych.ac.uk/mentalhealthinfoforall.aspx

CHAPTER 4

Inequalities in health

Introduction

Although on average we are living healthier and longer lives, health and life expectancy are not shared equally across the population. Despite overall improvements, there remain big – and in some communities increasing – differences in health between those at the top and bottom ends of the social scale. Some parts of the country have the same mortality rates now as the national average in the 1950s.

(Department of Health, 2004a, pp. 10–11)

The last century witnessed major improvements in the state of the nation's health. Statistical evidence shows a significant reduction in infant and childhood death rates and a rapid improvement in adult mortality rates, resulting in pronounced gains in life expectancy. Around 1900, for every 1,000 babies born nearly 150 died before the end of the first year of life, by 1990 this had fallen to just over 7 deaths per 1,000 live births. In 1994, the infant mortality rate was only 65 per cent of the 1984 rate (Dunnell, 1995). The improvement in infant survival rates continued into the twenty-first century; in 2006 the infant mortality rate stood at 5 per 1,000 live births (Office for National Statistics, 2007a, p. i). There were also marked improvements in life expectancy. In 1901, life expectancy at birth was 45 years for men and 49 years for women; the comparable figures for 2005 were around 77 years and just over 81 years respectively. Furthermore, it is forecast that life expectancy at birth will continue to increase for both sexes and by 2021 will be over 80 years for men and nearly 84 years for women (Office for National Statistics, 2007b, p. 88). Thus, there has been a significant change in the age of death. Whereas 63 per cent of all deaths over a five-year period between 1911 and 1915 were of people under the age of 60 years, only 12 per cent of deaths in 1991–1995 were accounted for by people in this age group. Infectious and parasitic diseases used to be a major cause of premature death. In 1880, such diseases accounted for around one in three deaths; by the end of the twentieth century this figure was nearer to one in every six deaths (Hicks and Allen, 1999, p. 9).

As the above figures testify, there is no doubt that over the years there has been a general improvement in the health of the population. However, what the aggregated national-level data do not tell us is whether the improvement has been uniform across social groups, geographical regions and local communities. The purpose of this chapter is to explore the relationship between social and economic circumstances and health experiences. This entails not only considering the impact of social class position, ethnic origin and gender on health but also involves examining the implications of unemployment, poverty and poor housing conditions for the health and well-being of adults and children.

Different ways of measuring health

> Mortality is unambiguous and, because death must be recorded by law, the data are generally complete. But as societies evolve, health problems alter in salience and new health indicators must be chosen to reflect changing health issues.
>
> (McDowell, 2006, p. 11)

A major problem encountered when attempting to establish the nature and extent of the relationship between people's social position and their health, is how to measure 'health'. The main measures used to measure the health of a population are life expectancy, mortality rates and morbidity rates.

Life expectancy

Historically, life expectancy has been viewed as a key indicator when assessing a population's health. Expectation of life at birth increased steadily for both sexes throughout the last century. During the latter part of the century, life expectancy for adults also began to show signs of a continuous improvement. For example, between 1971 and 2005 life expectancy for men aged 65 years increased by 4.6 years, compared to an increase of only 1.7 years between 1901 and 1971 (Office for National Statistics, 2007b, p. 88). However, given the growth in longevity, life expectancy at birth has become too crude an indicator for measuring a population's health, as it does not take into account the fact that as people live longer they are more likely to experience chronic disease and disability. Consequently, healthy life expectancy (HLE) is calculated (Bone *et al.*, 1995). This is the measure of the balance between length of life and quality of life, and as such embraces a much broader and positive definition of health by focusing on the 'quality-of-life' experienced by the individual, rather than concentrating on the mere presence or absence of disease. It is, therefore, more in tune with the view of health held by the World Health Organisation, which sees health 'as a resource for everyday life . . . a positive concept emphasising social and personal resources as well as physical capacities' (WHO, 1984). HLE is a composite measure. It combines life expectancy and population data with data on self-reported health status to provide an estimate of how many years are lived in good health over the lifespan. Self-reported poor heath is strongly associated with mortality and the utilisation of health services. The calculation of HLE is based on data from large-scale sample surveys. The annual British General Household Survey routinely measures two types of HLE, namely general HLE and life expectancy free from limiting long-term illness. Both are based on the responses of survey participants. In the case of the former, respondents are asked whether they consider their health over the previous twelve months to have been 'good, fairly good or not good'. As for the latter, survey respondents are asked if they have any 'long-standing illness, disability or infirmity'. The survey also includes questions designed to ascertain if individuals have any physical or health-related conditions that prevent them from participating in such day-to-day activities as working or engaging in leisure activities. Evidence of more severe disability is sought by questions asking about the extent to which individuals are capable of performing routine tasks of daily living such as dressing and shopping. These data can be used to calculate disability-free life expectancy (DFLE).

The GHS, which is based on a representative sample of the population, is a cross-sectional survey that questions a different group of people each year. As such, it provides a snapshot at one point in time, and is unable to capture the rates at which specific individuals move in and out of states of disability and dependency. In order to achieve such an insight it is necessary to conduct a longitudinal study, which recruits a sample of respondents and follows them over time. The English Longitudinal Study of Ageing is one such survey (Marmot *et al.*, 2002).

Summary health measures, such as HLE and DFLE, take into account not only the length of life but also its quality. People are living to older ages, when they are more likely to experience a long-standing illness or disability. As Table 4.1 illustrates, although there was a noticeable increase in life expectancy between 1981 and 2001, there was a slight fall in the proportion of life that was considered to have been spent in 'good' or 'fairly good' health. In other words,

Table 4.1 Trends in life expectancy and healthy life expectancy at birth: 1981 to 2001

Year	Women		Men	
	1981	*2001*	*1981*	*2001*
Life expectancy	76.8	80.4	70.9	75.7
General Healthy Life Expectancy	66.7	68.8	64.4	67.0
% life in 'good' or 'fairly good' health	86.9%	85.6%	90.0%	88.5%

Source: Parliamentary Office of Science and Technology, 2006, p. 1

people are living longer, but there is also an increase in the number of years spent in poor health. In the period 1981 to 2002 this was particularly the case amongst men, for whom the expected number of years spent in poor health rose from 6.4 to 8.8 years. The comparable figures for women were 10.1 to 10.6 years (Office for National Statistics, 2007b, pp. 88–9).

Clearly, it is important to know whether people are living longer, healthier lives or are experiencing increased levels of disability and suffering more chronic ill health. Using measures like HLE and DFLE can be useful when it comes to monitoring changes in the nation's health, identifying inequalities in health, targeting health promotion initiatives and ascertaining the impact of policies and strategies to improve health. To take one example, the Department of Health's National Service Framework for older people includes increasing HLE amongst its targets. However, while self-rated HLE and self-reported DFLE represent quick and easy ways of measuring health, disability and dependency in the population there are some issues surrounding this form of measurement:

- We need to know if the reported variation in self-reported health observed between different social groups is a reflection of real differences in health or is a product of different cultural expectations.
- There is a need for improved data, particularly in relation to disability and dependency. Current social surveys only provide us with a partial picture, as they underrepresent certain groups in the population (e.g. the very old, people living in long-term institutional care and minority ethnic groups).
- It cannot be assumed that HLE will remain at present levels. Indeed, '. . . some academics predict that rising obesity levels will cause future decreases in HLE, whereas improvements in medical technologies such as joint replacements could contribute towards lower disability rates and higher HLE' (Parliamentary Office of Science and Technology, 2006, p. 3).

Mortality

The infant mortality rate (which is expressed as the number of deaths of infants under one year old per 1,000 live births) provides one of the most sensitive

Box 4.1 Definition

Types of infant mortality

- *Perinatal* mortality:
  - stillbirths and deaths occurring during the first week of life.
- *Neonatal* mortality:
  - deaths during the first four weeks of life.
- *Postneonatal* mortality:
  - deaths after the first 28 days but before the end of the first year of life.

aggregate measures of the health of a population. There was a marked reduction in infant mortality during the early part of the last century. In the UK, the number of deaths per 1,000 live births fell from 140 in 1900 to 63 in 1930 (Hicks and Allen, 1999, p. 8). This was one of the major contributing factors to the increase in life expectancy during the early part of the last century. Infant mortality has continued to decline but at a slower rate. In the mid 1950s there were 24.4 infant deaths per 1,000 live births; by the end of the century the comparable figure was 5.6 deaths per 1,000. The downward trend has persisted and in 2005 there were 5.1 infant deaths per 1,000 live births. It is predicted that this rate will fall to 4.5 by 2021 (Office for National Statistics, 2007a, p. 90).

In compiling infant mortality statistics a distinction is made between perinatal, neonatal and postneonatal mortality (see Box 4.1). Generally, the perinatal mortality rate is seen as being largely influenced by the physiological state of the mother and infant and thus a reflection of the circumstances surrounding the birth of a child. In contrast, the neonatal and postneonatal rates are considered to be determined more by the socio-economic circumstances of the parents and the physical environment experienced by the young infant. Trends in neonatal and postneonatal deaths, for England and Wales, over a 31-year period are illustrated in Figure 4.1.

During the period 1976 to 2006:

- the total number of recorded infant deaths fell from 8,334 in 1976 to 3,368 in 2006;
- there was a 65 per cent drop in the infant mortality rate from 14.3 deaths to 5.0 deaths per 1,000 live births;
- the neonatal and postneonatal rates fell by 64 and 67 per cent respectively;
- the perinatal infant mortality rate fell by nearly 55 per cent;
- the stillbirth rate fell by 44 per cent from 9.7 to 5.4 per 1,000 live births.

Whereas neonatal deaths fell at a steady rate, the postneonatal death rate showed a marked decrease, particularly between 1989 and 1992 (Schuman, 1998). This decline in the postneonatal rate can be attributed to a marked fall in the incidence of Sudden Infant Death Syndrome ('cot death') (Macfarlane *et al.*, 2000).

England and Wales

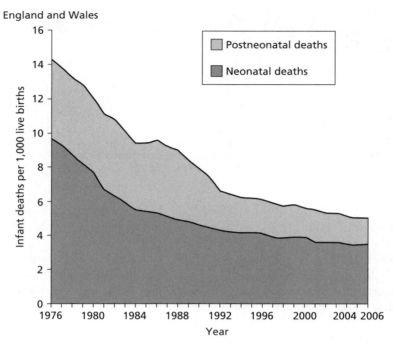

Figure 4.1 Infant mortality rates: 1976–2006

Source: Office for National Statistics, 2007a, p. ii

In advanced modern societies the majority of deaths occur to people aged 75 years and over. Figures for England and Wales show that in 2005 nearly three-quarters of all female deaths and just over one-half of all male deaths occurred after the age of 74 years (Wheller *et al.*, 2007, p. 9). Using information available from death certificates, a crude death rate, which is the simplest form of mortality rate, can be derived by dividing the number of deaths for an area by the population of that area. The area in question may be a country, city, town or local electoral ward or administrative district. However, as mortality rates generally increase with age, the crude death rate will be affected by the age structure of a population. Consequently, a simple mortality rate does not provide a useful means for making comparisons between the populations of different countries or between sub-groups within a given country or geographical zone. In order to address this problem, direct age-standardised mortality rates are calculated. Rates are usually standardised using the European Standard Population and usually presented per 100,000 or per million population. For example, mortality statistics for England and Wales for 1999 to 2003 show that age-standardised death rates per 100,000 population for all circulatory diseases in the age group 0–74 years were 69 for females and almost 152 for males (Romeri *et al.*, 2006, p. 25). Figure 4.2 shows the downward trend in all age mortality rates for the period 1996 to 2006. Over this period rates decreased by 18.1 per cent for females and 24.3 per cent for males.

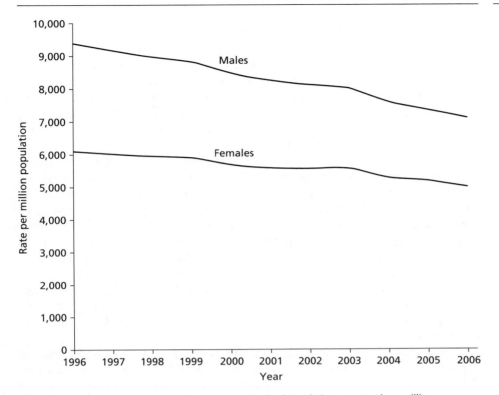

Note: These rates are standardised to the European Standard Population, expressed per million population; they allow comparisons between populations with different age structures, including between males and females and over time.

Figure 4.2 Age-standardised mortality rates (per million population) all causes by sex, 1996 to 2006

Source: *Health Statistics Quarterly*, 34, Summer, Web Supplement, 2007, p. ii. Found at: http://www.statistics.gov.uk/downloads/theme_health/Death_registration_2006.pdf (accessed 5 July 2008)

In order to compare mortality experience in a particular region to the national average, standardised mortality ratios (SMR) are calculated. The SMR for a given region represents the ratio of the *observed* number of deaths in an area to the number of deaths *expected* if the age-specific death rates for the standard population (e.g. the whole country) applied to the population of the region. Following this procedure the SMR for the standard population is fixed at 100. The formula is presented as follows:

$$SMR = \frac{Observed\ Deaths}{Expected\ Deaths} \times 100$$

Using ward-level data for deaths of persons under 85 years of age in England and Wales during the period 1999 to 2003, the SMR for Broughton in Salford is calculated as follows:

$$\text{SMR} = \frac{530}{267} = 1.985 \times 100 = 199$$

Regions with an SMR greater than 100 can be considered to have higher than average mortality, while regions with a figure of less than 100 have mortality rates lower than that for England and Wales as a whole. SMRs for all persons for selected government regions are as follows: South West (89), London (100), West Midlands (104), Wales (107), North West (113) and North East (115) (National Statistics Online, 2008).

Addressing the major causes of early death is a well-established key public health policy objective (Department of Health, 1999a). This has led to a focus on avoidable mortality and how healthcare services can prevent premature deaths. In this context a distinction can be made between two broad types of avoidable mortality, namely *amenable* mortality and *preventable* mortality (Wheller *et al.*, 2007). The former refers to those conditions where death can be avoided through medical treatment following diagnosis. Examples include cancer of the colon, breast cancer and leukaemia. Whereas preventable mortality refers to deaths from causes that are considered to be potentially preventable by changes in individual behaviour or public health service provision, but are not necessarily amenable to medical intervention once diagnosed. Two examples here are lung cancer and Hepatitis B.

There is no common consensus among health researchers concerning the definition of the concepts of premature and avoidable mortality. The fact that death cannot be avoided indefinitely raises the question as to how premature mortality is defined. In some studies premature mortality is defined as death before 65 years of age (Acheson, 1998), while in others the age threshold is taken as 75 years (Wheller *et al.*, 2006). There is also considerable debate surrounding the selection of statistical measures as indicators of avoidable mortality. Wheller *et al.* (2007), in a study of mortality in England and Wales, used age-standardised mortality rates as an indicator of avoidable mortality and found that between 1993 and 2005:

- mortality from amenable causes decreased significantly for both males and females;
- mortality from preventable causes decreased more among males than females;
- smoking-related diseases and alcohol-related diseases were the major causes of preventable deaths in both males and females;
- deaths from smoking-related diseases had declined over the period, while deaths from alcohol-related disease showed a marked increase.

Morbidity

Unlike the case with mortality, there are no comprehensive morbidity statistics available regarding the nature and distribution of illness within the population. Data collected as part of the routine monitoring of the provision of healthcare services are of limited usefulness when it comes to attempting to ascertain changes in the health of the population. When interpreting morbidity data careful consideration needs to be given to the purpose for which the information was originally collected. Statistics relating to consultations with general practitioners, visits to hospital outpatient departments, attendance at specialist clinics and admissions to hospital are sometimes used to describe the incidence and prevalence of illness and disease. However, as Blaxter (1989) notes, problems are encountered when attempting to use statistics on people's use of the health services as measures of morbidity. For example, only those conditions brought to the attention of medical personnel are counted, and because the figures are based on the use made of available clinical and medical services they are a reflection of the nature and type of services available in a particular locality. This is not to suggest that such information does not have its uses, but merely to point out that such statistics do not provide a satisfactory measure of health status and are of limited value when it comes to making comparisons between different geographical regions and administrative areas.

Blaxter (1990) suggests that it may be more useful in certain circumstances to define health in terms of its consequences. This requires not only establishing if an individual suffers from a disease or impairment, but also involves ascertaining the degree to which the condition is considered to have an impact on the quality of life experienced by the individual. Health surveys provide a useful source of information in this respect. A good example is the Health Survey for England (there are separate surveys for Wales and Scotland), which is a continuous sample survey that has been conducted annually since 1991. Originally it was based on a nationally representative sample of all adults over the age of 16 years living in private households in England. In 1995 the sample base was extended to include children of 2 to 15 years. The primary purpose of the survey is to provide baseline data in order to monitor trends in health and ascertain the extent to which national health targets relating to conditions such as blood pressure and obesity are being met. A variety of data are collected including information regarding health behaviours, lifestyle choices and risk factors associated with specific health conditions.

Some sample surveys not dedicated to health issues include questions relating to health and general social well-being. The General Household Survey, mentioned above, is a prime example. This survey, which covers Great Britain, has been running almost annually since 1971 and samples around 13,000 addresses each year. In each household that takes part all individuals aged 16 years or over are interviewed. Questions cover a variety of topics including health and the use of health services and alcohol consumption and smoking. In the 2005 survey, 62 per cent of respondents rated their health as 'good', 26 per cent considered their health to be 'fairly good', and 12 per cent described their health as 'not good' (Ali *et al.*, 2006, p. 5). Over the years there has been an increase in the prevalence of reporting a long-standing illness in adults and children: from 21 per cent in 1972 to 35 per cent in 2002. Respondents reporting a limiting long-standing illness increased from 15 per cent in 1975 to 21 per cent in 2002.

However, care needs to be exercised when interpreting these figures, as they are based on self-assessments and as such may be a reflection of a change in the expectations people have about their health rather than an indication of a change in actual levels of sickness (Office for National Statistics, 2004).

There are a number of standardised questionnaire scales used to measure subjective health status (Bowling, 2005). The various scales differ in terms of their scope and content; some are designed to measure general health status and cover a number of aspects of functioning and social and emotional well-being. The most frequently used health status instruments are the Nottingham Health Profile (Hunt *et al.*, 1986), the Functional Limitations Profile (Patrick and Peach, 1989) and the 36 Health Survey Questionnaire (Ware *et al.*, 1993). By concentrating on subjective well-being these scales tap into the patient's point of view. While health status measures can be used to monitor the health of a population (Ware, 1992), they also have a role in evaluating healthcare interventions and medical treatments, where they can be used as outcome measures (Jenkinson and McGee, 1997).

Determining social class

> How are people *objectively located* in distributions of material inequality? In this case, class is defined in terms of material standards of living, usually indexed by income or, possibly, wealth. Class, in this agenda, is a *gradational* concept; the standard image is of rungs on a ladder, and the names for locations are accordingly such things as upper class, upper middle class, middle class, lower middle class, lower class, under class.
>
> (Wright, quoted in Lareau, 2008, p. 13, emphasis in original)

Social class is the most commonly used indicator of the socio-economic circumstances of individuals and families. Up until 2001 two social classifications were widely used in official statistics: the Registrar General's Social Class schema (RGSC) and Socio-economic Group (SEG). The former first appeared in 1911 and the latter was introduced in 1951. These classifications of occupations were adopted in official surveys and censuses as the basis for determining social class. They were widely used to measure and report differences in mortality and health between sub-groups in the population. The occupational groupings used in the Registrar General's classification system are outlined in Box 4.2. This scale distinguishes between manual and non-manual work and reflects differences in skill levels. However, in 2001 an attempt was made to harmonise the RGSC and SEG scales by creating a third classificatory system, the National Statistics Socio-economic Classification (NS-SEC). This incorporates information regarding occupation, employment status and the size of the establishment in which the person works. There are a number of different versions of this scale. The one described in Box 4.3 incorporates a three-class version, which enables a distinction to be made between advantaged and disadvantaged groups in a similar way to the manual/non-manual divide characteristic of earlier occupational classifications such as RGSC and SEG. This makes it possible to examine the relationship between inequalities in mortality and morbidity and socio-economic status.

> **Box 4.2   Definition**
>
> **Registrar General's social class classification of occupations**
>
> **Non-Manual**
>
> | | | |
> |---|---|---|
> | I | Professional | Lawyers, doctors, chartered accountants, professionally qualified engineers. |
> | II | Intermediate | School teachers, managers, senior administrators. |
> | IIIN | Skilled non-manual | Clerks, shop assistants, cashiers. |
>
> **Manual**
>
> | | | |
> |---|---|---|
> | IIIM | Skilled manual | Plumbers, electricians, bricklayers. |
> | IV | Partly skilled | Security guards, care assistants, postal workers. |
> | V | Unskilled | Labourers, cleaners, porters. |

Using occupation as a general guide to social position and socio-economic status is not without its problems. Although all working men, whether married or single, are assigned to a particular social class category according to the nature of the job they do, only unmarried working women living alone are classified according to their own occupational status. More often than not, married women who work outside the home are classified on the basis of their husband's occupation. For many years, child health and mortality statistics have been compiled using the social class of the father and not the mother. The fact that social class classifications based on measures of occupation are gender-biased is well-documented (Abbott and Sapsford, 1987). According to Whitehead (1988) this male-centred approach to the social categorisation of women gives rise to three major problems.

1 As over half of married women are engaged in either full-time or part-time paid employment, by classifying them according to their husband's occupation valuable information concerning the health risks associated with their own employment is lost.

2 Failure to acknowledge the actual occupational status of married women makes it impossible to compare the health of this group with women who are not actively engaged in the labour market (e.g. 'housewives' and unemployed workers).

3 Working women make a contribution to family finances, and in some cases they may be the main or dominant income earner, this is not taken into account if the husband's occupation alone is used to establish the social position of the family.

Measures of social class based purely on the occupation of the husband do not necessarily accurately reflect the circumstances and experiences of other members of the household. It has been suggested that other ways of establishing the social position of individuals, and family units as a whole, need to be explored. According to the Black Report, produced by the Working Group on Inequalities

Box 4.3 Definition

National Statistics Socio-economic Classification (NS-SEC) – analytic classes

Condensed analytic class	Analytic class	Examples of occupations included
1 Managerial and professional occupations	1 Higher managerial and professional occupations	
	1.1 Large employers, higher managers	Senior officials in national and local government; directors and chief executives of major organisations; officers in the armed forces
	1.2 Higher professionals	Civil engineers, medical practitioners, physicists, geologists, IT strategy and planning professionals, legal professionals, architects
	2 Lower managerial, professional	Teachers in primary and secondary schools, quantity surveyors, public service administrative professionals, social workers, nurses, IT technicians
2 Intermediate occupations	3 Intermediate	NCOs and other ranks in the Armed Forces, graphic designers, medical and dental technicians, Civil Service administrative officers and local government clerical officers, counter clerks, school and company secretaries
	4 Small employers and own account workers	Hairdressing and beauty salon proprietors, shopkeepers, dispensing opticians in private practice, farmers, self-employed taxi drivers
3 Routine and manual	5 Lower supervisory and technical occupations	Bakers and flour confectioners, screen-printers, plumbers, electricians and motor mechanics employed by others, gardeners, rail transport operatives, supervisors of van, bus and coach drivers, labourers, scaffolders
	6 Semi-routine occupations	Pest control officers, clothing cutters, traffic wardens, scaffolders, assemblers of vehicles, farm workers, veterinary nurses and assistants, shelf fillers
	7 Routine occupations	Hairdressing employees, floral arrangers, roundsmen and women, sewing machinists, van, bus and coach drivers, labourers, hotel porters, bar staff, cleaners and domestics, road sweepers, car park attendants

Source: White et al., 2008, p. 20

in Health (DHSS, 1980), the occupational status of both husband and wife need to be considered when analysing the relationship between social factors and a variety of health conditions. The Working Group recommended that occupation-based classification systems should be made more objective by taking into account current income, projected financial earnings, job security and fringe benefits. In this way a fuller picture of the significance of occupation in determining the social and economic circumstances of individuals and families can be obtained. Indeed, as Blaxter notes, occupation constitutes a 'summary measure' which 'can best be regarded simply as a starting point for the investigation of social circumstances and health' (1990, p. 61).

Social class, life expectancy and mortality

> The overall picture is one of falling death rates across the social spectrum, but with the sharpest declines in non-manual classes, leading to an overall widening of the social class divide.
>
> (White *et al.*, 2003, p. 26)

People from all social classes are living longer. However, there are variations in life expectancy at birth between the different social classes. For example, the life expectancy of a male child born into social class V in the mid-1990s was over nine years less than that of a child born into social class I. The pattern for females was similar but not as extreme (House of Commons, 2001). Figures for 2002–2005 show males in the professional social class to have a life expectancy of 80 years, compared to 72.7 years for those in the unskilled manual category; the comparable figures for females are 85.1 and 78.1 years respectively (see Table 4.2). Despite the improvement in life expectancy in all social classes, class differentials persist and there is evidence that the gap between social classes I and V has actually widened over the years. For example, the difference in life expectancy

Table 4.2 Life expectancy by occupational class

	1972–1976		2002–2005	
	Male	*Female*	*Male*	*Female*
Non-manual				
Professional	71.9	79.0	80.0	85.1
Managerial/Technical/Intermediate	71.9	77.1	79.4	83.2
Skilled non-manual	69.5	78.3	78.4	82.4
Manual				
Skilled manual	70.0	75.2	76.5	80.5
Partly skilled	68.3	75.3	75.7	79.9
Unskilled	66.5	74.2	72.7	78.1

Source: Data taken from News Release, Office for National Statistics (2007d), 24 October 2007. Also available at: http://www.statistics.gov.uk/pdfdir/le1007.pdf (accessed 14 July 2008)

between men in social class I and V widened from 5.5 years in the period 1972 to 1976 to 7.4 years in 1997–1999 (Department of Health, 2002, p. 17). Thus, while it can be concluded that there has been a general improvement in all social groups, those situated at the top of the social hierarchy have benefited from a faster rate of improvement in life expectancy.

There is clear evidence of a well-established relationship between social class and mortality in the UK. Research suggests that socio-economic status is a major determinant of health status throughout the life course (Wilkinson and Marmot, 1998) and has an impact on mortality rates even after account is taken of other factors such as health-related behaviours (Jones *et al.*, 2000). There is a voluminous research literature recording the inverse social class gradient in mortality and the magnitude of the differences in mortality rates between the different social class groupings (Fox *et al.*, 1990; Blane *et al.*, 1990). In recent years attention has been turned to trying to establish whether or not the observed inequalities in mortality experience are increasing, decreasing or have stabilised.

As described above, infant mortality has displayed a consistent downward trend. However, despite this general improvement there is evidence that class differences remain. In 1984, the perinatal death rate for classes IV and V was 159 per cent of the rate for classes I and II; the comparable figure for the postneonatal death rate was 178 per cent (Whitehead, 1988, p. 259). Although a clear social class gradient is not evident in the infant mortality figures for England and Wales in 2005 (see Table 4.3), there is evidence of a marked disparity between certain occupational groupings. For example, the infant mortality rate for babies born to married couples in which the father is in a semi-routine occupation is twice

Table 4.3 Infant mortality by socio-economic classification 2005

England & Wales	Rates per 1,000 live births[3]	
	Inside marriage	Outside marriage[4]
Large employers and higher managerial occupations	2.7	3.1
Higher professional occupations	3.8	3.6
Lower managerial and professional occupations	3.4	3.9
Intermediate occupations	5.0	5.4
Small employers and own account workers	3.9	4.3
Lower supervisory and technical occupations	3.4	4.3
Semi-routine occupations	6.1	6.8
Routine occupations	5.8	6.2
All occupations	4.3	5.5

1 Deaths within one year of birth.
2 Based on father's occupation at death registration of the child. See Appendix, Part 7: National Statistics Socio-economic Classification (NS-SEC).
3 Figures for live births are a 10 per cent sample coded for father's occupation.
4 Jointly registered by both parents.
Source: Office for National Statistics, 2007b, p. 90

that found in cases where the father is in a higher managerial occupation in a large-scale organisation (6.1 and 2.7 deaths per 1,000 live births respectively). Furthermore, when comparing the neonatal and postneonatal periods, social class differences in infant mortality rates are more marked in the latter rather than the former. A study of the inequalities in infant mortality over the period 1976 to 2000 concluded that: 'Postneonatal mortality rates for babies with fathers in Social Classes IV and V were persistently higher than those for babies with fathers in manual occupations' (Maher and Macfarlane, 2004, p. 22).

Occupational class is not the only factor associated with infant mortality. The risk of death during the first twelve months of life is related to the age of the mother, the number of previous births (referred to as 'parity'), marital status at the time of the child's birth and low birthweight. Perinatal and infant mortality rates are highest for babies born to mothers under 18 years of age and lowest among babies born to mothers aged 30 to 34 years (Maher and Macfarlane, 2004). However, when account is taken of maternal age and parity, class inequalities in death rates at birth and during the first year of life remain. It would appear that age and the number of previous births is of significance when considering the wives of manual workers. Wives whose husbands are in professional and managerial occupations have a lower risk of stillbirth irrespective of their age or parity. The majority of infant deaths occur to low birth-weight babies, that is babies weighing under 2,500 grams at birth. Statistics show that mothers in households in which the main wage earner is a manual worker are more likely to give birth to low-weight babies than mothers from non-manual households. A social class effect is not only apparent in the incidence of low birth-weight; the survival rate of low-weight babies is also class related. Within each birth-weight category babies born to mothers in social class V are more likely to die than babies born to mothers in social class I. The 1985 perinatal mortality rate for babies weighing less than 1,500 grams was 283 in social class I compared to 389 in social class V (Coleman and Salt, 1992, p. 319). As observed by Whitehead: 'The inescapable conclusion is that occupational class differences are *real* sources of difference in the risk of infant mortality' (Whitehead, 1988, p. 115; emphasis in original).

The percentage of births occurring outside marriage has risen sharply since the 1970s. In 1975 9 per cent of live births in the UK occurred outside marriage, this rose to 31 per cent in 1992 and 43 per cent in 2005 (Office for National Statistics, 2007b, p. 22). In social class V stillbirth rates and postneonatal mortality rates have been found to be higher among unmarried women than married women (Macfarlane and Mugford, 1984). According to more recent data, postneonatal mortality rates are higher for those babies registered by their mothers only than for babies born within marriage or jointly registered by both parents (Maher and Macfarlane, 2004).

Although the childhood mortality rate per 1,000 population aged 1 to 14 years has fallen from 1 in 1954 to 0.2 in 2000, class differentials are evident. Children from families with fathers in class IV and V are twice as likely to die as their counterparts in class I and II families (OPCS, 1988). There is also evidence of a significant social class gradient in mortality throughout the first ten years of life

(Petrou *et al.*, 2006). Differences in mortality between classes I and V can be largely attributed to accidents and respiratory diseases (DHSS, 1980; Townsend and Davidson, 1982). Accidents account for the largest single cause of death in childhood and their higher incidence in the lower classes may be attributed to poorer environmental conditions and lack of material resources.

Class inequalities in health are not restricted to childhood but persist throughout adult life. The existence of social inequalities in mortality, particularly among men of working age, is well-documented. For example, in 2001–2003 the age-standardised mortality rate for men aged between 25 and 64 years in routine occupations was 2.8 times greater than the rate for men in higher managerial occupations: 513 and 182 per 100,000 population respectively (White *et al.*, 2007, p. 16). Despite evidence of a general reduction in mortality risk across the social spectrum, the rate of decrease has been more pronounced among professional workers and managers. In some cases the gap in mortality has widened, suggesting an increasing inequality in mortality risk by socio-economic position. In 1970–72 the SMR for males of working age in class V was 1.8 times that for class I, by the early 1990s this had risen to almost threefold (Drever *et al.*, 1996; Drever and Whitehead, 1997). A sense of the scale of the inequality in mortality can be obtained by comparing age-specific death rates. As noted by White *et al.*, '. . . in 1991–93, men in unskilled occupations aged 20–24 had a higher rate of death than professional men aged 40–44' (2007, p. 7). The existence of a clear social gradient in risk of premature mortality can be observed from a glance at Figure 4.3.

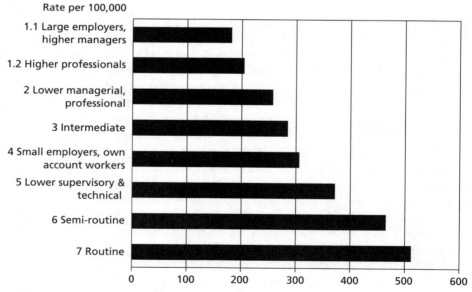

Figure 4.3 Age-standardised mortality rate by NS-SEC: men aged 25–64, England and Wales 2001–2003

Source: http://www.statistics.gov.uk/cci/nugget.asp?id=1899 (accessed 5 July 2008)

Differentials in mortality rates and ratios by occupational class or socio-economic grouping are more marked for some causes of death than others. Using data for men and married women, Marmot and McDowall (1986) conducted a study of adult mortality rates for specific causes of death. Their findings showed that in the early 1980s the disease-specific SMRs were consistently higher for manual workers: non-manual workers had a lower risk of death than manual workers. For example, for men in the 20 to 64 year age group, the SMRs for lung cancer for non-manual and manual workers were 65 and 129 respectively. In the same age group the manual classes also showed an above average SMR for coronary heart disease, 114 compared to 87 for the non-manual group. These findings suggest that as regards some major diseases the manual working classes are affected more than the non-manual middle classes. Whitehead (1988) makes the point that diseases which have often been associated with affluence or 'executive stress', such as coronary heart disease, appear to be more common in the manual classes. The significance of the influence of wider social factors and economic circumstances on mortality rates is indicated when she states, 'Clearly in this country nowadays "diseases of affluence" have all but disappeared and what is left is a general health disadvantage of the poor' (Whitehead, 1988, p. 232).

Social inequalities in mortality are also evident in more recent studies of cause-specific deaths using the NS-SEC to ascertain social class (White et al., 2008). Table 4.4 presents the age-standardised mortality rates for men aged between 25 and 64 years. This shows that across all major causes of death the mortality rates in both the higher managerial/professional class and the intermediate class were lower than the average for all men in England and Wales. The findings also reveal evidence of a continuation of an inverse social class gradient for a number of causes of death.

While death rates have declined substantially in all social classes, the sharpest falls have occurred in the non-manual classes. This has led to an overall widening of social class differences in mortality. As far as major causes of death are concerned, the largest ratios of mortality rates between the most and least disadvantaged social groups have been found for ischaemic heart disease, lung cancer, liver diseases and chronic lower respiratory diseases.

Table 4.4 Age standardised-mortality rates[1] for selected causes by NS-SEC, men aged 25–64, England and Wales, 2001–2003

NS-SEC analytic class	Circulatory disease	Respiratory disease	Digestive disease	Malignant neoplasms	Accidents
1. Managerial and Professional	741	98	164	918	94
2. Intermediate	976	149	229	1,052	154
3. Routine and Manual	1,522	292	368	1,491	206
All men	1,187	219	296	1,211	191

[1] Directly age-standardised rate using the European standard population, quoted per million population.
Source: White et al., 2008

Social class and morbidity

As can be seen from the above, patterns and trends in mortality rates are a reflection of a relationship between socio-economic status and inequalities in health. However, it is not only longevity that is of importance but the whole-life health experience. Indeed, as observed by Blaxter, '[i]nequalities in health may not be the same as inequalities in death' (Blaxter, 1990, p. 7). In other words, ill health is not only studied in relation to mortality rates but can itself provide a useful measure of health status. Given that people are now living longer and mortality rates in the early and middle years are generally low, state of health is considered to be a more significant indicator of inequality than death rates. As noted at the beginning of this chapter, health expectancies can be measured not simply in terms of the length of life but also in relation to the health-related quality of life. Measures based on self-reported healthy life expectancy and disability-free life expectancy can be used to monitor changes in the nation's health. By using data collected by the GHS and HSE it is possible to establish chronic and acute sickness rates for various groups in the population.

The data reveal that male manual workers are much more likely to suffer from chronic illness than are their non-manual counterparts. Furthermore, the difference between the classes is particularly marked for the 45- to 64-year-old age group (OPCS, 1992, p. 107). A similar age and social class distribution can be observed for women. As might be expected the experience of long-standing illness is strongly associated with age. When the effect of age is removed the relationship between morbidity and class is clearly visible. For men and women there is a marked gradient from the professional group, in which the prevalence of chronic sickness was lower than expected, to the unskilled manual class in which prevalence was higher than would be expected on the basis of age alone (OPCS, 1991, p. 105). The class gradient is at its steepest when considering limiting long-standing illness, which is defined as chronic illness that individuals feel restricts their activities in some way. Limiting long-standing illness rates in the unskilled manual class are reported to be more than double those found in the professional class for both men and women (OPCS, 1991, p. 110). Figure 4.4 shows self-reported illness by socio-economic group. Although the class gradient is not a smooth one, the incidence of reporting limiting long-standing illness is clearly higher in the routine and manual groups than in the professional and managerial groups. Differences between the socio-economic groups are particularly marked for adults aged 45 to 64 years, as illustrated in Figure 4.5.

Health surveys have consistently recorded higher rates of self-reported illness among manual classes than among non-manual groups (Blaxter, 1985). Using the Nottingham Health Profile, Hunt et al. (1985) observed a class pattern; people lower on the occupational scale reported poorer health in terms of experiences of pain, lack of energy, sleeping problems, emotional distress and physical mobility. One national survey of self-perceived health found 12 per cent of men in class I believing their health to be fair or poor, the corresponding figure for unskilled manual workers was 36 per cent (Cox et al., 1987). In this study a number of

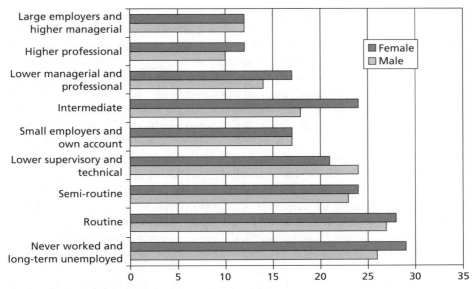

Figure 4.4 Percentage in different socio-economic groups reporting limiting long-standing illness: Great Britain, 2005

Source: General Household Survey, 2005, Table 7.5, reproduced at http://www.wmpho.org.uk/resources/MPHMM09.pdf

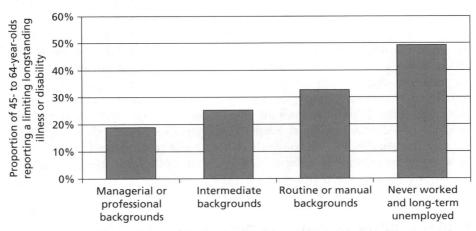

Figure 4.5 Adults aged 45–64 in routine and manual occupational groups are much more likely to have a limiting long-standing illness or disability than those from non-manual groups

Source: http://www.poverty.org.uk (accessed 7 July 2008)

different measures of health were used and Blaxter states that, 'at all ages, and for each dimension of health, there was a tendency for experience to be poorer as social class declined' (Blaxter, 1990, p. 63).

The evidence for social class gradients in self-reported morbidity is fairly substantial. However, as Asthana *et al.* (2004) point out the relationship between social class and health varies according age and gender. Research shows that social inequalities are particularly marked among infant populations but not among young people (West *et al.*, 1990; West, 1997) and that class-based inequality generally increases with age from the mid-thirties onwards (Rahkonen *et al.*, 1995). Accordingly, Asthana *et al.* warn against taking a simplistic view that class by itself is a valid and robust indicator of poor morbidity. By constructing a measure of 'relative class effect' they demonstrate that a demographic gradient can be identified for many health conditions. Consequently, they assert that relying on socio-economic position as a surrogate for poor health can lead to over-estimating the prevalence of poor mortality in the lower socio-economic classes while underestimating the levels of morbidity in elderly age groups.

People's sense of well-being and subjective assessments of their own health and fitness are undoubtedly influenced by cultural norms, values and expectations. However, the class differences noted in self-report studies are repeated when the distributions of objective health-related indicators, such as low birth-weight, height and tooth decay, are considered. Low birth-weight is one of the single most important determinants of perinatal mortality and can have implications for the future health and well-being of the young child. Poor maternal nutrition is believed to be responsible not only for higher infant mortality but also for increased vulnerability to chronic sickness and disease in later life. Birth statistics show that two-thirds of low-birth-weight babies are born to working-class mothers (Smith and Jacobson, 1988). In the first half of the last decade the percentage of low-birth-weight babies in social class V, in England and Wales, was 8.2 per cent; the comparable figure for social class I was 5.4 per cent (Macfarlane *et al.*, 2000). Height is considered to be a good indicator of general health and nutritional status. Social class differences in adult height are attributed to factors in early life such as inadequate interuterine growth or nutritional deficiency. Knight (1984) found that in most age groups men and women from the non-manual classes were taller on average than those from the manual classes. However, there is evidence to suggest a recent narrowing of inequalities in childhood height (Li *et al.*, 2004). As regards dental health, although there is evidence of an overall improvement in all age groups, surveys indicate that levels of tooth decay are unacceptably high and are class related (Jones *et al.*, 1997).

Regional differences in mortality rates

> The analysis of male deaths in 2001–03 shows that substantial socio-economic gradients in mortality existed within Wales and all regions of England. The size of these gradients varied significantly between regions. They were greatest in the North East, North West and Wales and least in the South East, South West and the East of England. Differences between regions were small for the most advantaged classes and greatest for the least advantaged.
>
> (Siegler *et al.*, 2008, p. 16)

Regional variations in mortality and life expectancy in the UK, which reflect the existence of a 'North–South divide', are well documented (Griffiths and

Table 4.5 Regional standardised mortality ratios for all causes of death, males and females, England and Wales, 1999–2003

Region	SMR	
	Males	Females
North East	115	115
North West	113	113
Yorkshire and the Humber	106	104
East Midlands	100	101
West Midlands	105	103
East of England	90	93
London	102	99
South East	89	91
South West	107	107

Source: National Statistics Online, 2008

Fitzpatrick, 2001). Table 4.5 shows the regional SMRs for all causes of death for both men and women in England and Wales. The mortality ratios for both men and women are lower in the South and East than in the North and West.

Studies of health inequalities in smaller areas, such as electoral districts, illustrate that variations in mortality rates can be found *within* the broad geographical regions. For example, Fox *et al.* (1984) discovered that areas with significantly high SMRs for adult males were characterised by an abundance of poor quality older houses, a large proportion of inner city, multi-occupancy dwellings and urban council estates. Areas with relatively low SMRs tended to be suburban residential districts. Thus low status areas were characterised by high mortality rates, while high status areas experienced low mortality rates. Similarly, the Health and Lifestyle Survey (Blaxter, 1990) identified regional differences in health. On the whole, those respondents living in the South and East experienced better health than those living in the Midlands and the North. Moving from regional to small-area analysis revealed that the health of people living in high status areas was better than average, irrespective of the geographical location of the area. People living in industrial districts or inner city areas reported the worst health. Women living in cities reported particularly high levels of illness. Thus, to talk in terms of a simple national North–South divide is to ignore the differences within the regions. Small-area analysis helps to pinpoint these differences and explore the implications local environmental characteristics have for health and well-being.

One characteristic which clearly has an impact on health inequalities is the level of deprivation. The link between poverty and poor health is well established and the fact that materially and socially deprived areas have higher mortality rates than less deprived areas is well known (Drever and Whitehead, 1995; Woods *et al.*, 2005). The Carstairs Morris deprivation index is widely used in health research to measure relative material deprivation across small areas such as electoral wards (Morgan and Baker, 2006). The index is a composite measure based on the following four census variables:

Unemployment: unemployed males aged 16 years and over as a proportion of all economically active males aged 16 years and over.

Overcrowding: persons in households with one or more persons per room as a proportion of all residents in households.

Car Ownership: residents in households with no car as a proportion of all residents in households.

Low Social Class: residents in households with an economically active head of household in social class IV or V as a proportion of all residents in households.

The deprivation score is calculated by standardising the four variables and then incorporating them in a common scale. Wards (neighbourhoods) are ranked from the 'least deprived' to the 'most deprived' and divided into quintiles (fifths), deciles (tenths) or twentieths according to ward population size, so as to ensure that each deprivation category contains approximately the same number of people. This method makes it possible to compare regions with regards to the proportion of the population estimated to be living in relatively deprived circumstances. For example, using deprivation quintiles and 2001 ward population estimates, Romeri *et al.* (2006, p. 21) show that at the beginning of this century 42 per cent of the population of London lived in the most deprived fifth of wards, whereas in the South West the corresponding figure was only 4 per cent.

Studies investigating the link between health inequalities (as measured by mortality, the expectation of life without disability and expectation of life in good health) and deprivation in England and Wales have reported the following key findings:

- The gap in disability-free life expectancy at birth between the least and the most deprived twentieths of wards was 14.1 years for males and 12.8 years for females. The corresponding gap in life expectancy was 7.6 years and 4.8 years respectively (Rasulo *et al.*, 2007).
- Males in Blackpool have a life expectancy eight years less than males in Kensington and Chelsea (Department of Health, 2006a).
- Male healthy life expectancy at birth ranged from 49.4 years in the most deprived wards to 66.2 years in the least deprived wards, a difference of 16.9 years. For females the comparable figures were 51.7 and 68.5 years, respectively, a difference of 16.8 years (Bajekal, 2005).
- Death rates were higher for people living in deprived areas than for those living in less deprived areas. The all-age mortality rate for males in the most deprived wards was 1.7 times higher than that in the least deprived wards. The death rate for females was 1.5 times higher (Romeri *et al.*, 2006).
- The relationship between deprivation and mortality was stronger at younger ages than for all ages. In the 15- to 64-year age group, the death rate for men

in the most deprived wards was 2.8 times greater than in the least deprived wards. The comparable figure for females was 2.1 times higher (*ibid.*).

- The fifth of the population living in the least deprived wards tended to display similar mortality rates irrespective of their geographical location (*ibid.*).

- Inequalities in health at birth were the widest in the North West, North East and Wales, and narrowest in the East of England and the South West (Rasulo *et al.*, 2007).

While individual characteristics clearly play a very important part in explaining the health inequalities observed between people, geographical setting is also of some importance (Curtis and Jones, 1998). As described above, it can be concluded from longitudinal studies and the examination of area-level data that the socio-economic composition of a neighbourhood is one of the primary factors influencing health outcomes.

Explaining health inequalities

> Inequalities in health exist, whether measured in terms of mortality, life expectancy or health status; whether categorised by socioeconomic measures or by ethnic group or gender.
>
> (*Independent Inquiry into Inequalities in Health*, Acheson Report, 1998)

Data from both epidemiological studies and health-related social research clearly demonstrate the existence of associations between social position and health and illness. While the existence of inequalities in health are well documented, readily acknowledged and relatively undisputed, the same cannot be said of the causes of these inequalities. When it comes to explaining the differential distribution of mortality and morbidity rates a number of causal explanations have been advanced. This section will focus on those explanations that deal with social and economic factors.

There is such an extensive body of literature dealing with class differences in health that it would be unrealistic to attempt a detailed and critical review here. Instead a general overview of the main types of explanations will be provided. Following the Black Report (Townsend *et al.*, 1992), explanations of health inequalities can be divided into four broad categories: artefactual explanations; theories of natural and social selection; structural/material explanations; cultural/behavioural explanations.

Artefact

One form artefactual explanations take is to deny the very existence of class-based inequalities by claiming that the health inequalities observed are not real but artificial; they are a construct of the measurement process (Jones and Cameron, 1984). In other words, the inequalities do not require an explanation because they are, in fact, an effect produced by trying to measure something which is more complicated than the tools of measurement can handle. According to this view social class is not easy to define or determine, and consequently there are inaccuracies in the way in which it is recorded. This creates problems when trying to draw inferences from mortality tables about the link between class position and mortality risk.

Some proponents of artefactual explanations claim that the apparent association between social class and health is not indicative of a link between material resources and physical well-being, but is a reflection of the changes which have taken place in the occupational structure in contemporary Britain. It is argued that in recent years there has been a decline in the number of people employed in manual occupations and an increase in the numbers engaged in non-manual work. This is seen to cause two problems. Firstly, changes in the size and composition of the Registrar General's occupational class categories makes comparisons between mortality rates for the different groups over time meaningless. Secondly, social class V is contracting and contains a disproportionate number of older workers. Given that both mortality risk and the incidence of chronic sickness increases with age, social class V can be expected to produce relatively high death rates and sickness rates.

In considering this explanation the Black Report draws attention to the fact that standardised mortality ratios are age-specific, thus allowing for the differences in age distributions in the different social class categories. Furthermore, it is among the younger age groups that inequality is most pronounced and there is evidence that inequality reduces with age. The Report concludes that the observed differences in mortality and morbidity rates between the classes are real and cannot be discounted as a measurement artefact. However, it has been suggested that the authors of the Black Report gave insufficient consideration to artefactual explanations and underestimated the relative importance of such explanations in accounting for the persistence of class-related inequalities in health (Bloor et al., 1987).

Social selection

Unlike most artefactual explanations, social selection explanations accept the existence of inequalities in health. It is argued that the concentration of poor health in the lower classes is a reflection of the effects of health on social mobility. Observed social class differences in health are interpreted as a result of the healthy becoming upwardly mobile and the unhealthy becoming downwardly mobile (Stern, 1983). In this type of account class position is a consequence of health status rather than vice versa. Poor health is viewed not only as a predictor of what is sometimes termed downward occupational drift, but is also seen as preventing or restricting upward social mobility. The overall result is that the high social class groups shed their unhealthy members and gain healthy individuals who have risen from the lower social classes. As a result of this process of social mobility, groups at the top end of the social scale can be expected to have more favourable mortality and morbidity rates.

A few research studies have identified health as a determinant of mobility chances. Quoting data from the National Survey of Health and Development, Wadsworth (1986) shows how unhealthy people are more likely to experience downward social mobility. He describes how those men who had been seriously ill during childhood appeared to be more likely than others to have experienced downward mobility by the time they reached their mid-twenties. However, extensive research on the causal relationship between health and mobility indicates that selection processes have a very small effect on mortality differentials (Fox *et al.*, 1986; Wilkinson, 1986).

Materialist and structuralist explanations

Although there are problems in defining and determining social class, research has shown time and again how class position relates to many other aspects of life such as level of income, type and quality of accommodation and degree of exposure to physical and environmental hazards. Materialist and structuralist explanations of health inequalities focus on how working-class people, because of their position in the social structure, tend to have limited opportunities and poorer access to financial and material resources than their middle-class counterparts. By examining material deprivation and social disadvantage these explanations explore the part played by structural factors in determining life circumstances and influencing the life chances of individuals. In exploring aspects of deprivation and disadvantage emphasis will be placed on income, housing and unemployment.

Income

> At the low end of the scale, individual incomes matter for health because of their link with both material deprivation and restriction on social participation and opportunity to exercise control over one's life.
>
> (Marmot, 2002, p. 44)

Income is one of the main determinants of the general living standards enjoyed by individuals and families. While sufficient income is required in order to secure the physical and material conditions essential for biological survival, income is still important once a basic subsistence level has been reached. There is evidence that income inequality within a society is associated with differences in health (Lynch *et al.*, 2000). In a study of the relationship between income and mortality, Wilkinson (1986) has shown that those occupational categories which experienced the fastest rise in income also recorded the fastest fall in death rates; whereas those occupational groups displaying the slowest rise in income also experienced the slowest fall in mortality rates. However, care needs to be taken when investigating the relationship between income, class and health.

Firstly, data on income distribution by social class reveal that average income differences between classes do not follow a simple downward gradient from class I to class V. Classes I and II have the highest average income of all the groups and class V has the lowest, but the comparable figure for class III (manual) is higher than that for class III (non-manual). There are a number of reasons for the income differences between manual and non-manual workers in class III. The non-manual category includes many low-grade salaried clerical and administrative staff who are relatively low paid and the manual group includes more highly paid skilled workers who can increase their basic pay by working overtime. The difference in average income between classes IV and V is negligible.

Secondly, income differentials can be found within occupational class categories. As Coleman and Salt have observed from the statistical evidence available:

> Doctors in social class I whose incomes on average are about twice those of university lecturers (also I) and schoolteachers (II), and perhaps three times those of clergymen (I), none the less have substantially higher mortality.
>
> (Coleman and Salt, 1992, p. 340)

Inconsistencies such as these would suggest that successive rises in income do not automatically produce health gains and falling mortality rates.

Thirdly, as with class and health, attention needs to be drawn to the measurement problems encountered when dealing with income. To take earnings from employment as the sole measure of income is to ignore other important sources such as 'fringe benefits' and realisable capital gains. Consideration needs also to be given to the unit being considered. If the focus of study is the health, lifestyle and consumption patterns of family members then details of the total income for the family or household are more appropriate than simply knowledge of the income of the principal earner in the family group, be they men or women.

There are practical and technical difficulties encountered in attempting to obtain accurate information on the level of income and degree of access to material resources enjoyed by individuals and families. Bearing in mind these difficulties, and the overlap in the social class distribution of incomes, research has tended to concentrate on those at the bottom end of the income scale. Research clearly illustrates that low income is strongly associated with poor health, and there is evidence that the health gap between the rich and poor has widened during the second half of this century (Smith *et al.*, 1990; Townsend, 1990). Recent figures also reveal that income inequality generally increased over the period 2004/05 to 2006/07, with a particular increase in the gap between wages for skilled and unskilled workers (Office for National Statistics, 2008a).

Housing

> Recognition of the link between poor housing and ill health started in the 1800s, so it is appalling that in the 21st century we are still raising concerns about this issue. . . . Poor housing can cause psychological and physical health problems, and the best way to reduce health inequalities in this country is to improve living standards. We are worried about children growing up in overcrowded, substandard bed and breakfast accommodation and about the elderly living alone in poor housing conditions.
>
> (Dr Vivienne Nathanson, head of science and ethics, BMA, quoted in the *British Medical Journal*, 10 May 2003)

The existence of a relationship between housing and health has been recognised for many years. Since the publication in 1842 of Chadwick's report on the insanitary conditions found in urban working-class areas research studies have established that overcrowding, poor ventilation and damp houses help to spread infectious diseases and thereby increase mortality rates (Preston, 1978). While improvements in general living conditions, along with the rise in the quality and standard of houses, have helped to reduce the incidence of infectious diseases there is still evidence of a link between housing and health.

Infections, cot deaths and accidents are the main causes of post-neonatal mortality. A disproportionate number of these infant deaths occur in households in which basic amenities are lacking, people are living in overcrowded conditions or facilities are shared with other families (Fox and Goldblatt, 1982). In a study of the quality of accommodation and health, Platt *et al.* (1989) describe how both physical health can be impaired by damp living conditions. They discovered that adults and children living in damp housing reported more respiratory symptoms than those living in dry surroundings. Furthermore, they found these differences persisted even when factors such as income, overcrowding and the incidence of smoking were taken into account. Poor living conditions are not only associated with increased ill health and mortality; research has discovered links between housing and general social and psychological well-being. Brown and Harris (1978) and Gabe and Williams (1986) describe how cramped living accommodation, lack of privacy, inadequate facilities and other housing problems can produce stress and in some cases can be contributory factors in the onset of clinical depression.

The location of housing is also important. Where a person lives determines access to a range of amenities and resources. In some inner city areas there is a lack of recreational facilities and safe play areas for children. Council housing estates on the outskirts of towns and cities may not allow for easy access to shops or healthcare services. The physical and social isolation produced by large housing estates should not be overlooked (Freeman, 1984). In a study of the health of council tenants Byrne *et al.* (1986) concentrated on housing estates with 'difficult to let' houses. These estates where in unattractive settings, had a high proportion of poorly maintained dwellings and lacked recreational facilities. When compared with residents on other council estates those living in 'difficult to let' accommodation reported more ill health.

A broad range of housing issues have an effect on health outcomes but it is difficult, for a number of reasons, to establish clear causal links between poor quality accommodation and ill health. For example, it is not possible to isolate the impact of poor housing conditions as these often exist alongside other forms of deprivation (such as inadequate income, unemployment or social isolation), which also have adverse consequences for the physical and mental well-being of individuals (Taske *et al.*, 2005). Where research has reported that housing tenure and dwelling type have some association with specific aspects of health, the association has been found to be fairly modest (Grainger and Robinson, 2004).

For some people access to suitable accommodation is the problem. Statutory homelessness statistics show that in 2007 there were nearly 100,000 households accepted as homeless in England. However, pressure groups like Shelter claim that official figures seriously underestimate the true nature and extent of the homeless problem as they do not include the 'hidden or concealed homeless', that is those people who live in substandard, overcrowded housing. It is estimated that in England there are approximately 554,000 overcrowded households (Department for Communities and Local Government, 2007, p. 2) and more than one million children living in bad housing (Shelter, 2006). The living conditions and health problems experienced by individuals and families living in temporary accommodation have been well documented in surveys conducted and commissioned by professional bodies and pressure groups. Particular emphasis has been placed on the physical and mental impact on children. There are reports of high accident rates among children living in temporary accommodation and an increased incidence of emotional, behavioural and developmental problems (Connelly and Crown, 1994; Vostanis, 2002).

Unemployment

> Employment plays a fundamental role in our society. People are often defined, and define themselves, through what they do for a living. Sociological studies emphasise that not only is employment a primary source of status in industrialised countries like Britain, but it is also significant in providing purpose, income, social support, structure to life and a means of participating in society.
>
> (*Independent Inquiry into Inequalities in Health*, Acheson Report, 1998)

When discussing the impact of unemployment it is possible to distinguish between the material, physical and psychological aspects of job loss. The first and most obvious effect of unemployment is the marked drop in income as earnings are replaced by unemployment benefit. Poverty is a common feature in the lives of the unemployed and their families. As Berthoud (1986, p. 2) has observed: 'With the possible exception of the down-and-out homeless, direct measures of hardship show there is no poorer group of people than unemployed couples with children'. From the evidence available there is no disputing the fact that the unemployed and their dependants suffer considerable financial hardship and material deprivation. For some, unemployment is a temporary and short-term phase; for the less fortunate it can last for years.

The physical effects of unemployment cannot be as easily determined. The problem is one of distinguishing between cause and effect: does poor health lead to job loss or does the experience of unemployment cause deterioration in physical health? (Bartley, 1987, 1994). Data from studies of death rates indicate that unemployment might play a significant causal role. A longitudinal study of the mortality records and employment histories of men over a ten-year period from 1971 to 1981 found that those men who were unemployed and actively seeking work in 1971 had higher mortality rates than those men who were in continuous employment throughout the period. As the study excluded men who were unemployed as a result of chronic sickness the findings can be seen to support the view that raised mortality was a consequence of unemployment rather than the result of pre-existing poor health. The wives of unemployed men were also found to have relatively high mortality rates, a possible indication that unemployment has an impact not only on the unemployed themselves but also on other family members (Moser *et al.*, 1984). A three-year follow-up study based on men out of work in 1981 identified a similar mortality pattern for men but no significant excess mortality was observed in the sample of wives (Moser *et al.*, 1987).

A strong association between male unemployment and mortality has also been found by Carstairs and Morris (1991) in an analysis of data on health and deprivation in Scotland. They dismiss the explanation that higher death rates are a direct consequence of unemployment: unemployment 'appears to form part of a complex of adverse social conditions and poor life chances' and as such 'rather than having an independent influence probably acts to exacerbate other stresses already present' (Carstairs and Morris, 1991, p. 222).

Morbidity rates also appear to be higher among the unemployed. Using data on self-reported limiting long-standing illness from the General Household Survey, Arber (1987) has calculated age-standardised illness ratios. These show that compared to all men, employed men were 20 per cent less likely to report limiting chronic illness whereas unemployed men were over 40 per cent more likely to report such illness. Chronic illness ratios for unemployed women were 16 per cent above the average for all women. There is also evidence that children in families hit by unemployment have poorer health and development (MacFarlane and Cole, 1985).

Both the physical and psychological effects of unemployment on the unemployed and their families have been addressed in an in-depth case study of 22 families (Fagin, 1981; Fagin and Little, 1984). At the outset of the study a distinction was made between those families in which health problems were present prior to unemployment and those in which health problems occurred following unemployment. Unemployment was identified as a cause of stress in all the families and it was this stress which was seen as a possible mechanism by which job loss leads to illness. The authors point out the difficulties of disentangling the effect of unemployment from other stress-producing life events which may be experienced at the same time, such as the death of a member of the family or marital separation.

The study found that following unemployment spouses with a record of poor health had a tendency to suffer a reoccurrence of their previous illnesses. In a number of cases the unemployed reported an increase in some physical symptoms, such as headaches and backache, which may be triggered by psychological mechanisms. Job loss is viewed as setting in motion certain psychological changes, which for some produce feelings of hopelessness, loss of self-esteem and violent outbursts of temper. The effects of unemployment can be felt by all members of the family. Children in families where the father had been out of work for a long time experienced more health and behavioural problems.

Not all the unemployed in Fagin and Little's study showed signs of poorer physical and mental health following unemployment. Indeed in one or two cases there were noticeable improvements in health during unemployment. This was particularly true when the job had been the cause of stress in the first place. An investigation by Ramsden and Smee (1981) into the health status of workers made redundant did not show any net deterioration in health over a two-year period following redundancy.

Adopting a social psychological perspective, Hayes and Nutman (1981) describe how individuals respond to unemployment. They refer to stages in the transitional cycle of unemployment. The initial response is one of shock coupled with a tendency to treat the forced inactivity as a welcome break. The situation is seen as a temporary one; an unexpected opportunity to take a holiday. However, once this holiday phase is over individuals are faced with organising their daily routine. The prospects of obtaining employment are considered to be good, the individual is optimistic about the future and much time is spent searching for work. Eventually the failure to secure employment gives rise to pessimism; nevertheless the individual goes through the motions of applying for jobs but with reduced hope and little enthusiasm. It is at this stage in the cycle that individuals begin to encounter difficulties in their relationships with family and friends. For the long-term unemployed the final stage in the transitional cycle is characterised by a fatalistic attitude towards the future. The individual feels helpless and powerless and becomes resigned to accepting a life without work. The various ways in which unemployment can damage mental health have been well documented and are outlined in Box 4.4.

A number of studies have confirmed a relationship between suicide or para-suicide (non-fatal deliberate self-harm, i.e. attempted suicide) and unemployment. Data from the OPCS Longitudinal Study indicate a two- to threefold increase

---

Box 4.4   Research findings

Nine characteristic features of the unemployed person's role which are thought to contribute to a reduction in psychological well-being

1 Reduced income produces worries about money and causes stress;

2 Separation from the workplace and inability to afford leisure activities results in a marked reduction in social contacts;

3 Fewer goals to achieve;

4 Lack of scope for decision-making. Although in one sense there is more freedom of choice this is in the main limited to a number of small repetitive decisions about routine, mundane daily activities; there is little scope for long-term decision-making and planning;

5 Loss of opportunities for exercising existing skills and acquiring new ones;

6 Increase in psychologically threatening activities such as facing continued rejection in the search for work or being treated as a second-class citizen or welfare scrounger;

7 Increased uncertainty and anxiety about the future;

8 A decline in the quality of interpersonal contacts and relationships;

9 Loss of social position to the extent that on becoming unemployed an individual comes to occupy a less valued social position in a society which judges people by their occupation.

Source: Warr, 1983; Smith, 1985

in suicide among the unemployed in England and Wales (Moser *et al.*, 1987). Research from other countries also supports a link between unemployment and suicide (Chan *et al.*, 2007). Blakely *et al.* (2003) found that being unemployed was associated with almost a threefold increase in the relative risk of death by suicide. However, it is difficult to establish the influence unemployment itself has on the suicide rate. The causes of suicide are complex and multi-factorial and no single factor can fully explain any observed trends in suicide mortality. At the individual level, the presence of mental illness is an obvious risk factor. Nevertheless, analysis of aggregate data can be used to identify how societal changes are associated with changes in the incidence and prevalence of suicide. The impact of particular social changes on suicide risk may vary for different stages of the life course. In an analysis of suicide in England and Wales during the second half of the last century, Gunnell *et al.* (2003) found that trends and patterns varied according to age. For example, the suicide rate rose for young men between the ages of 25 and 34 years but fell for those aged 60 years and over.

Research into the effects of unemployment on health has consistently shown that the material well-being and psychological health of unemployed people tends to be significantly below that of people in full-time employment. However, while the fact that unemployment can lead to deterioration in mental health has been well documented, the role of unemployment as a causal factor in the onset of physical ill health is less well established.

Cultural and behavioural explanations

Increasingly health policy initiatives have come to focus attention on the need to address individual behaviour and lifestyle factors as a way of improving the health of the nation. The Government sees its role as one of providing people with opportunities for making informed, healthy lifestyle choices. This is encapsulated in the following:

> We are clear that Government cannot – and should not – pretend it can 'make' the population healthy. But it can – and should – support people in making better choices for their health and the health of their families. It is for people to make the healthy choice if they wish to.
>
> (Prime Minister, Tony Blair in Department of Health, 2004a, p. 3)

Behavioural explanations of the observed inequalities in health focus on the way in which individuals from different social groups lead their lives. Attitudes, values, beliefs, knowledge and behaviour are the focus of attention. Smoking, alcohol consumption, diet, exercise and the utilisation of healthcare services are usually highlighted in this perspective for these are considered to be areas of activity and decision-making in which individuals make free choices.

The contribution of behaviour to health is clearly evident in the case of cigarette smoking. Nearly 80 per cent of lung cancer mortality is directly related to tobacco smoke and it is estimated that one in six of all deaths may be attributed to smoking. There is also growing evidence that breathing other people's tobacco smoke can be a health hazard. For example, a study of respiratory health among primary-school children found that those children whose parents were moderate smokers were more likely to develop bronchitis than the children of non-smokers (Somerville *et al.*, 1988). Other research has shown deaths from lung cancer to be higher among non-smoking spouses of smokers than non-smoking spouses of non-smokers (Wald *et al.*, 1986). In the medical literature there is extensive documentation of the health risks encountered by smokers.

There has been a marked decline in cigarette smoking in Britain since the early 1970s. In 1974 51 per cent of men and 41 per cent of women smoked, by 2005 these figures had reduced to 25 per cent and 23 per cent respectively (Office for National Statistics, 2007b, p. 94). This reduction can be largely accounted for by an increase in the number of people giving up smoking rather than to young people avoiding taking up the habit in the first place. Much of the decline occurred during the 1970s and early 1980s. Despite the general downward trend there are still differences in smoking prevalence rates between socio-economic groups. Data for England show that in 2005 29 per cent of those people in manual occupational groups were cigarette smokers, compared to 19 per cent of managerial and professional workers (Goddard, 2006). A social gradient is also visible when considering smoking by women during pregnancy (see Table 4.6).

Department of Health guidance on alcohol consumption recommends daily benchmarks of 3 to 4 units for men and 2 to 3 units for women. Findings from the 2005 General Household Survey reveal that just over one-third of men and one-fifth of women reported exceeding the recommended limit on at least one day during the week prior to interview. When taking socio-economic group into account, the survey data show that '. . . over many years . . . there is little difference in usual weekly alcohol consumption between those in non-manual and manual households. Where differences do exist, it has been those in the non-manual categories who tend to have the higher weekly consumption' (Goddard, 2006, p. 50).

Table 4.6 Cigarette smoking by women during pregnancy by social class

United Kingdom				Percentages
			Year	
	1985	1990	1995	2000
Professional	8	8	7	4
Managerial	18	13	12	8
Intermediate	19	16	14	11
Skilled Manual	31	29	23	20
Semi-skilled Manual	32	34	28	21
Unskilled	46	39	37	26
All women	30	28	24	20

Source: Infant Feeding Survey data found at http://www.statistics.gov.uk/STATBASE/ssdataset.asp?vlnk=5231 (accessed 10 March 2009)

The National Food Survey provides a wealth of information on patterns of domestic food consumption in the British Isles (MAFF, 1985). Class and regional differences in diet are clearly evident. For example, households in the lowest-income groups purchase less fresh green vegetables, fresh fruit and wholemeal bread than higher-income households. Generally the diets of social classes IV and V have a higher sugar content and a lower fibre content than diets typically found in social classes I and II. Diet has been identified as a contributory factor in accounting for the higher rates of coronary heart disease among the manual working classes (Marmot *et al.*, 1981).

There are regional differences in food preparation and consumption. Regional contrasts can be marked: 'Generous Northern breakfasts are a revelation to Southerners increasingly used to insipid muesli, and the traditional "Ulster Fry" looks like a particularly defiant rejection of nutritional rationality' (Coleman and Salt, 1992, p. 364). The existence of regional variations in diet has led some observers to argue that eating habits are determined more by attitudes and taste than by income. When she was a Junior Minister for Health in the mid-1980s Edwina Currie claimed that Northerners were 'dying of ignorance and chips', while '*Independent* and *Guardian* readers have bean sprouts coming out of their ears' (quoted in Graham, 1990, p. 204).

Cultural or behavioural explanations view consumption patterns as a reflection of cultural differences in the way individuals live their lives. Lifestyles are thought to be shaped by the traditional values and socially accepted patterns of behaviour found within the wider communities in which individuals and families live. Subcultures may be deemed to be reluctant to embrace health-enhancing attitudes and individuals may be perceived as either unwilling or unable to change their behaviour. The fact that low income might constrain food choices is either ignored or rejected. It is assumed that the observed health choices are a product of individual irresponsibility, ignorance or irrationality. This is contrary to research findings on poverty and diet, which maintain that behaviour is shaped more by income than by attitudes and taste. Studies of food choices show that families in receipt of low incomes are aware of what constitutes a healthy diet but they are unable to afford such a diet (Lang *et al.*, 1984; Cole-Hamilton and Lang, 1986).

Those who support cultural or behavioural explanations clearly see individual actions and choices as causal factors in the production of health inequalities. Certain behaviours are known to increase the risk of poor health, therefore individuals who pursue an unhealthy lifestyle and fail to take heed of the advice contained in health education programmes are seen as having only themselves to blame. What this line of reasoning fails to appreciate is that the behaviour may be a response or reaction to the cumulative material deprivation faced by an individual or family over many years. By emphasising voluntary behaviours cultural explanations draw attention away from the external constraints which may have a negative influence on people's daily lives. As Marmot (2004) describes, the socio-economic circumstances in which people find themselves conditions the very way in which they live and work. Individuals may not always be in a position to exercise a free choice, but may find that the behavioural options available are limited due to lack of resources or the existence of constraints imposed by wider social, economic and political circumstances. Thus it can be argued that:

> . . . social class, throughout the life course, has a powerful influence on behavioural, social and psychological variables. Health-related and psycho-social behaviours are never truly 'voluntary'; they are a product of, and embedded in structures of society. Therefore, the unit of analysis is not the individual but the socio-cultural context that shapes the individual.
>
> (Singh-Manoux and Marmot, 2005, p. 2130)

From a structural or material perspective individuals make behavioural choices but these are, in large part, conditioned by wider social experiences and economic circumstances. In a sense the cultural or behavioural perspective only provides a partial explanation of inequalities in health. As Blane asserts, 'The behaviour/ culture type of explanation . . . can go some way towards accounting for social-class differences in health, although such behaviours need to be seen in their material context and uncertainty remains about their importance relative to materialist explanations' (1991, p. 125). Thus, structural/materialist and cultural explanations are not mutually exclusive and the way forward may be to find the right balance between these two types of explanation (Macintyre, 1986).

The link between material living conditions and lifestyle has been explored by Graham (1987, 1990) in her study of women's experiences of health behaviour in poverty. In order to understand the problems women face in trying to pursue a healthy lifestyle she claims that it is necessary to appreciate how poverty within families structures health behaviour. She points out that women are not only expected to perform the role of 'housekeeper', but are also assigned the role of 'health-keeper'. The former role carries responsibility for the domestic budget, particularly in respect of the purchase and preparation of food. The latter role is concentrated on the day-to-day provision of childcare. Graham describes how in families in poverty mothers and children can spend a considerable amount of time alone at home. The immediate physical and social environment can be a cause of stress and it is necessary to develop strategies to cope with the material and psychological deprivation. Some of the coping strategies adopted can in fact be a threat to good health; cigarette smoking is a typical example. From interviews with mothers living in poverty Graham describes how smoking is both a luxury and necessity. Expenditure on tobacco occupied a significant place in the family budget and women would cut down on food for themselves rather than go without cigarettes. For these mothers, smoking provided a way of reducing stress. It gave them a little time to themselves when they could have a break from the daily struggle of living in poverty. Under conditions such as these Graham observes that:

> . . . smoking can be both necessity and luxury: a necessity that enables a woman to maintain her role as family health-keeper and a luxury that symbolizes her participation in the lifestyle of the wider society. Cigarettes offer moments when, however temporarily, the experience of relative poverty is suspended.
>
> (Graham, 1990, pp. 216–7)

The women also described how smoking was a reward for sacrificing their own wants and needs in order to ensure they had sufficient money to provide the best they could for their families. In fulfilling their domestic and health-keeping roles the women were jeopardising their own health.

Another aspect of behaviour is the use made of health services. There is ample evidence that the working classes make less use of a wide range of services; this is particularly noticeable in preventive medicine. For example, middle-class women are more likely to attend antenatal classes and well-woman clinics. Those who favour cultural or behavioural explanations see this pattern of unequal use in terms of differences in sub-cultural lifestyles and attitudes to health. It is assumed that the low take-up rates among the lower classes are a result of ignorance or the inability or unwillingness to adopt a long-term perspective. However, in a review of the literature on the utilisation of health services, the Black Report concludes that: 'Severe under-utilisation by the working-classes is a complex result of under-provision, of costs (financial, psychological) of attendance, and perhaps of a lifestyle which profoundly inhibits any attempt at rational action in the interests of future well-being' (Townsend and Davidson, 1992, p. 80).

With reference to the provision of healthcare, Tudor Hart has postulated the 'inverse care law' which states that 'the availability of good medical care tends to vary inversely with the need of the population served' (Hart, 1971, p. 412). Areas with high mortality and morbidity are less well served by hospitals and have more overworked general practitioners than healthier areas. A consequence of the uneven distribution of some healthcare resources is that some groups receive fewer resources than their needs would appear to merit. Research shows that the middle classes tend to be the main beneficiaries of the National Health Service (Cartwright and O'Brien, 1976).

Whereas behavioural explanations tend to blame the individual for failing to recognise the benefits to be gained from the services offered, structuralist or materialist explanations place emphasis upon the conditions under which people live and work, and the nature and organisation of healthcare provision. According to the structuralist perspective the low take-up rates among working-class groups is not a reflection of a lack of interest in protecting health. The health behaviour observed is not an expression of values and norms peculiar to the working class, but can be considered a realistic response to the lack of resources and external constraints characteristic of working-class life. It has also been suggested that healthcare institutions and professionals need to recognise the importance of cultural and lifestyle differences when organising or delivering healthcare. There is evidence that some women fail to use the services because of the attitudes of professionals or because of practical problems such as the lack of suitable facilities for young children (Graham, 1984).

Within the inequalities in health literature it is difficult to clearly identify within the materialist argument the mechanism(s) by which material conditions (as determined by social class location) produce health outcomes. Macintyre (1997) suggests that it is helpful to distinguish in this context between a 'hard' and 'soft' version of the materialist argument. The former holds that differences in material circumstances (mainly the level of income and amount of accumulated wealth) are sufficient to explain observed social class gradients in mortality and morbidity rates. In contrast, the 'soft' version of the argument contends that the conditions of life which are determined by structural forces include psycho-social factors and social as well as economic capital. 'Social capital' is a very broad social concept with a wide range of meanings, which has increasingly been used in health research as a way of linking inequality and health (Hawe and Shiell, 2000). In a generalised sense, it refers to a feature of social structure and is considered to be a property or characteristic of a group or social network. Social capital constitutes a social resource. From a social-support perspective, social networks are central to people's objective and subjective well-being. It is through personal involvement in a web of cooperative relationships that individuals develop a sense of interpersonal trust, acquire access to a broad range of resources and enjoy the individual and collective benefits stemming from social cohesion. Empirical research from more than one country shows a link between social capital and better health. A number of ecological studies have found social capital to be a good predictor of mortality and self-reported health status at neighbourhood, regional and national levels (Barefoot *et al.*, 1998; Kawachi *et al.*, 1997, 1999). In an analysis of data from the Health Survey for England, Poortinga (2006) found that personal levels of social support contributed to a better self-reported health status.

While cultural and behavioural approaches have succeeded in identifying real differences between the classes in health-related behaviours, these approaches can be criticised for failing to take account of the fact that some forms of behaviour cannot be fully understood without reference to the social and material circumstances in which people lead their lives. In order to understand the social determinants of health it is necessary to integrate the structural, material, cultural and behavioural explanations. There is a strong case to be made for not focusing exclusively on individual differences and seeing health behaviours as simply a consequence of individual choices. Consideration needs to be given to the interrelationship between social structural factors and behaviours that are either potentially health-promoting or health-impairing. As observed in the following:

> . . . social class, throughout the life course, has a powerful influence on behavioural, social and psychological variables. Health-related and psycho-social behaviours are never truly 'voluntary'; they are a product of, and embedded in structures of society. Therefore, the unit of analysis is not the individual but the socio-cultural context that shapes the individual.
>
> (Singh-Manoux and Marmot, 2005, p. 2130)

The socialisation process is presented as the mechanism by which individual behaviour is shaped and particular attitudes, beliefs and behaviours are acquired. During childhood the individual is influenced by key agents of socialisation such as parents, teachers and peers. However, Singh-Manoux and Marmot also draw attention to the fact that an individual's socio-economic environment conditions how they live and work and thus has a socialising influence throughout the life course. Introducing a socialisation perspective in this way illustrates the importance of explaining group behaviour as opposed to individual behaviour. Elaborating on the ideas of Bourdieu (1984) they hold that there is a link between social structures and ways of thinking and acting, which they refer to as the 'structure–disposition–practice' schema. In brief, within social structures characteristic dispositions are generated that facilitate the successful performance of social practices. These practices serve to reinforce and reproduce the structural principles that gave rise to them in the first place. Social perceptions and strategies for negotiating the life course are influenced by an individual's general social position and socio-economic circumstances. Thus, dispositions are socially generated through a process of socialisation and transmitted from one generation to the next. This explains the existence of a uniformity of lifestyle and behaviours within a particular structural context. Social norms in relation to healthy behaviour are determined and conditioned by socio-economic circumstances and thus variations are found between different social classes. By addressing macro-structural processes of socialisation this approach attempts to integrate social, psychological, behavioural and material factors in explaining the relationship between socio-economic position and health.

Gender inequalities in health

Over their lifetime, on average males in England spend 59.1 years in good health and 15.9 years in poor health and females 61.4 and 18.6 years. . . . Hence, although women live longer than men, they also spend more years in sub-optimal health.

(Bajekal, 2005, p. 21)

It is accepted as 'almost an article of faith among epidemiologists and health professionals that gender differences exist in patterns of health and illness' (Macintyre *et al.*, 2005, p. 461). There is indeed evidence of gender differences in both mortality and morbidity rates. When investigating gender specific patterns of health, illness and disease it must be remembered that gender differences reflect biological differences between the sexes as well as differences in social and economic circumstances. Official statistics show a continual improvement in life expectancy for both women and men. Although women have a significantly longer life expectancy than men, the gap between women's and men's average life expectancy has reduced in recent years from 6.4 years in 1974 to 4.4 years in 2004. While women live longer than men they spend more years in poor health or with a disability.

As regards mortality, the stillbirth rate is higher for male foetuses than female foetuses and, following birth, males have higher death rates than females in every age group. The difference in average life expectancy between men and women is largely accounted for by differences in mortality in the older age groups. Mortality rates for circulatory diseases, which constitute the most common cause of death in the UK, have declined in recent decades. In 1971 age-standardised death rates stood at 6,900 per million males and 4,300 per million females; by 2004 the

Rates per 100,000 population

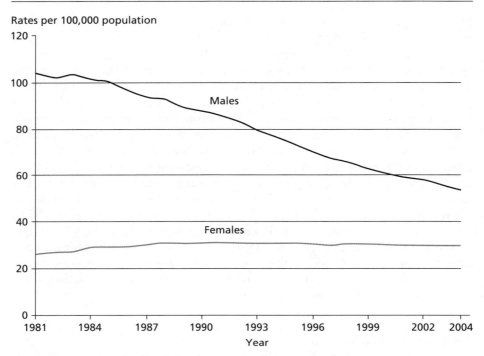

Figure 4.6 UK standardised death rates for lung cancer by sex
Source: Office for National Statistics, 2006

comparable rates had declined to 2,800 and 1,800 respectively. Cancers represent the second most common cause of death for both men and women. Death
rates in this category have declined for both sexes over the last twenty years and
in 2004 were 2,300 per million for men and 1,600 per million for women.
As illustrated in Figure 4.6 there has been a particularly marked decline in the
lung-cancer death rate for men, which is attributed to the decline in smoking
(Office for National Statistics, 2006).

Men have higher mortality rates than women, but some health surveys reveal
that women tend to report more illness than do men. The Health and Lifestyle
Survey used physiological measures and self-reports of psycho-social well-being,
in addition to self-reported physical illness, disease and disability, to construct
an overall measure of health. The survey found that in all age groups women
experienced more illness than men and had poorer psycho-social health (Blaxter,
1990). However, this gender difference is not significantly marked in all studies.
As shown in Table 4.7, the pattern of self-reported illness is similar for both males
and females across all age groups. As might be expected, the proportion of people
reporting a limiting long-standing illness increases with age. Gender differences
however do emerge when looking at particular health problems and diseases. While
prevalence rates for arthritis and rheumatism increase with age for both sexes,
in the 65- to 74-year-old age group women are nearly twice as likely as men to
suffer from these chronic conditions (Office for National Statistics, 2006). Arber

Table 4.7 Self-reported illness: by sex and age, 2005

	Long-standing illness	Limiting long-standing illness
Males		
0–4	140	46
5–14	181	72
15–44	175	90
45–64	401	233
65–74	554	342
75 and over	583	402
All ages	273	150
Females		
0–4	93	28
5–14	160	67
15–44	209	114
45–64	407	245
65–74	589	370
75 and over	545	401
All ages	282	163

Source: Office for National Statistics, 2007b, p. 89

and Ginn (1993) have noted that despite the fact that elderly people make greater use of health service facilities than any other age group little is known about the patterning of health inequalities in old age. Using data from the General Household Survey they report that, 'Women evaluated their own health only slightly less positively than men, but elderly women are seriously disadvantaged compared to men in terms of functional disability' (Arber and Ginn, 1993, p. 43).

One sociological explanation for the perceived gender differences in self-reported sickness and the utilisation of healthcare facilities focuses on the different social and economic conditions experienced by men and women. In particular, attention has centred on the characteristic features of the social roles assigned to women. Traditionally women's roles are largely structured around providing care for children and other family members. The housewife/mother role is presented as a natural full-time vocational activity, which women are supposed to find emotionally rewarding and psychologically satisfying. This is disputed by Gove and Tudor (1973) who describe some of the ways in which the nature of the social roles assigned to women increase the risks of mental illness. Similarly, feminists such as Oakley (1974) and Bernard (1976) maintain that the role of housewife has low status, involves monotonous work, serves to socially isolate women and can have adverse consequences for their physical health and mental well-being. There is evidence that women who are full-time housewives have higher levels of chronic sickness and poorer health in general than women who work in some capacity outside the home (Beral, 1987). In contrast, men's roles are not confined to the domestic sphere, they can be a major source of gratification and provide opportunities for exercising existing expertise and developing new skills. Paid work gives men financial independence and access to a wider social network of contacts. Brown and Harris (1978) in a study of clinical depression in women identified the lack of employment outside the home as one of four factors responsible for the greater susceptibility to depression of working-class women compared with middle-class women. This is supported by research which suggests that employment does have a positive effect on the health status of women (Nathanson, 1980).

Given the financial, social and psychological rewards accruing from work can it be assumed that paid employment will be beneficial for women's health? In other words, will the positive effects gained from working protect women from, or help them to overcome, the disadvantages associated with the role of house-wife? Arber *et al.* (1985) have studied the effects of employment on women's health and found that full-time employment had a detrimental effect on the health of women who were under 40 years of age, had children and were engaged in lower non-manual and manual occupations; little adverse effect was noted among women over 40 years of age, without children and in similar types of employment. Fulfilling the multiple roles of housewife, mother and employee can place a physical and mental strain on women and increase the risk of ill health. However, for some women role accumulation has its advantages. For example, women employed in professional and managerial occupations not only obtain the social and psychological rewards associated with these jobs, but they also have the financial resources which enable them to spread the burden of child-care and housework. The level of role strain created by occupying multiple roles will vary according to the woman's social position:

> . . . the adverse consequences of occupying the roles of mother, housewife, and full-time worker are less for women in more 'privileged' structural positions. Indeed there may be positive benefits of role accumulation for these women. For other women freedom to work may be a dubious freedom if it means that they have little time to do anything except paid work, unpaid domestic tasks, and routine childcare.
>
> (Arber, 1990b, p. 91)

Arber (1990a) argues that one of the problems with many of the studies dealing with the impact of role accumulation on women's health is that they have failed to give sufficient consideration to the material circumstances within which the roles are located. Not all work outside the home provides women with an escape route from the dull routine and monotony of housework. This is particularly the case for women who are already in a disadvantageous structural position. Economic necessity may force them into accepting work which is unskilled, tedious and offers no opportunity for personal development. The major difference between this kind of employment and housework is that it constitutes paid, as opposed to unpaid, labour. However, the level of pay is unlikely to be sufficient to enable them to buy the support services necessary to help them to fulfil their domestic roles. The same roles can have different consequences depending on the social and economic circumstances of women's lives. For example, fulfilling parental, marital and employment roles will not be the same experience for a mother working part-time, with an unemployed husband and living in shared accommodation, as it is for a part-time professional worker with children, married to a business executive and living in a large house in a residential suburban district.

In looking at the self-reported health status of women between 20 and 59 years of age, Arber (1990a) found that unemployed women and housewives in all age groups above 30 reported more illness than employed women, and in all but one age group unemployed women reported poorer health than housewives. Of those in full-time employment, manual workers reported poorer health than non-manual workers, with married women in non-manual occupations reporting the best health overall. Arber argues that as far as women's health inequalities are concerned occupational class alone is of limited explanatory value. In order to understand women's health status it is necessary to appreciate the combined influence of occupational class, parental roles, marital roles and employment status.

The view that women, on average, live longer than men but experience more acute and chronic sickness has come to be seen as something of an over-simplification. Patterns of gender differences in morbidity are complex and subtle and vary according to a number of factors including age, historical period, cultural setting and type of health assessment tool used (Macintyre et al., 1996; Hunt and Annandale, 1999). For example, research reveals an absence of, or reduction in, gender-based morbidity when comparing men and women with similar social, material and occupational backgrounds (Bartley, 2004). Also, care needs to be taken when examining the findings from patient surveys. Although women report more symptoms and make greater use of the health services, they may not actually suffer more ill health than men. Morbidity data, compiled from self-reported symptoms in health surveys and records of general practitioner consultations and hospital visits, requires careful interpretation. Firstly, it is possible that women are more willing to report symptoms to female interviewers conducting health surveys. As a result of gender role socialisation men are encouraged to take risks, display courage and be independent in both thought and action. In contrast women are socialised to be dependent on others and openly expressive about their feelings and emotions. Thus, men may not only be more reluctant to disclose details of any illnesses in a health-survey interview, but they may also be less likely to seek medical advice. Consequently there may be underreporting and underrecording of illness in the male population. Secondly, women consult their general practitioners more often than men do, but as Graham (1984) states this can be partly accounted for by the fact that it is usually mothers who take their sick children to the doctor. Finally, pregnancy and childbirth are natural events that are subject to increasing medical surveillance (Leesen and Gray, 1978). The fact that women come into frequent and regular contact with the health services during pregnancy can distort morbidity figures.

Ethnic inequalities in health

Ethnic health inequalities are demonstrable using virtually all classifications of race and ethnicity, and are usually sharpened by taking account of population heterogeneity and examining men and women separately. The differences between ethnic groups are often large, particularly for specific conditions e.g. prostate cancer, and less so for general measures of health e.g. life expectancy.

(Bhopal, 2007, p. 181)

Ethnicity is a complex, multi-dimensional concept, which differs from race and nationality. Individuals are usually considered to belong to a particular ethnic grouping on the basis of having one or more of the following characteristics in common:

- a shared ancestry or social background;

- a shared language or religious belief system;

- a distinctive set of social and cultural traditions that are passed down from one generation to the next and provide a sense of group identity.

On official documents and in health and social surveys individuals are usually asked to choose their ethnic identity from a list of standardised, predefined categories. Box 4.5 lists the ethnic categories used in the 2001 Census. There are, however, problems in using ethnicity as a variable in epidemiological research. For example, the populations identified are not homogenous and conceal large within-group differences (Senior and Bhopal, 1994). Also the size and proportion of the ethnic minority population varies greatly across the regions and where the numbers are small there is limited potential for analysing the data. Furthermore, there are also issues surrounding the quality of the data. Death certificates record country of birth and not ethnicity, which means that when attempting to assess the impact of ethnicity on premature death country of birth is used as a proxy measure of ethnicity.

Notwithstanding the lack of routinely collected, ethnically coded health statistics, the official data that are available on the health patterns of ethnic

---

Box 4.5   Definition

Ethnic categories used in 2001 Census

A **White:** includes British, Irish, 'Other' (e.g. Polish).

B **Mixed:** includes White and Black Caribbean, White and Asian, White and Black African.

C **Asian** or **Asian British:** Indian, Pakistani, Bangladeshi and other Asian backgrounds.

D **Black** or **Black British:** Caribbean, African, Indo-Caribbean.

E **Chinese** or **other ethnic group:** e.g. Kurdish, Iraqi.

Table 4.8 Infant death rates by mother's country of birth, England and Wales, 2006

	Stillbirth[1]	Perinatal[1]	Neonatal[2]	Postneonatal[2]	Infant[2]
UK	5.4	7.4	3.3	1.4	4.6
Bangladesh	6.3	9.3	4.0	1.5	5.5
India	8.9	10.8	3.4	1.4	4.9
Pakistan	8.8	13.2	5.9	3.5	9.4
Caribbean	8.7	14.1	7.1	1.6	8.8

[1] Deaths per 1,000 live births and stillbirths.
[2] Deaths per 1,000 live births.
Source: Adapted from Table 4, *Health Statistics Quarterly*, 36, Winter, 2007, p. 87

minorities in Britain indicate that ethnicity is a relevant dimension of health inequality. This is evident with regards to infant mortality. In 2005 Asian and Black ethnic groups accounted for 11 per cent of live births in England and Wales and 17 per cent of infant deaths (Office for National Statistics, 2008b). Although there has been a decline in infant mortality rates in all ethnic groups, differentials still remain. For example, during the period 1986 to 1988 the perinatal mortality rate was 16.4 deaths per 1,000 live and stillbirths for babies of mothers from Pakistan, compared with 8.8 for infants of UK-born mothers. By 2006 the perinatal mortality rate had fallen to 13.2 in the Pakistani group and 4.6 in the UK group (see Table 4.8). The overall infant mortality rate for babies born to mothers from Pakistan and the Caribbean was double that for the White British group.

Studies show that black and minority ethic groups generally experience worse health than the overall population. However, some ethnic groups fare worse than others and patterns of inequality vary depending on the health condition concerned. Some of the major findings regarding ethnic health inequalities are summarised in Box 4.6.

The causes of ethnic health inequalities are complex and it is difficult to determine the impact of any one particular characteristic on morbidity and mortality rates. Indeed, there is considerable debate about the interplay between genetic, biological, environmental, socio-economic and cultural/lifestyle factors in influencing the health of members of minority ethnic communities. Socio-economic position is clearly an important determinant of health outcomes. Many minority ethnic groups experience higher rates of material deprivation and social disadvantage than the White British population (Platt, 2007). The poor self-assessed health of minority ethnic groups can be partly explained by the relatively poor standard of living they experience (Nazroo, 1997). Cooper (2002) found adult male and female morbidity ratios greater among black and minority ethnic groups than among whites. Pakistanis and Bangladeshis displayed the greatest health disadvantage. A substantial proportion of the observed inequality in health was attributed to socio-economic factors, particularly level of education, employment status and material deprivation. However, while socio-economic factors were seen

Box 4.6   Research findings

Ethnic health inequalities

- Ethnic differences in health vary across age groups, between generations, men and women and geographic areas.
- Health surveys reveal that the percentage of the population reporting their health as 'not good' is highest among the Pakistani and Bangladeshi populations.
- Standardised mortality ratios for all-cause mortality are higher than the national average for people born in Ireland, Scotland, West Africa and East Africa and lower for people born in Hong Kong and China.
- Black and minority ethnic groups have higher rates of cardio-vascular disease than White British people but lower cancer rates overall.
- Across most regions there is a higher prevalence of diabetes in Black Caribbean and South Asian groups.
- South-Asian-born men are 50 per cent more likely to have a heart attack than men in the general population.
- Minority ethnic groups can feel excluded from 'mainstream' White society and health and support services.

Source: Erens *et al.*, 2001; Fitzpatrick *et al.*, 2005; Parliamentary Office of Science and Technology, 2007; Salway *et al.*, 2007 and Wild *et al.*, 2007

to contribute to an understanding of ethnic health inequalities, the existence of health differences across ethnic groups was not reducible to socio-economic position alone. Research suggests that other forms of inequality, such as the experience of racism, plays a part.

Racism can have a negative impact on health in two main ways. First, racial harassment and discrimination can result in educational and employment opportunities being restricted to such an extent that certain individuals and groups come to occupy a disadvantaged socio-economic position that is associated with poor health outcomes. Second, the direct experience of racism itself can have a negative impact on both the quality of life and feelings of general psychological well-being. According to Karlsen and Nazroo (2002), perceptions of racial discrimination and experience of racial harassment both make a contribution to health independently of socio-economic position. They found that individuals who reported that their property had been the target of racially motivated vandalism or that they had been the victim of a physical attack, were twice as likely as non-victims to describe their health as 'poor' or 'fair'. In a more recent study, Kelaher *et al.* (2008) report that while discrimination affected anxiety, worry and depression there was no observable association between discrimination and self-assessed health status. As they assert, 'This may be due to the fact that self-assessed health status taps into both mental and physical aspects of health and most studies of racial discrimination and physical health outcomes have had null findings' (Kelaher *et al.*, 2008, p. 1633). However, the combined effects of economic marginalisation and racism can impair help-seeking behaviour (Ahmad and Bradby, 2008).

The term 'direct racism' refers to situations in which people are treated less favourably (i.e. discriminated against) because of their race or ethnic background. 'Indirect racism' occurs when services that are supposedly provided equally to all people are actually provided in a way that favours some ethnic groups at the expense of others. The phrase 'institutional racism' describes endemic indirect racism in an organisational setting where ignorance, prejudice or negative stereotyping becomes a feature of institutional processes and procedures. This is clearly of relevance in the context of access to healthcare facilities and the delivery of health services. Bhopal (2007, p. 168) maintains that minority ethnic groups may receive poorer health service provision for any of the following reasons:

- an individual health worker may treat a patient unequally because of racial prejudice;
- health policies based on the needs of the ethnic majority may fail to address the needs of patients from minority ethnic backgrounds;
- specialist resources necessary for meeting the needs of minority groups may not be available;
- existence of discriminatory employment practices.

Ethnic health inequalities are the result of numerous interlinking factors, of which material deprivation is one of the most important. However, not all minority ethnic groups are uniformly disadvantaged with regards to socio-economic position relative to white groups. As Cooper (2002) shows, the poor health reported by Indian men was not a consequence of their socio-economic status: there were more similarities than differences in socio-economic position between the two ethnic groups. Ethnic health is affected by a complex combination of factors including biological susceptibility, environmental factors prior to and following migration, lifestyle behaviours and cultural differences, poverty and social deprivation, experiences of racial discrimination and ethnocentrism in service planning and delivery. It is essential that any policy to tackle ethnic health inequalities is not only based on an understanding of how different forms of socio-economic disadvantage are experienced by minority ethnic groups, but also displays an awareness of the various ways in which racism impacts upon physical health and mental well-being.

Tackling inequalities in health

If future inequalities in health are to be reduced, it will be essential to carry out a wide range of policies to achieve both a general improvement in health and a greater impact on the less well off. By this we mean those who in terms of socioeconomic status, gender or ethnicity are less well off than average in terms of health or its principal determinants – such as income, education, employment or the material environment.

(*Independent Inquiry into Inequalities in Health*, Acheson Report, 1998)

Early in 1998 the Government produced a consultation paper entitled *Our Healthier Nation: A Contract for Health*, which acknowledged a need 'to improve the health of the worst off in society and to narrow the health gap'. Later the same year the *Independent Inquiry into Inequalities in Health* was published; the Inquiry's report contained a review of the evidence relating to health inequalities and identified 'priority areas for future policy development' (Acheson, 1998). In subscribing to a social model of health, only three of the report's 39 substantive policy recommendations were specifically aimed at the health service. Given the wide-ranging nature of social determinants of health, it was recognised that policy action was required across a broad front in order to improve overall health status and narrow the health inequalities gap. This is reflected in what the Inquiry identified as the three highest priority areas:

1 The need to ensure that all policies likely to have implications for health are made subject to 'health impact assessments' to determine their potential impact on health inequalities. Furthermore, such policies should be formulated in such a way that by favouring the less well off they would, wherever possible, reduce such inequalities.

2 A high priority should be given to policies aimed at improving health and reducing health inequalities in women of childbearing age, expectant mothers and young children.

3 The introduction of policies to reduce income inequalities, and improve the living standards of households in receipt of social security benefits.

By commissioning the Independent Inquiry in 1997 the incoming New Labour Government made tackling health inequalities a major policy priority. The Inquiry's report raised the general profile of the inequalities debate and according to Exworthy *et al.* (2003) made an initial impact by:

• prompting new policies;
• engendering a climate of opinion favourable to the introduction of policies to tackle health inequalities;
• introducing a health inequalities dimension to existing policies;
• providing a useful source of information regarding the nature, extent and patterning of inequalities in health.

The early years of the first decade of the twenty-first century witnessed considerable activity on the policy front. The promotion of public health measures to tackle the underlying causes of poor health and the introduction of policy initiatives designed to reduce health inequalities represented a marked shift in focus from 'illness and sickness' to 'health and well-being'. The Government's national *Programme for Action* was informed by the findings of the Acheson Inquiry and specifically designed to tackle health inequalities. It was organised around four main themes: supporting families, mothers and children; engaging communities and individuals; preventing illness and promoting better treatment; dealing with the long-term underlying causes of health inequalities (Department of Health,

2003a). In the first three years the primary objective was to lay the foundations for reducing infant mortality in all social groups and raising life expectancy in the most disadvantaged and deprived areas at a faster rate than elsewhere by the year 2010.

Summary

- Life expectancy for both men and women has improved throughout the twentieth century. People are living longer, but there is also an increase in the number of years spent in poor health.
- Socio-economic status is a major determinant of health status throughout the life course and has an impact on mortality rates even after account is taken of other factors such as health-related behaviours. People in manual occupational groups have higher mortality rates than people in non-manual groups. Despite a general improvement in mortality rates, there is evidence of widening inequalities in health between the rich and the poor.
- The relationship between social class and health varies according age and gender. Social inequalities are particularly marked among infant populations but not among young people. Social class-based inequality generally increases with age from the mid-thirties onwards.
- The link between poverty and poor health is well established; materially and socially deprived areas have higher mortality rates than less deprived areas.
- It is necessary to integrate social, psychological, behavioural and material factors in order to reach a satisfactory explanation of the relationship between socio-economic position and health.
- There are gender differences in both mortality and morbidity rates. When investigating gender specific patterns of health, illness and disease it must be remembered that gender differences reflect biological differences between the sexes as well as differences in social and economic circumstances.
- The causes of ethnic health inequalities are complex and it is difficult to determine the impact of any one particular characteristic on morbidity and mortality rates. The health status of minority ethnic populations is the outcome of a complex combination of factors including biological susceptibility, environmental factors both prior to and following migration, lifestyle behaviours and cultural practices, poverty and material deprivation, exposure to racial harassment and discrimination and ethnocentrism in service planning and delivery.

Questions for discussion

1 What is health and how can it be measured?
2 How useful is occupation as a measure of social class when studying the relative health status of different social groups?

3 What evidence is there for a social gradient in mortality rates?

4 Evaluate the main explanations that have been advanced to account for social inequalities in health.

5 To what extent can gender differences in morbidity be explained by reference to the different social roles performed by men and women in society?

6 What factors influence ethnic health inequalities?

7 How might inequalities in health be reduced?

Further reading

Acheson, Sir D. (1998) *Independent Inquiry into Inequalities in Health: A Report*, London: Stationery Office. Available at: http://www.archive.official-documents.co.uk/document/doh/ih/ih.htm.

Ahmad, W. and Bradby, H. (2008) *Ethnicity, Health and Health Care: Understanding Diversity, Tackling Disadvantage*, Oxford: Wiley-Blackwell.

Bartley, M., Blane, D. and Davey Smith, G. (1998) *The Sociology of Health Inequalities*, Oxford: Blackwell.

Bartley, M. (2003) *Health Inequality: An Introduction to Theory, Concepts, and Methods*, London: Polity Press,

Bird, C. E. and Rieker, P. P. (2008) *Gender and Health: The Effects of Constrained Choices and Social Policies*, New York: Cambridge University Press.

Bhopal, R. (2007) *Race, Ethnicity and Health in Multicultural Societies: Foundations for Better Epidemiology, Public Health, and Health Care*, Oxford: Oxford University Press.

Graham, H. (ed.) (2000) *Understanding Health Inequalities*, Buckingham: Open University Press.

Marmot, M. and Wilkinson, R. G. (eds) (2005) *Social Determinants of Health*, 2nd edn, Oxford: Oxford University Press.

Townsend, P., Davidson, N. and Whitehead, M. (1992) *Inequalities in Health: The Black Report* and *The Health Divide*, in one volume, 2nd edn, Harmondsworth: Penguin.

Wilkinson, R. G. (2005) *The Impact of Inequality: How to Make Sick Societies Healthier*, Abingdon: Routledge.

Useful websites

Association of Public Health Observatories: http://www.apho.org.uk

British Heart Foundation Statistics Website: http://www.heartstats.org

Centre for Evidence in Ethnicity, Health and Diversity: http://www2.warwick.ac.uk/fac/med/research/csri/ethnicityhealth

European Portal for Action on Health Equity: http://www.health-inequalities.eu

General Household Survey: http://www.statistics.gov.uk/ssd/surveys/general_household_survey.asp

Health Challenge England: factsheets: http://www.dh.gov.uk/en/Publicationsandstatistics/Publications/PublicationsPolicyAndGuidance/DH_4139513

Health Survey for England: http://www.dh.gov.uk/en/Publicationsandstatistics/PublishedSurvey/HealthSurveyForEngland/index.htm

Living in Britain 2000: Information from the General Household Survey: http://www.statistics.gov.uk/lib/index.html

National Centre for Health Outcomes Development: http://www.nchod.nhs.uk/

Office for National Statistics, National Statistics Online: http://www.statistics.gov.uk/default.asp

Statistics on poverty and social exclusion: http://www.poverty.org.uk/index.htm

World Health Organisation: Commission on Social Determinants of Health: http://www.who.int/social_determinants/equity/en/index.html

CHAPTER 5

Childhood and adolescence

The study of ageing

> Aristotle may have been the first to codify theories of age; he ascribed humours to four stages of life, with youth being hot and moist and old age cold and dry.
>
> (Bengtson *et al.*, 2009, p. 6)

Age and stage theories

Ageing of the human individual can be described as a gradual process consisting of a complex series of changes that take place over the major part of the lifespan.

In the study of this process considerable emphasis has been placed on the biological, physiological and psychological changes associated with normal ageing. The life course is presented as a linear process starting with conception and ending with death. The early years of life are characterised by growth and development of the human organism. This is a period of maturation during which growth occurs as part of an orderly sequence and many bodily changes are regulated by a biologically determined time schedule. This is clearly demonstrated in the case of foetal growth. In the later years of life, following the attainment of maximum growth, there is a decline in the efficient functioning of the organism. From a biological perspective this reduction in the capacity for growth, coupled with functional loss, is part of the natural process of ageing which is referred to as senescence.

In this approach to the understanding of ageing, growing old constitutes a predictable passage through fixed stages marked by particular chronological ages. The concept of the *life cycle* is used to describe an orderly progression from infancy to old age. In a broad sense the main stages in the cycle are identified as infancy, childhood, adolescence, adulthood and old age.

The identification of stages or phases in the life course is a feature of developmental psychology. An example of a stage theory is Piaget's theory of intellectual development in which cognition is described as developing through four main stages as children mature. The first stage is the sensorimotor, which covers the first two years of life. In this stage the child develops an awareness and knowledge of its environment. The second stage is the pre-operational; this lasts from the ages of two to seven and is when the child begins to use language. Between seven and twelve years of age the child experiences the third stage of cognitive development which Piaget termed the concrete operational. This is when children become capable of logical thought. The fourth and final stage is the formal operational and covers the period of adolescence. In this stage individuals display a capacity to grasp highly abstract ideas. Whilst the first three stages are universal not everyone reaches the fourth stage.

In an introduction to the psychology of human ageing Bromley (1974) distinguishes between two phases of the life-path: the juvenile and the adult. Within each of these phases a number of sequential stages are identified. He distinguishes seven stages of adult life as follows: early adulthood (20 to 25), middle adulthood (25 to 40), late adulthood (40 to 60), pre-retirement (60 to 65), retirement (65 to 70), old age (70) and the terminal stage (Bromley, 1974, pp. 18–25). Bromley uses these chronological age categories as a general guide in order to describe the relative impact of biological, psychological and social aspects of ageing at different stages in the life course. He acknowledges their arbitrary nature and recognises the existence of individual differences.

From the perspectives of biology and psychology the human life cycle is viewed as a natural, universal and continuous process incorporating growth, maturation and degeneration. Whilst not denying the relevance of biological and psychological facts sociologists have drawn attention to the social and cultural aspects of age categorisation. As Berger and Berger (1976) have remarked with respect to childhood:

It is no doubt possible for the biologist to provide a definition of childhood in terms of the degree of development of the organism; and the psychologist can give a corresponding definition in terms of the development of the mind. Within these biological and psychological limits, however, the sociologist must insist that childhood itself is a matter of social construction. This means that society has great leeway in deciding what childhood is to be.

(Berger and Berger, 1976, pp. 69–70)

The idea that social and cultural factors play a part in the definition of childhood can be extended to other stages in the life course. Adopting a sociological perspective such as this is not intended to discount the relevance of biological and psychological factors; it merely serves to illustrate that although these stages may be timed in relation to biological growth and psychological development they are also socially defined. Sociologists are not concerned with the systematic physical and psychological changes associated with ageing; their primary concern is with how the relations between individuals and groups are regulated by age differences. The aim is to identify the social norms and roles characteristic of people in different age groups and determine whether or not there is an unequal distribution of rights and rewards according to age group.

In all modern societies there are age-status systems operating in which rights, obligations and rewards are differentially distributed. For example, in England and Wales a child can have a savings account opened in their name at birth, drink alcohol in private when they reach 5 years of age and enter a public house at 14 years of age but not purchase or consume alcohol. They must attend full-time education between the ages of 5 and 16. At 10 years of age a young person can be held fully responsible for a crime; at the age of 16 they can get married (with the consent of one parent, a guardian or a court). Boys may join the armed forces at 16 providing they have parental approval. At 18 years of age young people can marry without parental consent and are also entitled to vote.

Age-related rules such as these reflect a belief that chronological age is a good indicator of competency. At the age of 18 the young person is considered sufficiently mature to be granted adult status. However, this apparent reliance on the index of chronological age does not mean that age-norms are fixed. Age-norms, whether formalised through legislation or informally expressed through established customs and traditions, are responsive to social and economic change. Consequently, age-related rules and age-appropriate behaviour can vary both between societies at any one time and within a single society over time.

Life cycle or life course?

Recently some social scientists have rejected the notion of a life cycle in favour of the concept of the life course. As previously indicated, the term life cycle has been used to describe the process whereby individuals pass through a number of rigid, clearly defined age-based stages. Critics of this approach maintain that it is unrealistic to assume such a measure of uniformity in the way people pass through life (Cohen, 1987; Hockey and James, 1993). The concept of the life course does not imply such a rigidly prescribed movement from one age grade to the next. As Cohen has commented:

> The term 'life course' is used here rather than the more familiar 'life cycle' as the latter implies fixed categories in the life of the individual and assumes a stable social system, whereas the former allows of more flexible biographical patterns within a continually changing social system.
>
> (Cohen, 1987, p. 1)

She suggests the life course can be likened to a bus journey in which the various stages are represented by boarding and embarkation points. While the bus always follows the same route the location of the bus stops may alter. 'The boarding and embarkation points for childhood, youth and mid-life have either lengthened or shortened over time and vary according to region and culture' (Cohen, 1987, p. 3). As in the life cycle approach, at each stage in the journey through life individuals take on different roles and statuses, but there is recognition of the fact that the length and patterning of the stages are influenced by individual, social, economic and cultural factors. In the context of the study of old age Hockey and James (1993, p. 50) maintain that a life course approach '. . . allows us to see how the status of an elderly person is gradually taken on through a progressive withdrawal from certain aspects of social life which varies between individuals'. Arber and Evandrou also recommend the adoption of a life course perspective because it 'provides a dynamic framework which focuses on change and continuity' (1993, p. 10).

It is claimed that the concept of the life course reflects the cultural diversity, individual differences and historical variation characteristic of the ageing process. As Featherstone and Hepworth (1989) note:

> Unlike the term 'life cycle', which implies fixed categories in the life of the individual and assumes a stable system, the term 'life course' suggests more flexible biographical patterns within a continually changing social system.
>
> (Featherstone and Hepworth, 1989, p. 154)

However, not all share this view. Bernard and Meade (1993) see life course analysis as assuming a rigid structuring of life stages and providing an inflexible and deterministic picture of ageing.

Burgoyne (1987) has identified five typical stages in the life course, as illustrated in Box 5.1. In each of these stages there are crucial 'turning points' when individuals experience changes that have implications for the way in which they organise their lives. On a practical level marriage or cohabitation leads to changes in living arrangements and with the onset of parenthood the structure and composition of the household changes. New roles and responsibilities acquired during the life course produce changes in the pattern of close relationships which results in individuals acquiring new social identities, for example becoming a grandparent. Childhood and adolescence are two stages of the life course covered in this section; later adulthood is dealt with in the next chapter.

The social construction of childhood

> Childhood is a social creation and, although 'truths' about childhood may appear to have the status of objective fact, in reality they reflect specific social and political preoccupations and concerns.
>
> (Murphy, 2007, p. 105)

The emerging concept of childhood

Ideas about when childhood ends, and how it differs from adulthood, have changed considerably down the centuries. These ideas are important because they have influenced the status accorded to children and determined their subsequent treatment by adults. Much has been written about what it is to be a child; however, most of this consists of 'adults imagining childhood, inventing it, in order to make sense of their world' (Cunningham, 2006, p. 12). As Cunningham observes, given that we have inherited so many conflicting views of childhood from the past, it is not surprising that we struggle to provide a coherent and positive conceptualisation of childhood in the present. When considering the contemporary image of childhood, he maintains that this should not be viewed as the natural outcome of some form of historical progress. He points out that the age at which a person is deemed to be criminally responsible has often been taken as marking the end of childhood. While this was set at 12 years of age in the Middle Ages he comments that: 'It is therefore something of a shock to move forward to the eighteenth century and find a girl of seven in Norwich being hanged for stealing a petticoat. It tells us, if nothing else, that the history of childhood is not, as has sometimes been thought, a simple story of progress' (Cunningham, 2006, p. 13).

In contemporary Western societies childhood is generally recognised as a clear and distinct stage in the life course. It is a period characterised by natural growth and increasing maturity. As such it is often perceived as a transitory phase, 'a place of waiting' with emphasis being placed upon the '"not-yet-adult" qualities' of the child (Burgoyne, 1987, p. 40). The tendency is to stress the differences between adults and children rather than focus on the similarities. However, this view has not always prevailed; historical evidence suggests the concept of childhood is a recent invention. In a book entitled *Centuries of Childhood*, the French demographic historian Philippe Ariès argues:

> In medieval society the idea of childhood did not exist; this is not to suggest that children were neglected, forsaken or despised. The idea of childhood is not to be confused with the affection for children: it corresponds to an awareness of the particular nature of childhood, that particular nature which distinguishes the child from the adult . . .
>
> (Ariès, 1962, p. 128)

Ariès' analysis of the historical transformations of childhood is informed by a study of paintings, literature, letters and journals. He claims that up until the end of the thirteenth century children were seen as very much a part of adult society. According to Ariès a concept of childhood began to emerge between the fourteenth and eighteenth centuries. He describes how changes occurred in the rules of social etiquette governing the relationship between adults and children and how children acquired a social identity different from that of adults. This emergence of childhood as a separate social category is reflected in changes in the styles of dress. Ariès illustrates how there was little variation in medieval dress to distinguish the child from the adult, but by the end of the sixteenth century childhood was viewed as a separate entity with a specialised costume.

There are two important features in this growing awareness of childhood. The first refers to the special treatment accorded to children within the family. As Ariès notes: 'A new concept of childhood had appeared, in which the child, on account of his sweetness, simplicity and drollery became a source of amusement and relaxation for the adult' (Ariès, 1962, p. 129). This new attitude towards children first emerged among the property owning and professional classes. Once children were singled out as constituting a distinct social group it was not long before they were seen as being in need of care and protection. The second feature of the new view of childhood refers to children not as 'charming toys' but as creatures requiring training and disciplining. Ariès portrays seventeenth-century churchmen, moralists and pedagogues as presenting an image of children as 'fragile creatures of God who needed to be both safeguarded and reformed' (Ariès, 1962, p. 133). In order to understand this approach to childhood it is necessary to appreciate the philosophical and intellectual climate in which it arose. The Puritan doctrine of the seventeenth century, with its belief in Original Sin, had a particular view of the child. Children were seen as uncontrolled and irrational beings; they were in a natural state of sin. The only way this innate sinfulness could be overcome, and the individual child enter a state of grace, was by training both the body and the mind.

The history of childhood presented by Ariès has not gone unchallenged. Pollock (1983) argues that although it is possible to detect changes in attitudes to childhood over the centuries these changes have not formed part of a smooth, continuous process as suggested by Ariès' thesis. Other critics have claimed that in concentrating on cultural and ideological aspects insufficient attention is paid to the influence of economic factors and the salience of social class. Thane (1981) describes how the growth of a capitalistic economy in Europe during the fifteenth to eighteenth centuries created a demand for adult workers with professional and commercial skills. Thus it was in the interests of the entrepreneurial class to ensure that future generations had the skills and attitudes deemed necessary for commercial success. However, criticisms such as these do not detract from the fact that historical trends in the social construction of childhood can be identified (Cunningham, 1995).

In a review of the historical research, Jenks (1996) outlines two clearly distinct images or discourses of childhood: the Dionysian and the Apollonian. The image of the child presented in seventeenth-century Puritanism (as described above) is an example of the former. Children were seen as having a tendency towards evil rather than good. Consequently, their behaviour needed to be regulated and controlled, thus producing an approach to child-rearing that 'saw socialisation as almost a battle but certainly a form of combat where the headstrong and stubborn subject had to be "broken", but all for their own good' (Jenks, 1996, p. 71). In contrast, according to the Apollonian discourse on childhood, children possess a natural goodness and a primary aim of child-rearing is to provide an environment in which children are protected and nurtured in such a way as to enable them to reach their full potential as human beings.

To argue that childhood is a social construct serves to draw attention to the role of cultural factors. The physical immaturity of childhood is undoubtedly a biological fact of life but the ways in which this immaturity is understood is a fact of culture (La Fontaine, 1979). Thus unlike biological immaturity the concept of childhood is neither a natural nor universal feature of life. It is the '. . . ways in which the immaturity of childhood is conceived and articulated in particular societies into culturally specific sets of ideas and philosophies, attitudes and practices which combine to define the "nature of childhood"' (James and Prout, 1990, p. 1). Consequently, definitions of childhood can differ between societies at any one time, as well as vary within any one society over time. Hendrick (1990) illustrates this historical variability of childhood when he describes the changing meaning of childhood in Britain over the last two centuries. His analysis suggests that the way childhood is defined is influenced by social, economic and political factors. During the course of the Industrial Revolution working-class children provided a cheap source of manual labour. Throughout the greater part of the nineteenth century social reformers campaigned on behalf of working children. They were not opposed to child labour as such but wanted to see an end to the employment of very young children and a restriction placed on the length of the child's working day. During the course of the century, legislation was passed which extended legal protection to children and improved children's employment in a range of industries. For example, the Factory Acts from 1833 onwards reduced children's working hours and introduced compulsory part-time schooling for children employed in factories. For Hendrick, the introduction of this regulatory legislation marked the beginning of the gradual transformation of the working child into the school pupil.

The early decades of the nineteenth century saw increasing social and political unrest. Some reformers held the view that by educating the young it would be possible to shape a new society. Education was seen as the vehicle for transmitting dominant social values thereby ensuring that future generations were nurtured on the values of industry, diligence and respect for authority. Thus in the latter part of the century '. . . the school played a pivotal role in the construction of a new kind of childhood' (Hendrick, 1990, p. 46). It was the emphasis on schooling, rather than the restrictive factory legislation, which effectively reduced the nation's commitment to the extensive use of child labour. This served further to separate children from the adult world of work. The end of schooling and the start of work became the age at which childhood was considered to end and adulthood begin. Ultimately this had implications for the status of children. Prior to being excluded from the workplace they had been engaged in paid employment which enabled them to make a contribution to the family income. Once children were prevented from engaging in such activity they came to be seen as dependants. Hendrick maintains that while compulsory schooling freed children from the pain of employment the new concept of childhood reduced the child's sense of usefulness. Zelizer (1985) has described the process as one of growing economic worthlessness.

It was by the second decade of the twentieth century that what is commonly recognised as a 'modern' notion of childhood began to take shape. This was heavily influenced by psychological explanations of child development which came to dominate the study of childhood as the century progressed. According to Prout and James (1990), the psychological approach emphasised naturalness, universality and rationality. Childhood was depicted as a period of natural growth: a biologically determined stage in the transition to adulthood. Early studies by developmental psychologists presented childhood as a single universal phenomenon and paid little, if any, attention to cultural factors. The differences between the child and the adult were stressed. Whereas the adult was seen as being capable of rational thought and action the child was not. It was through a process of natural growth, characterised by, for example, increasing cognitive ability and language development, that the child was seen as progressing from a state of dependence to independence. Childhood was now open to extensive examination by experts. Specialists in the study of children searched for new and better ways of monitoring physical growth, intellectual development and the acquisition of cognitive skills. Consequently it was possible to identify certain levels of ability and attainment as normal. Hendrick refers to this as the 'psycho-medical construction of childhood' (1990, p. 47).

What emerged from all this was a view of the child as being vulnerable and in need of protection. Hendrick describes how this gave rise to the concept of the 'welfare child'. In his account of the social construction and reconstruction of British childhood he claims that the concepts of the psycho-medical child and the welfare child have been dominant throughout the twentieth century.

While it is generally accepted that constructions of childhood have shifted over time, and that a more child-centred approach to child-rearing has emerged, care should be taken not to assume that there has been a simple historical progression, in which the Dionysian model has replaced the Apollonian model as part of a process of enlightenment. As Jenks (1996) maintains, despite the marked difference between these two images of childhood, they can be found to co-exist. Thus, elements of both images may be found in contemporary debates about children and childhood. According to Murphy (2007), 'one might argue that the Dionysian image of the child, with its associated demand for parental control and constraint, is clearly discernible in recent UK policy developments such as parenting orders, which may, for example, require parents to ensure that their children are at home at certain times or do not visit specified places' (Murphy, 2007, p. 108). Furthermore, while the social experiences of children may vary from one historical period to the next, the models or images of childhood provided by psycho-historians may not capture the true complexity of what it means to be a child in a particular era. This may lead to making false assumptions about the uniformity of childhood. It is essential to distinguish between children's own experiences of being children and the prevailing attitudes towards childhood. Some writers suggest that there is a dissonance between the two, which suggests that childhood is not a natural, unified category but refers to a temporary state without any natural boundaries. Consequently, it is claimed that it makes more sense to think in terms of a *plurality of childhoods* (Jordanova, 1990; Mayall, 1994a) or a *proliferation of childhoods* (Jenks, 2004).

A brief critique of the functionalist view of primary socialisation

The notion of childhood as a training ground for adulthood permeates early psychological approaches; it also appears in the accounts of sociologists, particularly when referring to the process of primary socialisation (Dreitzel, 1973). As noted by Rogers and Pilgrim (2005, p. 104), 'there is a strong consensus across theoretical positions in both sociology and psychology that childhood is a special part of the life span'. It is during the period of primary socialisation, covering infancy and the early years of childhood, that children are expected to learn the norms and values of the society into which they have been born. This is a critical stage in their social development. It is by learning the culturally acceptable modes of behaviour, and the importance of conforming to rules, that children become well-adjusted adult members of society. For functionalist sociologists, childhood is a preparatory phase in the development of the individual; it is a time when children are prepared for their future integration into society. Parsons (1956) describes how parents, either consciously or unconsciously, encourage the child to adopt those values, beliefs and personality characteristics associated with success in adult life. This functionalist perception of childhood as a transitory phase is clearly captured in the following:

> an individual's most important functions for society are performed when he is fully adult, not when he is immature. Hence society's treatment of the child is chiefly preparatory, and the evaluation of him mainly anticipatory (like a savings account).
>
> (Davis, 1940, quoted in Qvortrup, 1991, p. 14)

Ultimately, it is this socialisation process which ensures social stability by producing individuals willing to accept behavioural norms and conform to societal expectations. The assumption is that if anything happens to disrupt this early learning process, then conformity will be difficult to develop in later life. The functionalist approach can be challenged on a number of counts.

1 **It presents an 'oversocialised' picture of the individual.**
   As Wrong (1961) asserts socialisation refers to both the 'process of becoming human' and the 'transmission of culture'. All individuals are socialised in the former sense, in so far as they acquire uniquely human attributes as a result of interaction with others. However, he claims it is wrong to assume individuals are passive recipients of a particular set of cultural values and beliefs. The child should not be viewed as a pre-social being, completely moulded according to a predetermined pattern of norms and roles considered essential for ensuring the smooth functioning of society.

2 **It represents child socialisation as a one-way process.**
   The emphasis on the preparation for adult roles and the learning of socially acceptable forms of behaviour leads to a conceptualisation of child socialisation as a one-way process. This has been criticised as a one-sided view which studies childhood from the point of view of the parents and neglects the experiences of children themselves. According to McKay (1973), conventional views of socialisation tend to view childhood from the vantage point of the dominant group, that is, parents. Thus, children and child-rearing are viewed as 'problems'; the management of children becomes the central concern. This representation of childhood as a special state is based on a conception of children as essentially deficient. The skills and competencies necessary for successful integration into adult society are seen as being learned from parents and other adult role models. This is not a criticism peculiar to functionalist approaches. Dominant adult ideologies of childhood have influenced the thinking of researchers and professional practitioners across a range of disciplines. The result is that the focus of study has been the experience of parenting rather than the experience of childhood (Leonard, 1990). By neglecting to acknowledge the child's world as a distinct culture in its own right it is claimed that some researchers have failed to recognise that children are capable of behaving in socially competent and rational ways (Denzin, 1970). Once it is accepted that children are not pre-social beings then socialisation can be seen, not as a one-way process, but as a two-way affair in which there is reciprocal interaction between adult and child.

3 **It focuses too narrowly on the differences that separate childhood and adulthood.**
   The functionalists' concern with the question of social order leads them to concentrate on childhood as a preparatory stage in the process of becoming an adult. Consequently, continual emphasis is given to the essential differences between adulthood and childhood. What is seen as in need of explanation is how the child develops into an adult. In this perspective the child is seen as

something of an outsider, needing to be integrated into society. However, for Qvortrup, this is only part of the picture, for it must be remembered that 'childhood persists as a part of the social structure' (1991, p. 14). In other words, we must not lose sight of the fact that the life circumstances of children are determined by the same social and economic forces that create the framework within which adults live their lives. Although it does not follow that the effects will be the same for both groups.

4 **It ignores the powerlessness of children.**
Traditional sociological approaches to the study of childhood have ignored the powerlessness of children. Only recently have researchers begun to investigate the ways in which children as a social group are socially marginalised and subjected to various forms of social control both in the family and in formal organisational settings. Childhood is fashioned according to rules and regulations imposed by adults. Consequently, the status assigned to children is clearly ascribed. Thus, functionalist theorists see childhood socialisation as a social learning process, in which adults are seen as playing a significant and instrumental role. As observed by Tucker (1977, p. 26), 'childhood may be lengthened and prolonged at some periods of history, and abbreviated at others, according to adult perceptions, needs and expectations'.

These identified shortcomings in the functionalist approach to socialisation should not be interpreted as a criticism of the concept of primary socialisation *per se*. The aim is merely to draw attention to the fact that children need to be viewed as 'active beings', as opposed to 'passive subjects', in this whole process.

A new paradigm for the sociological study of childhood

Looked at from a historical perspective, 'we might say that the development of modern childhood itself marks the movement of children from productive contributors to domestic economies to objects of more or less conspicuous consumption' (Hood-Williams, 1990, p. 160). As described above, during the Industrial Revolution children who engaged in paid employment outside the home were in a position to make a contribution to the family income. The introduction of restrictive legislation and compulsory schooling helped to form a realisation that children belonged to a distinct group with special needs. This helped to create a distance between adults and children and thereby alter the value attached to children. As Leonard states, 'late twentieth century children exist to be enjoyed by adults and to appreciate the childhood that is being provided for them' (1990, p. 68).

Hood-Williams (1990) uses the concept of 'age patriarchy' to explore the principal areas of control to which children are subjected in everyday life and the nature of the disciplinary procedures invoked when children fail to obey their parents. What he considers distinctive about the controls is the fact that they refer to space, body and time. Children's lives are spatially restricted, they may be expected to comply with adult demands to remain in a particular place or there may be areas from which they are excluded. Physical control may be exercised over the child's body. This is particularly the case in early childhood when parents play a significant part in determining the style of dress and physical appearance of their children. As for time, Hood-Williams maintains that childhood is a period of transition and parents can be seen as attempting to control the speed of the child's progression through childhood.

> Childhood is not only a continuous transition of ages and stages in the writings of psychologists but also in daily struggles with parents for different treatment . . . Many of the intergenerational struggles between children and their parents may be regarded as struggles over the rates of transition from one age stage to the next.
>
> (Hood-Williams, 1990, p. 167)

The concept of age patriarchy does not imply that the nature of the controls over children's space, bodies and time, and the disciplinary practices adopted by parents, are uniform throughout society. There is not only considerable variability in what constitutes acceptable conduct but there is also variation in the disciplinary methods used by parents. The concept helps us to appreciate that there is a hierarchy that permeates society and creates a distance between adults and children.

It is not only functionalist accounts of childhood that are guilty of ignoring the views of children themselves and proffer an image of the child as a passive social actor. In exploring the structure and organisation of family life sociologists have tended to concentrate on issues such as the changing nature of conjugal role relationships and the position of the nuclear family within the wider kinship system. In other words, according to Wagg (1992), little attention has been given to children and the patterning of parent–child relationships. In sociological studies of family life 'children are either invisible or they are bit-part players. Mostly they are *objects* – factors, primarily, in the activities or calculations of

---

Box 5.2 Definition

A new paradigm for the sociological study of childhood

- *Childhood should be seen as a social construction and not simply a biological fact.* Whereas physical dependence in the early years of life is considered a natural phenomenon, the ways in which this dependence is understood are a fact of culture. Resulting constructions of childhood are not natural but the product of specific structural and cultural forces.

- *Childhood is not a single universal phenomenon.* The way in which childhood is conceived varies according to social class, ethnicity and gender. The concept of childhood is culturally specific and not fixed or immutable.

- *Children's experiences of growing up are worthy of study in their own right.* Researchers need to pay more attention to the distinct culture of childhood.

- *Children need to be viewed as active members of families and other social groupings,* and not seen primarily as passive subjects on whom social forces exert an influence.

Source: Prout and James, 1990, p. 8

their parents' (Wagg, 1992, p. 10). Leonard (1990) also draws attention to this objectification when she comments on the apparent reluctance of sociologists to approach the study of childhood by interviewing the children themselves.

The critique of conventional approaches to the study of childhood produced a call for a new paradigm or conceptual framework to direct the sociological study of children. Four of the key features of this paradigm, as identified by Prout and James, are outlined in Box 5.2.

Towards a sociology of child health

> For whilst parents may be taught by health and education professionals and the media that children are to be regarded as socialisation projects, children themselves forcibly teach parents that children are people, who work towards control over the organisation of their lives.
>
> (Mayall, 1998a, p. 278)

Children as active participants in healthcare work

As discussed earlier in the chapter, traditional perspectives in sociology have tended to view the child as a pre-social being who is subjected to a process of socialisation. This process has been presented as a kind of developmental continuum, which is in keeping with the 'age and stage' theories of physical, psychological and moral development favoured by many psychologists. For many years the conceptualisation of socialisation as a form of linear progression or maturation dominated sociological approaches to the study of children and childhood. The primary purpose of the whole process was to ensure that children were prepared for adult society. They required nurturing and protecting by parents and other responsible adults, such as schoolteachers. According to this view, socialisation can be described as deterministic and adult-focused (Alanen, 1998). Children are depicted as 'passive socialisation vessels' (Prout, 1986, p. 113) or 'socialisation projects' (Mayall, 1998a, p. 269). As Christensen (1998) notes, there is in the Western cultural tradition an emphasis on children 'becoming' rather than 'being' a social person. The tendency has been to view them as objects of socialisation by adults, rather than as active participants in their own right in the socialisation process.

Sociological studies of childhood illness have tended to concentrate on adults' perspectives on child health issues, with the voice of children rarely being heard. Prout (1979) maintains that this is partly a result of the underdeveloped nature of the sociology of childhood, which up until fairly recently did not acknowledge children as active social participants capable of constructing and sustaining their own social worlds. The social worlds of children are separate from, but at the same time related to, the adult-constructed and controlled social worlds of home and school. It is through an understanding of children's social worlds that we can begin to appreciate the active role that children play in health care activity.

Mayall (1993, 1994b) undertook a study of the division of labour in healthcare-related activities between children, parents, teachers and other school employees. The research was conducted in a primary school in North London and involved classroom observation, informal discussions and individual interviews. The children studied were from the reception class (5-year-olds) and the fifth-year class (9-year-olds). The researcher describes that in focusing on ordinary day-to-day health maintenance activities and health promotion practices 'an important aim of the study was to do the research *for* rather than *on* the children' (1993, p. 468, emphasis added). To this end she concentrated on encouraging the children to provide accounts of routine daily events at home and at school. On the basis of these accounts, Mayall describes how children can be seen as actively interacting with adults in three main ways: negotiating an acceptable social position; establishing a measure of independence in their daily lives; and constructing a child domain for themselves. These activities are a fundamental feature of childhood in which children are seen as engaging with adults as they attempt to influence the major structuring features of their daily lives, namely, the character of child–adult relationships, the image adults have of the role of children and the nature of childhood (Mayall, 1998b).

The evidence obtained by Mayall (1993) suggests that both 5-year-old and 9-year-old children participate in the process of negotiating an acceptable social position for themselves both in the private sphere of family life and the public domain of school. As regards the home, it is here that children learn to take charge of their bodies and develop competence as healthcare actors. From the accounts the 5-year-olds gave, it is clear that they saw themselves as carrying out many routine daily health-related activities, such as cleaning their teeth. However, they did appreciate the fact that in performing these activities they were helped and supported by their mothers, who were the principal authorities on health maintenance at home. The idea of a division of healthcare labour between mothers and their 5-year-old children is evident in the following extract.

Child A:	(In the morning) I wash me first.
Interviewer:	Yourself?
Child A:	Yes. I get dressed. I have my breakfast. I put my shoes on, on my own. Get ready for school. I get my book. I remember it, to bring it back. Then we go to school. With my Mummy.
Mother:	She reminds me about giving her vitamins in the morning. And that she's supposed to do her teeth.
Child B:	I brush my teeth, but sometimes my Mum helps me, and when the toothpaste's stiff and I can't get it out, she helps.

(Mayall, 1993, p. 472)

In the accounts provided by the 9-year-old children, there was more evidence of negotiation taking place and an expressed desire to be in control and establish a separate domain. Whereas for the 5-year-olds the mother was the organiser and principal provider of healthcare, the older children saw her as more of an 'overseer and checker of routine health maintenance work'. Mayall concludes that:

The children's accounts indicate their understanding that the important health-related activities take place at home. Health care there is an enterprise lightly undertaken by them as actors, within the accepted context of maternal authority. It is, above all, an interactive enterprise, where the division of labour is constantly negotiated.

(Mayall, 1993, p. 474)

While the home is seen as an enabling environment, capable of providing holistic healthcare in a private domain where children have the opportunity to develop a sense of independence, the school is seen in a different light. The children interviewed did not see the school as offering them healthcare or health knowledge. Mayall observes that the school, as a formal institution, imposes an adult-focused model of childhood in which children are viewed as socialisation projects. In her opinion, the competence children develop as healthcare actors within the family setting is not fully acknowledged when they enter school. The lay healthcare system that operates within the school is more prescriptive than that found within the home. At school, children do not enjoy the same opportunities for negotiating with adults and establishing independence.

Laying claim to the sick role

As described in Chapter 2, a core feature of the sick role is that it legitimates temporary social withdrawal from a number of obligations. For example, adults whose sick role status is confirmed by others are absolved of certain responsibilities surrounding work and family life, whereas children are allowed to miss school and may be relieved of any domestic chores they are normally expected to undertake. The important point is that claims of illness can be contested and subjected to a process of evaluation. This may involve formal procedures, as in the case of medical certification by general practitioners, and/or informal assessments made by family members, friends, work colleagues or other adults. If a claim to illness is deemed to be false and the individual is not considered to be 'really ill', then the sick role status will be denied them.

Children's claims to illness are carefully scrutinised by adults, particularly parents and teachers, before they are taken seriously. Therefore, it is important to know something about adults' perspectives on children's claims to illness if we are to achieve a better understanding of the informal healthcare work undertaken by mothers and teachers. According to Christensen (1998), everyday interactions between adults and children about child illness are influenced by cultural assumptions based on a contrasting conception of adult competence and child incompetence.

In general adults constitute themselves as competent by drawing on 'rational' knowledge and mediating devices (such as a thermometer) to classify children's mental and bodily experiences as 'real' illness. This simultaneously entails that children's competence becomes suspended; their subjective experiences of their own bodies do not qualify them as 'speakers of fact'.

(Christensen, 1998, p. 190)

Where chronically sick children show competence in controlling their condition, as for example when they administer their own medication, adults do not necessarily see this display of competence as a general feature of childhood but interpret it as a quality that serves to set some children apart from the majority.

Without a doubt it is mothers who are chiefly responsible for the physical and emotional well-being of children. Not only are they the primary carers when their children fall ill, but the responsibility for much preliminary healthcare work, such as promoting good health and detecting and interpreting symptoms, also falls to them. Child health maintenance is such an integral feature of the cultural role assigned to the mother that it forms a core element in the very definition of motherhood. As Prout has pointed out, 'Illness in a child carries a prima facie implication of a deviation from good mothering . . .' (1986, p. 118). Consequently, some people may treat the decisions that mothers make on issues of health and illness as measures of 'good mothering'. Research shows that mothers are acutely aware of this and this knowledge influences how they react when their children say that they feel ill.

In an ethnographic study of sickness in an English primary school, Prout (1988) investigated how mothers decided whether or not to keep their children 'off school sick' when they complained of feeling unwell. From an analysis of the accounts the mothers gave, Prout was able to describe the decision-making dilemmas they faced. First of all, there was the matter of having to determine if the symptoms described by the child were real or whether the child was feigning illness. It is clear from the descriptions the mothers gave of their attempts at establishing the authenticity of claims to illness, that they saw themselves as engaging in a process of negotiation with their children. Many admitted that making decisions about feigning was not an easy task but because of the personal knowledge they had about their own child they felt they were usually successful at separating the genuine claims from the spurious ones. In order to decide whether their child was 'really ill' they looked for evidence of illness other than complaints about feeling unwell. The visibility, timing and duration of symptoms were all seen as important. Christensen (1998) also describes how adults perceive the duration of symptoms to be a significant factor when it comes to assessing a child's claim to illness. Adults know from experience that children may sometimes display symptoms that disappear after a couple of hours and do not develop into a 'real illness'. Thus, from an adult perspective, time is important in helping to decide whether or not a child's claim needs to be taken seriously.

Prout notes from the mothers' accounts that although they sometimes felt that a child's expression of illness lacked credibility, they did not always assume that the child was deliberately feigning illness in order to gain preferential treatment. Other explanations were advanced as to why a child might make a bid for the sick role. For example, some mothers expressed the view that a child who is anxious or emotionally upset may report symptoms like a stomach ache or a headache, when in fact there is nothing actually physically wrong with them. As one mother stated when explaining why she had kept her daughter off school for a day:

Last Friday she had a tummy ache. I thought she might be constipated, 'cos when she gets like this she feels too unwell to go to school. Nothing seemed to persuade her so I kept her at home. She was OK the next day. A lot of it is nerves with her. She builds herself up if something is coming up. It's either headache or tummy ache. Anxiety I suppose. They've had some exams to do recently. Also we're moving house in a fort-night so whether it's that? Rachel is very affected by it, very worried about her friends and that.

(A mother quoted in Prout, 1988, pp. 774–5)

Another reason why mothers did not treat all reported but unsubstantiated symptoms as attempts at feigning illness was that they subscribed to the view that some children were all too ready to make claims on the sick role no matter what their symptoms. This was not seen as intentionally manipulative behaviour, but a consequence of a lack of stoicism in the face of feelings of illness. The decision-making possibilities identified in the mothers' accounts by Prout are illustrated in Figure 5.1. As Prout emphasises, the diagram is not meant to

Figure 5.1 Decision-making possibilities present in mothers' accounts of everyday sickness
Source: Prout, 1988, p. 775

represent a decision-making flow chart but should be seen as depicting what he describes as a 'structural system of possibilities'. In evaluating particular children's claims to the sick role, mothers did not proceed in a systematic fashion through the pathways as outlined in the diagram but shifted from one possibility to another as and when they acquired new information.

As previously indicated, this decision-making process needs to be seen within the wider context of the social construction of motherhood. Despite the steady increase in the percentage of women in the labour force, women's primary social identity is still constructed around the roles of wife and mother. Although both parents have childcare responsibilities, mothers are by far the major providers of such care (Wyke and Hewison, 1991). This is particularly noticeable in the area of child health. Not only are mothers the main carers of sick children but they are also responsible for much of the day-to-day health promotion and health maintenance work that goes on in families (Mayall and Foster, 1989). As a result, having healthy children and responding appropriately when children report minor symptoms are two criteria used to define 'good mothering'. According to Prout, '. . . child illness requires mothers to execute complex manoeuvres in defence of their claim to be a "good mother"' (1988, p. 783). He describes how a number of the mothers he interviewed were well aware of the fact that decision-making around sickness absence from school was subject to the critical comments of other mothers and teachers. On the one hand, mothers did not want to appear overly protective towards their children by keeping them off school too often for trivial reasons. However, on the other hand they did not want to convey the impression that they were neglectful and uncaring by sending their children to school when they were genuinely unwell.

Adolescence

The teenage years are commonly characterised as a time of rebellion, emotional angst and careless risk-taking. Enduring portrayals of adolescents include the 'can't be bothered', sex-obsessed 'Kevin the Teenager' and the brooding, near psychotic Holden Caulfield from the *Catcher in the Rye*. These characterisations suggest that adolescence is a turbulent time and thus the phrase, 'storm and stress' first coined by psychologist G. Stanley Hall (1904) to describe this period appears as fitting today as it was 100 years ago.

(Asmussen *et al.*, 2007, p. 23)

Transition to adulthood

The physical dependency of babies and infants ensures that all human societies have some conception of childhood, even though in some cases this may be limited to a relatively short span of years. Pubertal change, involving growth to maturity and reproductive maturation, is a universal feature of adolescence, although its timing and the rites and ceremonies to which it gives rise are influenced by social factors, economic conditions and cultural beliefs. While there is some definition of adulthood in every society, the age at which adult status is ascribed is not the same in all societies. However, it is only in some societies that intermediary stages between child and adult are recognised and the transition to adulthood can be described as 'a continuous one throughout the mid-teens and early twenties' (Harris, 1988, p. 509).

In modern societies 'adolescence' and 'youth' have come to be defined as part of a distinctive developmental period in the transition from childhood to adulthood. It was at the beginning of the twentieth century when psychologists first identified adolescence as a new phase in the life course (Hall, 1904). The age limits of adolescence are not clearly defined, but it is generally assumed that it is a developmental stage, which begins with puberty and ends in the middle to late teenage years when physical growth is almost complete. Adolescence has been described as a discreet developmental period 'beginning with biology and ending in society' (Lerner and Galambos, 1998, p. 414). This conceptualisation of adolescence as a scheduled transition to adulthood characterises psychological approaches (Coleman, 1990). Given the nature and complexity of the biological, intellectual and social changes involved, those who study this stage of the life course do not conceptualise the period as incorporating a single transition. For example, Asmussen *et al.* (2007), following DeBord (1999), identify three distinct phases, as illustrated in Box 5.3. As Asmussen *et al.* (2007) assert, at an individual level there can be marked differences in the actual onset and length of these phases. Some young people may experience a lengthier period of middle adolescence than others. Also, it is not uncommon for some children to be economically and emotionally reliant on their parents in some shape or form well beyond their teenage years.

As Coleman and Hagnell (2007) assert, a good of way of understanding adolescence is to view it as one of the major transition points in the life course. This process of transition is characterised by:

- A feeling of anticipation for what is ahead.
- A sense of regret for the stage that has been lost.

Box 5.3   Definition

Three distinct phases of adolescence

- **Pre-adolescence** (9 to 13 years of age): Starts with the onset of puberty and is marked by a rapid growth spurt.
- **Middle adolescence** (14 to 16 years of age): The need for independence becomes more apparent and friends and peers come to have an increasing influence.
- **Late adolescence** (17 to 19 years of age): Teenagers begin to disengage from their families and there is a gradual shift towards economic and emotional independence.

Source: Asmussen *et al.*, 2007, p. 24

- Anxiety about the future.
- A major psychological readjustment.
- A degree of ambiguity of status during transition.

(Coleman and Hagnell, 2007, p. 3)

This transition can be understood from a number of different perspectives including the biological, psychological and sociological.

Concentrating solely on biologically based models of adolescent development only gives us a partial understanding of the transition to adulthood. In order to appreciate fully this aspect of the life course we need to consider the social, economic and cultural factors that help shape the lives of young people. The timing of life transitions, such as leaving school and starting work, are not determined by biological changes alone. As already noted, young people may continue to be economically dependent on their parents long after they have reached biological maturity, largely as a result of continuing in full-time education or being unable to find employment on leaving school.

From a sociological perspective, adolescence is viewed as a product of specific social, economic and cultural changes stemming from industrialisation and the subsequent introduction of compulsory education (Hurrelmann, 1989). The industrialisation process with its emphasis on mass production and highly specialised division of labour resulted in the removal of paid work from the home to the factory. Paid labour increasingly became an activity that occurred outside the home. This separation of work life and family life, along with legislation restricting the employment of children and introducing compulsory schooling, resulted in the establishment of different daily routines for adults and children. Over the years technological advances have created a need for a more highly trained workforce. The age at which compulsory education ceases has been increased and individuals encouraged to stay in full-time education or training beyond the age of 16 years in order to acquire appropriate skills. According to some observers this has led to the creation of 'youth' as a new stage of life between adolescence and adulthood (Keniston, 1970). The period of transition to adulthood appears to be getting longer. Coffield (1987) comments on how adolescence and youth are socially defined and can be extended or curtailed according to the needs of the economy. Consequently, given that 'adolescence . . . is prolonged in many societies, it has become a period of life itself, and not simply a transition from childhood to adulthood' (Hess *et al.*, 2006, p. 10).

Adolescence is a period when adult personal and social identities begin to take shape through the process of social interaction. However, not all theorists see the young person as an entirely passive recipient of biological influences or a victim of social structural forces. While they acknowledge the importance of biological and structural factors, they reject overtly deterministic explanations in favour of a view that considers adult identity formation as the outcome of a process of negotiation that takes place throughout adolescence. The young person is depicted as having an active rather than passive role to play in setting his or her future goals and is described as a 'productive processor of reality'

(Hurrelmann, 1988). However, it is acknowledged that this negotiation takes place within the limits imposed by structural factors.

The transition to adulthood is characterised by leaving school, entering employment, leaving the parental home and establishing a separate household (Harris, 1988). Leaving home is considered to be of particular importance as it symbolises '. . . leaving the private world of family relations and encountering the public world and formal relations of housing markets, labour markets and other adult institutions' (Jones and Wallace, 1992, p. 93). In order to ensure a successful transition to adulthood, employment and income are essential. Indeed, engaging in paid work is generally perceived as a significant phase in the socialisation process during adolescence. It provides a context in which young people have opportunities for interacting with people from outside their families and friendship groups. Consequently, they acquire a sense of independence and learn to take on responsibility. Furthermore, their new status as 'income earners' means that they can be seen to make a direct contribution to the family finances, which effectively reduces their sense of financial dependence upon others.

Clearly, the work role is a major role in adulthood. Unfortunately, it 'is outside the purview of many adolescents' given the nature of labour markets in many post-industrialised societies (Hess *et al.*, 2006, p. 4). Data from the Labour Force Survey on youth unemployment (i.e. people aged between 16 and 24 years) in the UK reveal that over recent decades youth joblessness has been an issue of considerable concern and that in proportionate terms the level of unemployment found among adolescents tends to be two to three times greater than that found among adults. In the early 1980s in some regions of Britain, as many as a third of all school leavers faced the prospect of long-term unemployment (Roberts, 1984). The lack of suitable employment opportunities for young people led to the claim that 'youth has increasingly become a stage of "redundancy"' (Coleman and Husen, 1985, p. 9). Although the youth unemployment rate showed signs of a decline during the closing years of the last century (down from around 14 per cent in 1997 to 12 per cent in 2001), it began to rise again towards the end of the first decade of this century and in the last quarter of 2008 stood at just over 16 per cent. The impact of unemployment on the health and general well-being of young people is well established. In general, jobless young people experience more health problems than their employed counterparts and enjoy a poorer quality of life (Lakey, 2001, 2002). It is therefore within this wider social and economic context that the health-related behaviours and health status of young people are best understood.

Health and lifestyle

During the period of early adolescence, friendship groups and peer groups come to play an increasingly important role in the lives of many young people. As children move through adolescence, there is a decline in parental influence and an increase in opportunities for them to develop relationships with people of a similar age outside the family. Being part of a group of like-minded

Box 5.4   Definition

Focal concerns of adolescence

- developing a sense of self-identity in the light of physical changes;
- developing and maintaining a gender identity;
- gaining a degree of independence from parents;
- accepting or rejecting adult values;
- acquiring and adjusting to an occupational role or coping with an unemployed role;
- establishing and developing friendships and adult relationships.

Source: Coleman and Hendry, 1999

individuals with shared values and common interests helps to create a sense of identity and a feeling of belonging. This identification with a peer group may go some way towards countering the sense of powerlessness that can be experienced by young people. Feelings of powerlessness may be seen to emanate from the apparent mismatch between the level of competence displayed by young people and the degree to which they can be considered to have control over their own lives (Graham, 2004).

During the adolescent phase of the life course young people face a number of major 'focal concerns' (Box 5.4). It is in the pursuit of these focal concerns, and in negotiating the physical, cognitive and psycho-social transitions referred to above, that risks associated with the teenage years are encountered (Kelly *et al.*, 2004). Indeed, adolescence is often portrayed as 'an age of particular risk . . . a particularly problematic age' (Coleman and Hagnell, 2007, p. 2). Risks associated with sexual activity include teenage pregnancy and sexually transmitted diseases. In the case of the former, the UK has the highest teenage pregnancy rate in Europe. Although conception rates for under 18-year-olds declined from 46.3 per 1,000 in 1998 to 41.5 per 1,000 in 2004 (Coleman and Schofield, 2007), the figure for 2007 shows a slight rise to 41.9 per 1000. As regards sexually transmitted infections, new cases of Chlamydia among 16- to 19-year-olds treated at UK clinics increased more than threefold over a ten-year period from the mid-1990s to 2005 (Coleman and Schofield, 2007). Adolescence is also a period when young people are likely to indulge in a variety of risk-taking behaviours such as drinking alcohol, smoking and experimenting with recreational drugs. In a national survey of 11- to 15-year-olds in England in 2005, 22 per cent admitted to having consumed alcohol in the last seven days, 9 per cent described themselves as 'regular smokers' and 19 per cent claimed to have taken illegal drugs in the last year (Information Centre, 2006).

Much useful information about the health, lifestyle and socialisation experiences of young people can be obtained from both national and local social surveys. Questionnaires can be used to elicit information about a range of activities and health-related behaviours such as participation in leisure pursuits, the consumption of alcohol, smoking, diet and the use of illicit drugs. Drawing on questionnaire data from a sample of over 2,000 young people attending secondary school in Scotland, Glendinning *et al.* (1995) describe the importance of the family, school and peer group in the socialisation of adolescent health behaviours. In examining how young people in middle adolescence, that is 15 to 16 years of age, interact with the social environment, they identified four key themes:

- disaffection with school;
- integration into peer groups;
- relationships with parents;
- attitudes to adult authority.

From the pattern of questionnaire responses three broad types of young people were identified: conventional, school- and family-oriented youth; peer-oriented youth; and disaffected, peer-oriented youth. Links were found between these types and various health-related behaviours, particularly smoking and the consumption of alcohol.

As the researchers note, an 'unhealthy' lifestyle was associated more with young people in the 'disaffected' group than it was with those in the 'conventional' youth category. For example, on comparing the responses from these two groups it was found that regular smoking and drinking featured more commonly in the adolescent lifestyle characteristic of 'disaffected' youth. In conclusion, the researchers claim that,

> . . . our findings indicate that adolescent health behaviours are very much bound up with patterns of social integration, and associated attitudes to adult authority, where these may be viewed as aspects of lifestyle which reflect the individual's wider personal and social contexts.

(Glendinning *et al.*, 1995, p. 247)

What is more, these lifestyle factors have implications for health in later adolescence and early adulthood.

Many studies of health lifestyle factors in adolescence pay scant attention to young people within the context of the household. A notable exception is a study undertaken by Brannen *et al.* (1994) of a sample of young people and their parents living in West London. In focusing on health, illness and health-related behaviour of young people, the researchers sought to explore how parents and young people negotiate responsibility for health maintenance during middle adolescence. The study used a multi-method research design, incorporating self-administered questionnaires and semi-structured, in-depth interviews. A total of 843 questionnaires were completed by a sample of 15- to 16-year-olds drawn from both state and private sector schools. This schools survey provided quantitative information on health-related activities and general health characteristics of the respondents. The household interviews generated data on how social relationships were negotiated between parents and young people and provided an insight into what goes on in families with respect to young people's health. A total of 142 interviews were conducted with young people and their parents.

There is a general assumption that, by and large, teenagers represent a fairly healthy section of the population and consequently they are not seen as being among the major users of health services. However, this is not supported by the survey findings. Almost four in ten respondents reported having a long-term illness or recurrent health problem. In the twelve months prior to the start of the study, nearly one in ten of the young people had been in hospital, just over a third had had cause to visit a hospital casualty department and 84 per cent had visited their general practitioner at least once.

As regards responsibility for young people's health, the findings confirm the central role played by mothers. Mothers usually detect the early signs of illness and are instrumental in encouraging young people to seek professional advice and treatment. Brannen *et al.* found that when health problems were felt to be serious, mothers tended to accompany their teenage children on visits to the doctor. However, the researchers observed that, 'Where illness is relatively minor or involves follow-up GP appointments, parents and young people negotiate intermediate strategies. These enable young people to exercise autonomy in managing their own illnesses' (Brannen *et al.*, 1994, p. 99). In order to understand the process of negotiation that goes on between parents and young people concerning matters of health, it is necessary to have some idea of wider parental perspectives on adolescence as well as knowledge of the rules which govern what parents expect of their teenage children.

Interviews with the parents revealed the existence of two broad contrasting normative views of adolescence. Some parents described adolescence as a time when young people strive to achieve independence and a sense of individual autonomy; others viewed it more as a stage in the life course in which young people learn to take on the responsibilities and obligations associated with adulthood. These two perspectives are associated with different approaches to parental control and regulation of young people's behaviour. Where parents see adolescence as 'a progressive quest for independence', they lay emphasis on the need for renegotiating the parent–child relationship. Young people may be granted a certain amount of autonomy or freedom from direct parental control but there is an expectation on the part of parents that they will provide them with information in return. For example, parents may allow their teenage children to stay out late, as long as they inform them where they are and whom they are with. In this context, young people's status transitions are individually achieved. This is in marked contrast to the other adult perspective on adolescence, which sees the changes in status as normatively ascribed and not a subject for negotiation between young people and their parents. This view was particularly prevalent amongst those parents who were born and raised in countries in Asia and the Middle East.

Gender emerged as an issue in the final analysis in a number of ways. As Brannen *et al.* affirm, 'gender is a strong differentiator of young people's health beliefs, health status and health behaviour' (1994, p. 211). Young women and mothers were less likely than young men and fathers to see health as being something over which they had some individual control. As regards self-reported health-related behaviours, young women were more likely than young men to admit to smoking. While there was no difference between young men and young women with regard to the reported frequency of drinking, it was young men who reported consuming larger quantities of alcohol. Gender was also relevant in terms of the renegotiation of relationships between parents and young people that characterises the transition to adulthood. Mothers not only saw it as their task to establish a 'talking relationship' with their teenage children but they also performed the role of 'mediators' between young people and their fathers.

For many parents the central challenge is one of striking the right balance between care and control as relationships are renegotiated. Parental strategies of control and regulation differ in accordance with parents' particular normative views on adolescence. Some mothers used communicative strategies in an effort to regulate the activities of their teenage children. This was particularly the case with middle-class mothers and was more successful with daughters than with sons. When interviewed, mothers in this category described how they used talk as a way of cultivating 'closeness' and 'openness' in the mother–daughter relationship. For these mothers, as young people moved towards achieving independent adult status, direct forms of parental control, such as the strict enforcement of rules and regulations, no longer seemed appropriate. Control was exercised by more covert means. In return for granting their teenage children a measure of independence, parents expected to be kept informed as to their activities.

This was not the dominant mode of control reported by working-class parents. They saw adult status as being ascribed rather than achieved. In their view, the transition to adulthood was governed by age-related norms; it was not open to negotiation. The assumption was that once young people reach the age of economic independence they are no longer subject to the norms imposed on younger age groups. Thus, by and large, in working-class households parental control is more likely to be exercised overtly through the enforcement of normatively prescribed rules; whereas in middle-class families it is more common to find maternal communication strategies used as a covert means of regulating young people's behaviour.

Studies of the health beliefs and health status of young people can provide important information for those involved in delivering healthcare, designing health education programmes and organising health promotion activities. As Brannen *et al.* assert, 'The state of the nation's health in the future depends upon the fitness of today's teenagers. If young people are to lead healthier lives, strategies are required which match the complexity of their lives' (1994, p. 214). Healthcare professionals need to understand how the responsibility for young people's health is shared between parents and their teenage children, and how gender, culture and social class can influence the health status of young people.

Childhood and adolescence: the contemporary context

The state of childhood is one of the recurring topics of our times. Today's children and young people live in an era of rapid change, which poses particular challenges for their growth and development. In this climate, there is growing concern about the health and well-being of our children. Politicians, academia and the media alike ponder how best to bring up the nation's children.

(Children's Society, 2006, p. 4)

Childhood lifestyles and electronic media

In September 2006 the Children's Society published a report launching a national inquiry into childhood in the UK. The report recorded findings from a 2005 national survey of over 8,000 young people, between the ages of 14 and 16 years, living in England. The two principal aims of the survey were to explore young people's views on the quality of their lives and identify what issues and problems caused them most concern. In the context of health, social welfare and general well-being, Bob Reitemeier, Chief Executive of the Children's Society, made the following observation in the foreword to the launch report:

> Our children and young people suffer from higher incidences of mental and physical ill-health than their European contemporaries. As a society we share a damaging ambivalence towards children: preoccupied with protecting our own children from harm, we often fail to reach out to those who need our attention most. And all the while our young people are continually subjected to pressure to achieve, behave and even consume like adults at an ever earlier age.

(Children's Society, 2006, p. 2)

The survey findings formed the backdrop to the national Good Childhood Inquiry and helped to inform the purpose, focus and thematic structure of the exercise.

An independent panel of experts was commissioned to conduct the inquiry and its members were drawn from a number of disciplinary backgrounds including child health, child psychiatry, social policy, economics and education. The panel considered evidence from a wide variety of sources such as expert reviews of the research literature, opinion polls and sample surveys, focus groups and specially commissioned research studies. Evidence was gathered from over 30,000 individuals, at least two-thirds of whom were children and young people. Emphasis was focused on the following aspects of childhood: family; lifestyle; values; schooling; mental health; inequality. The findings describe some of the major changes in family and social life over the last 50 years and how these have impacted upon children. Some of the main points are summarised in Box 5.5.

It is within the general context of these wider social changes that the lifestyles of individuals and groups are fashioned. The concept of lifestyle embraces the general manner in which people live their lives; it encompasses their interests, attitudes, activities and actual behaviour. It is a feature that is focused upon when assessing the quality of life. However, there is no single lifestyle that is characteristic of childhood or adolescence. Lifestyles have complex origins and manifest themselves in a variety of ways. They are influenced by a range of factors including family background and upbringing, social class location, cultural milieu and religious affiliation. At the same time, lifestyles are also shaped by the

Box 5.5   Research findings

The Good Childhood Inquiry

Family

- The majority of women now work outside the home. In Britain 70% of mothers with 9–12 month old babies now do some paid work. The comparable figure twenty-five years ago was 25%.
- As a result of increased family break-up, a third of British 16 year olds now live apart from their biological father.

Lifestyle

- Compared to fifty years ago, children today have more money, more leisure time and access to new technologies. They inhabit a 'new youth culture'.
- On average children spend 17 hours a week watching television and four hours a week playing video games or using a computer. An estimated 80% of 5 to16 year olds have their own TV and 70% have access to the internet. Two out of every three children have their own mobile phone.
- Levels of obesity are rising. It is estimated that if current trends continue, by 2023 there will be a 54% rise in Type II diabetes and by 2051 life expectancy will fall by five years.

Values

- A perceived decline in a sense of, and commitment to, the notion of social obligation means that confidence in values such as generosity and fairness has been eroded. These values are more difficult to foster in a climate of excessive individualism where the underlying belief is that everything will work out all right if everybody looks after themselves.

Schooling

- Educational inequality is evident in the school system. In 2006 only 28% of children in the most deprived quarter of schools gained five or more good GCSE passes at A*-C. The comparable figure in the least deprived quarter of schools was 67%.

Mental Health

- One in ten 5–16 year olds now has clinically significant mental health difficulties (ranging from anxiety, depression, attention deficit hyperactivity disorder and anorexia through to conduct disorders such as uncontrollable or destructive behaviour).
- Only a quarter of children with mental health difficulties get any specialist help.

Inequality

- In Britain 22% of children are poor (i.e. defined as living below 60% of the typical income). This compares to 8% in Sweden and 10% in Denmark. Thirty years ago the figure for Britain was only 13%.
- Poverty in childhood is one of the five most powerful and consistent predictors of subsequent disadvantage in later life.

Source: Layard, R. and Dunn, J. (2009) *A Good Childhood: Searching for Values in a Competitive Age*, © The Children's Society 2009 availability of, and access to, new technology. The lifestyles of children and teenagers in the contemporary era have been strongly influenced by the expansion of the electronic media, which has led to the emergence of digital lifestyles. A survey of video-game use in the UK found that 95 per cent of ten 6- to 10-year-olds and 98 per cent of 11- to 15-year-olds reported playing such games at least a few times a week. In the latter age group, an average video-game session lasted 2.2 hours (Pratchett, 2005). In the US, Gentile *et al.* (2004) quote average figures for computer game playing of 5 hours and 13 hours per week respectively for adolescent girls and boys.

Growing use of the electronic media and the availability of computer games featuring violence have served to raise concerns in various quarters about children and young people gaining access to potentially harmful or inappropriate material. With respect to the damaging effects of computer games on behaviour, there is a body of psychological research that suggests exposure to violent video games can lead to displays of aggression in real-life situations (Anderson, 2004). Gentile *et al.* (2004) found that teenagers who played violent video games for extended periods were more likely to be confrontational with their teachers, engage in fights with their peers and show signs of a decline in their overall academic performance. However, much research claiming to have established a causal link between computer game-playing and actual behaviour has been criticised on methodological grounds. For example, it has been suggested that the body of research is relatively small, the findings are contradictory, the measures of aggression used are crude, and specific causal factors have not been identified (Boyle and Hibberd, 2005). Establishing causation is crucial in this type of research and careful consideration needs to be given to the design of specific research studies. Researchers need to be able to establish whether it is the case that children display more aggressive behaviour after playing computer games with a violent content or whether children who are already predisposed to behaving in an aggressive manner are more likely to choose to play such games in the first place. A recent review of the research literature on the harmful effects of computer games depicting violence concluded that 'this research has been significantly disputed on methodological and theoretical grounds: it does not amount to a definitive or persuasive body of evidence' (Buckingham *et al.*, 2007, p. 4).

As illustrated in Figure 5.2, reviews of research into the effects of computer games on children report positive as well as negative outcomes (Harris, 2001). Playing computer games can be a cognitively demanding activity and not simply an idle leisure pursuit. According to some researchers, this type of game-playing promotes the development of key cognitive skills such as strategic thinking, hypothesis-testing and problem-solving (Taylor, 2006). A survey conducted in the US explored the correlation between the amount of computer game-playing activity and scores achieved on measures of positive mental health, positive school engagement, engagement in recreational activities and family interaction (Durkin and Barber, 2002). The researchers found that on average those individuals whose game-playing was classified as 'moderate' scored more highly on the aforementioned measures than their counterparts who did not play computer games.

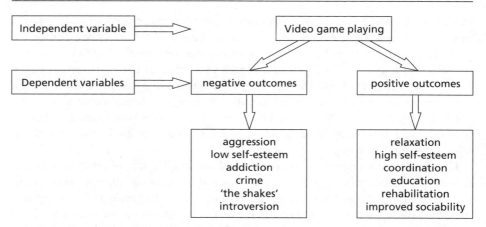

Figure 5.2 The positive and negative effects of computer games on young children
Source: Harris, 2001, p. 13

Furthermore, children and young people who reported a high level of computer game-playing scored no worse on the measures than non-players. The researchers also noted that the majority of young computer game players only played for relatively short periods of time. Consequently, they suggested that playing computers could be viewed as one aspect of an active and well-adjusted lifestyle.

Research to date into the potential harmful consequences or possible beneficial effects of computer games has not produced any definitive and conclusive findings. Indeed, the evidence presented is far from scientifically robust and the research methods employed have their limitations (Freedman, 2002). For example, the relevance of laboratory experiments is questionable when it comes to establishing causal relationships between phenomena in real-life contexts. Where survey methods are used, researchers have to rely on the truthful and accurate reporting of respondents. The research literature is replete with contradictory findings. The situation has been described as one in which '. . . the evidence about effects is weak and inconclusive – and this applies both to positive and negative effects. Of course, this does not in itself mean that such effects do not exist. However, it is fair to conclude that directly harmful effects are significantly less powerful and less frequent than they are often assumed to be, at least by some of the most vocal participants in the public debate' (Buckingham *et al.*, 2007, p. 4).

Computer games represent only one aspect of the electronic media. In recent years attention has be drawn to children's and young people's use of the internet. There is evidence that this use is widespread and growing. Official figures reveal that in 2008 the internet was available in 16 million households in Great Britain (National Statistics Online, 2008). It is estimated that eight out of ten 7- to 16-year-olds in the UK have access to the internet at home and 25 per cent of this group can access the internet in their own room (ChildWise, 2008). By using the internet it is possible gain instant access to a wealth of information, view websites, download music and video images, play multi-player games online and share material with other users. As a medium of communication it offers individual users a degree of anonymity. While these characteristics offer benefits in terms of both providing opportunities for learning and facilitating communication, they are also seen as being potentially harmful and posing a threat to children's safety. Thus, children and young people 'are seen as "the digital generation", being in the vanguard of new skills and opportunities, yet also vulnerable and potentially at risk' (Livingstone and Bober, 2003, p. 5).

In terms of risks, two commonly expressed concerns by parents are that children may access material of a pornographic or violent nature via the internet or come into contact with unknown adults who pose a threat, such as paedophiles. In the case of access to undesirable images, despite the dearth of reliable empirical evidence, 'it would seem uncontroversial to claim that the internet has made it more likely that children will be exposed to pornographic or sexually explicit material' (Buckingham *et al.*, 2007, p. 36). One study in the US found a quarter of 10- to 17-year-olds reporting that they had accidently encountered pictures of a sexual nature when online (Mitchell *et al.*, 2003). Surveys in the UK also reveal that children come across potentially harmful or offensive material without their parents knowing (Livingstone and Bober, 2005). However, researching the impact this exposure has on children is not a particularly easy task for three main reasons. First, there is a difficulty in defining pornography. Not all sexually explicit images are necessarily pornographic. However, in the case of child pornography there is less ambiguity surrounding its definition (Taylor and Quayle, 2003). Second, it is important when determining impact to distinguish between an image causing offence and access to such material actually having harmful consequences in terms of the future behaviour of the individual viewer. Third, ethical and legal considerations restrict the type of research that can be undertaken using children as subjects (Thornburgh and Lin, 2002).

What research findings there are suggest that the majority of children who encounter pornographic images and sexually explicit material on the internet claim not be offended or particularly bothered by the experience (Millwood Hargrave and Livingstone, 2007). Indeed, whether pornographic websites are seen as being problematic by young people is not immediately apparent (Sutter, 2000). However, a significant minority do report that if they accidently or inadvertently encounter pornographic images when online they feel offended, distressed or disgusted. In one survey in the UK around 25 per cent of 7- to 16-year-olds claimed to be upset by sexually explicit online materials; many rarely mentioned their experiences or feelings to an adult (Wigley and Clarke, 2000). Gender is an important issue in this context, as noted by Livingstone and Bober (2003, p. 21): 'While some respondents regard it (online pornography) as unwelcome, especially the younger teenage and mid teen girls, others, especially teenage boys, express curiosity about sexual matters and are not opposed to seeing it'. Consequently, there were mixed views as to whether or not access to pornographic materials should be restricted.

The risk of teenagers being the target of unwanted attention from adult strangers through internet contact is another frequently expressed concern in recent years. This needs to be seen within a wider socio-cultural context. Over the last two decades child safety issues and concerns about the risks and dangers children face during the course of their daily lives have become major issues for parents and society in general (Roberts *et al.*, 1995). For some social theorists this can be understood as part of a wider debate surrounding the social changes of late modernity that have produced the 'risk society' (Beck, 1992). Greater opportunities for individuals to exercise choice have resulted in a weakening of traditional social ties, growing social diversity and changes in institutional structures. As a consequence, social life has become more uncertain and individualised. The traditional supports that once structured a person's life course can no longer be taken as being stable and fixed. In the light of increasing individualisation and mounting uncertainty, 'life becomes in principle a risky venture' (Beck and Beck Gernsheim, 2002, p. 47). This produces feelings of insecurity and fear in relation to many aspects of modern life, which ultimately influences people's behaviour. For example, parents have become increasingly anxious over the safety of their children and in recent times there has been a marked increase in fear over the likelihood of children falling victim to paedophiles. This fearfulness has been fuelled by the publicity given to a small number of disturbing cases (Valentine, 2004) and, as described below, parents have taken action to protect their children from a widely perceived threat.

'While the actual incidence of attacks and abductions has not significantly increased, parents are now much more keen to confine their children to the home – and to furnish them with media and technology that will make the child's bedroom a more attractive alternative to the apparent dangers of the outside world. Ironically, in doing so they have created the possibility that "stranger danger" will now be imported into the apparent safety of the family home.'

(Buckingham *et al.*, 2007, p. 38)

Given that it is impossible to prevent children from being exposed to the potential harmful effects of the electronic media, it is necessary to develop strategies for dealing with the problem. While legislation can be used to control content and various technological devices employed to bar access to certain types of material, there has been a growing interest in recent years in 'media literacy' as a mode of intervention. This is defined as 'the ability to access, understand and create communications in a variety of contexts' (Ofcom, 2009). It is not an alternative to regulation, but an educational strategy in that it seeks to enable children to make informed choices on their own account. As Livingstone and Bober (2003, p. 4) note: 'Being able to make an informed evaluation of online sites and services is crucial if children are both to benefit from online opportunities and to avoid the dangers'. This requires ensuring that children develop a critical understanding of, and an ability to evaluate, media content. Research shows that parents can play an important role in this process by raising awareness of online safety issues (Cho and Cheon, 2005). However, media literacy is not only about teaching children how to make safe and productive use of new media technology, it also raises questions about inequalities in young people's access to the positive opportunities it offers. Research shows that there is a 'digital divide', in so far as access to the internet is stratified, and that the educational and social consequences of this exclusion require further research (Livingstone and Bober, 2003).

Mental health

Good mental health in childhood is about children having the ability to grow and develop emotionally, socially and intellectually in ways, and at a rate, which is considered normal for their age. The terms 'mental health problems' and 'mental health difficulties' are not particularly precise and are used to cover a wide range of conditions from anxieties associated with daily living to psychiatric disorders which impair normal functioning and cause distress. There are also differences in the way these terms are employed by the various professional groups involved in healthcare, social welfare and education. In its provision of guidance to healthcare professionals the British Medical Association distinguishes between a *problem*, a *disorder* and an *illness* as described in Box 5.6 below. While this tripartite definition is helpful for purposes of conceptual clarification, the term 'mental health problems' is often used generically to embrace all three definitions.

From a psychological perspective it is assumed that certain experiences in childhood can make a person more susceptible to mental health problems in later life. Thus it is important to have an understanding of the incidence and prevalence of mental health problems among children and young people. A national survey of child mental health in Great Britain in 2004 revealed an overall prevalence rate approaching 10 per cent, when it found that nearly one in ten children aged between 5 and 16 years had a clinically recognised mental disorder (Green *et al.*, 2005). A similar rate was reported in a national survey conducted five years earlier (Meltzer *et al.*, 2000). However, it is difficult to ascertain trends in prevalence rates over longer periods of time for three main reasons. First, as a result of advances in psychology and psychiatry, definitions of some mental disorders have changed and new methods of assessment have been developed so

---

Box 5.6   Definition

Defining mental health

Mental health **problems**: relatively minor conditions such as sleep disorders or excessive temper tantrums.

Mental health **disorders**: a marked deviation from normality, together with impaired personal functioning or development, and significant suffering.

Mental **illness**: severe forms of psychiatric disorder, particularly of the kind also found in adulthood, for example, schizophrenia, depressive disorders and obsessive disorders.

Source: BMA, 1999

as to render meaningful comparisons over certain time periods as problematic. Second, there has been an increase in the number of people seeking help with mental health problems as a result of the growth in public awareness of such issues. In earlier periods ignorance and the stigma associated with mental disorders may have led to a reluctance to disclose symptoms and seek professional help. Consequently, any observed increase in reported mental health problems may be partly attributed to changes in attitudes and help-seeking behaviour, rather than being seen as representing a 'real' increase in prevalence rates. Finally, not only have definitions of mental disorders changed over time, but there is some variation in the measures used in different surveys. This lack of uniformity in measurement makes trend analysis extremely difficult. The researchers who conducted the 2004 national survey, referred to above, clearly recognised these difficulties when they observed that:

> Estimates of the psychiatric morbidity among young people depend on the choice of concepts as well as how they are operationalised. These, in turn, depend on the particular purposes and aims of the study. This point needs emphasising because it means that estimates from this survey will not necessarily be comparable with those obtained from other studies using different concepts, sampling designs, assessment instruments or analytic methods.
>
> (Green *et al.*, 2005, p. 8)

However, it is possible to make meaningful comparisons between the findings of the two national surveys mentioned here as they employed an identical methodological framework.

Childhood mental disorders fall into three broad diagnostic categories:

1 disruptive disorders (e.g. attention-deficit hyperactivity disorder and conduct disorder);

2 emotional disorders and problems (e.g. depression, generalised anxiety disorder, separation anxiety, obsessive compulsive disorder and phobias);

3 somatic and developmental disorders (e.g. autistic spectrum disorder and eating disorders such as anorexia nervosa and bulimia nervosa).

In the 2004 survey, 6 per cent of children had a conduct disorder, 4 per cent had an emotional disorder and 2 per cent had a hyperkinetic disorder. In nearly 2 per cent of cases children had more than one type of disorder. In other words, among children with a disorder, one in five had two disorders. Overall, as shown in Figure 5.3, there was a gender difference in that boys were more likely to have a mental disorder than girls. The proportions in the 5- to 10-year-old age group were 10 per cent of boys and 5 per cent of girls: figures for 11 to 16 year olds were 13 per cent and 10 per cent respectively (Green *et al.*, 2005). However, patterns of gender disparity vary depending on the type of mental disorder. With regards to conduct problems and hyperkinetic disorders rates are invariably higher for males than for females. In the case of emotional problems there is evidence of a comparative increase in the proportion of girls reporting psychological distress (West and Sweeting, 2003) and low self-esteem (Maughan *et al.*, 2005).

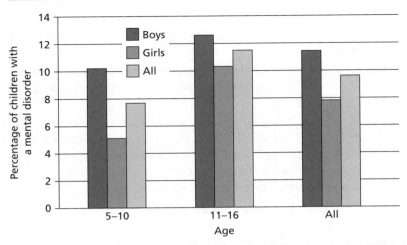

Figure 5.3 Prevalence of any mental disorder by age and sex, 2004, Great Britain

Source: Green *et al.*, 2005, p. 24

Studies have identified a large number of risk factors that increase the vulnerability of children and teenagers to experiencing mental health problems. Factors found to be independently associated with increased rates of childhood mental disorders include characteristics of the child (e.g. physical health problems), family background features (e.g. poor family functioning) and household circumstances (e.g. type of accommodation) (Meltzer, 2007). Material deprivation and social disadvantage are particularly important in this context (Wicks *et al.*, 2005) and a high prevalence of mental health problems is noted among the homeless (BMA, 2003). The relevance of family background factors and socio-economic circumstances is reflected in the results of the 2004 national survey, which found the following:

- Nearly 18 per cent of boys living in one-parent households had a mental disorder; the comparable figure for girls was 13 per cent.
- Children living in families where there were stepchildren (i.e. reconstituted families) were more likely to have a mental disorder than children living in families without stepchildren (the figures were 14 per cent and 9 per cent respectively).
- Twenty per cent of children living in families without a parent in paid employment had a mental disorder: this was more than twice the proportion found among families in which one or both parents were employed (the corresponding figures were 9 per cent and 8 per cent respectively).
- Children living in households where the main wage earner was in a semi-routine or routine occupation were three times as likely to experience mental disorder as children living in families where the householder was from a higher professional group.

- The proportion of children with a conduct disorder was five times higher in families in the routine occupational group than in families in the professional occupational category.
- Children living in rented accommodation (private sector or social housing) were twice as likely to have a mental disorder as those in owner-occupied accommodation.
- The proportion of children classified as having a mental disorder was twice as high among those living in 'hard pressed' areas (i.e. residential neighbourhoods characterised by low income and high levels of unemployment) as it was among children living in the more affluent residential areas classed as 'wealthy achievers' or 'urban prosperity'. (See Figure 5.4.)

The above findings are similar to those reported in an earlier national survey conducted in 1999 (Meltzer *et al.*, 2000).

Risk factors increase the probability of a child developing a mental health problem and the more severe the risk, the greater the likelihood of a negative impact on their quality of life and subsequent mental health. Furthermore, there is also evidence which suggests that such risks can be cumulative.

> If a child has only one risk factor in their life, their probability of developing a mental health problem has been defined as being 1–2%. However, with three risk factors it is thought that the likelihood increases to around 8%; and with four or more risk factors in their life this increases to 20%.
>
> (Department for Education and Skills, 2001, p. 3)

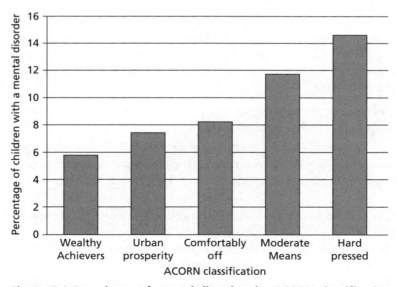

Figure 5.4 Prevalence of mental disorders by ACORN classification, 2004, Great Britain

Source: Green *et al.*, 2005, p. 31. For details of ACORN (A Classification of Residential Neighbourhoods) see http://www.caci.co.uk/ACORN/acornmap.asp (accessed 22 March 2009)

These risk factors may be located in the child, the family or the community, as outlined in Box 5.7 below.

While there is a wealth of research identifying the presence of risk factors and their association with the occurrence of mental health problems in childhood and adolescence, our knowledge as to exactly how these factors cause the mental health problems they do is less well established. Indeed, the risk factors may work in different ways depending on where they are located (i.e. in the child, the family or the wider community). For example, in the case of particularly young children who are dependent on their parents and do not have a network of contacts

---

Box 5.7 Research findings

Risk factors for child mental health

The Child

- Specific learning difficulties
- Communication difficulties
- Specific developmental delay
- Genetic influence
- Difficult temperament
- Physical illness especially if chronic and/or neurological
- Academic failure
- Low self-esteem

The Family

- Overt parental conflict
- Family breakdown
- Inconsistent or unclear discipline
- Hostile or rejecting relationships
- Failure to adapt to a child's changing needs
- Physical, sexual or emotional abuse
- Parental psychiatric diagnosis
- Parental criminality, alcoholism or personality disorder
- Death and loss – including loss of friendship

The Community

- Socio-economic disadvantage
- Homelessness
- Disaster
- Discrimination
- Other significant life events

Source: Department for Education and Skills, 2001, p. 4

outside the immediate family, risk factors centring on the family may prove to be of primary import. However, as children grow older, their experiences at school and in the wider community may come to have a greater influence in their lives and problems encountered in these areas will have more of a direct effect on them. There is also the question as to how, in cases where children face multiple difficulties, constellations of risk factors are identified around specific mental problems and disorders.

The risk factors identified above are not absolute. Not all children facing the difficulties described go on to develop mental health problems. There are marked differences in vulnerability that need to be taken into account. Vulnerability can be understood by considering what might be termed *protective* factors; these are those characteristics that serve to increase children's resilience in the face of risk. Research into resilience focuses attention on positive outcomes for individuals and explores those factors associated with overcoming adversities (Howard *et al.*, 1999). As such, the concept of resilience refers to a dynamic process whereby individuals display an ability to successfully function despite being faced with difficult and challenging circumstances. From a psychological perspective, childhood resilience represents the capacity of an individual child to progress at a normal rate through a sequence of developmental stages despite encountering one or more disruptive life events such as family breakdown. However, resilience is not perceived simply as a fixed personal attribute of an individual (although attributes of the child may act as internal protective factors). Account needs to be taken of the fact that risk alters in the light of changing circumstances (Rutter, 1990). As described above, resilience is not a static concept but is best understood from a dynamic perspective. Where there is an increase in the number of stressful life events experienced by an individual, there is a need for more protective factors to act as a counterbalance. Consequently, resilience can be perceived as 'a two-dimensional construct defined by the constellations of exposure to adversity and the manifestation of successful adaptation in the face of that risk' (Schoon, 2006, p. 7).

As with risk factors, protective factors cover the three broad areas of the child, the family and the community (see Box 5.8). From the perspective of the child, the important factors are having a sense of self-esteem, a belief in one's own self-efficacy, the ability to cope with change and the skills to solve problems (Rutter, 1985). These may be referred to as internal factors. Protective factors external to the child and located in the family include an emotionally stable home environment, an effective parenting style and adequate resources to enable parents to spend leisure time with their children (Howard *et al.*, 1999). As regards the wider community, relevant factors include having access to social support networks (formal and informal), experiencing a happy school life, enjoying a varied social life and having a close circle of friends (Barnes and Morris, 2007).

Although the concept of childhood resilience takes into account external protective factors (i.e. those relating to family and household circumstances and the wider community), there is a strong emphasis on the personal attributes of the individual child when it comes to explaining success in overcoming adversities.

Box 5.8   Research findings

Resilience factors for child mental health

The Child

- Secure early relationships
- Being female
- Higher intelligence
- Easy temperament when an infant
- Positive attitude, problem-solving approach
- Good communication skills
- Planner, belief in control
- Humour
- Religious faith
- Capacity to reflect

The Family

- A least one good parent–child relationship
- Affection
- Clear, firm and consistent discipline
- Support for education
- Supportive long-term relationship/absence of severe discord

The Community

- Wider social network
- Good housing
- High standard of living
- High morale school with positive policies for behaviour, attitudes and anti-bullying
- Schools with strong academic and non-academic opportunities
- Range of positive sport/leisure activities

Source: Department for Education and Skills, 2001, pp. 5–6

The danger here is that it is all too easy to view resilience as a personal trait, rather than seeing it as a capacity for adaptation that is the result of a complex, dynamic process involving a variety of internal and external factors. Focusing on the characteristics of the individual can lead to a victim-blaming perspective, which fails to appreciate the significance of protective factors associated with socio-economic circumstances and access to social support networks in the community (Luthar and Zelazo, 2003). There is clearly a need for research that is directed at levels of analysis other than the individual. As Mohaupt states in her review of the concept of resilience, in order to obtain a better understanding of how

Box 5.9 Policy

What the outcomes mean

Be healthy

- Physically healthy
- Mentally and emotionally healthy
- Sexually healthy
- Healthy lifestyles
- Choose not to take illegal drugs

Parents, carers and families promote healthy choices

Stay safe

- Safe from maltreatment, neglect, violence and sexual exploitation
- Safe from accidental injury and death
- Safe from bullying and discrimination
- Safe from crime and anti-social behaviour in and out of school
- Have security, stability and are cared for

Parents, carers and families provide safe homes and stability

Enjoy and achieve

- Ready for school
- Attend and enjoy school
- Achieve stretching national educational standards at primary school
- Achieve personal and social development and enjoy recreation
- Achieve stretching national educational standards at secondary school

Parents, carers and families support learning

Make a positive contribution

- Engage in decision-making and support the community and environment
- Engage in law-abiding and positive behaviour in and out of school
- Develop positive relationships and choose not to bully and discriminate
- Develop self-confidence and successfully deal with significant life changes and challenges
- Develop enterprising behaviour

Parents, carers and families promote positive behaviour

Achieve economic well-being

- Engage in further education, employment or training on leaving school
- Ready for employment
- Live in decent homes and sustainable communities
- Access to transport and material goods
- Live in households free from low income

Parents, carers and families are supported to be economically active

Source: Adapted from Department for Education and Skills, 2004, p. 9

people cope with adversities there is a need for 'more research with different levels of analysis such as networks, organisations and policies' (Mohaupt, 2008, p. 67).

Policy context

Child health and welfare issues have been at the forefront of childcare policy in recent years. The Government's policy strategy in this regard reflects a commitment to the general principles and basic health and welfare articles contained in the United Nations Convention on the Rights of the Child. In 2003 the Green Paper *Every Child Matters* was published. In this document the Government expressed its commitment to improving social, economic and welfare outcomes for all children and young people, especially those considered to be disadvantaged. The following year the Government published *Every Child Matters: Change for Children*, outlining a national framework for building services around the needs of children and young people (Department for Education and Skills, 2004). Five broad outcomes were regarded as being central to the well-being of children and young people from birth to 19 years of age:

* being healthy;
* staying safe;
* enjoying and achieving;
* making a positive contribution;
* achieving economic well-being.

What these outcomes mean and the types of support children need from parents, carers and families in order to achieve them are outlined in Box 5.9. The outcomes were given legal force in the Children Act 2004. In the case of England, the Act placed a duty on key agencies and service providers to safeguard and promote the welfare of children. Furthermore, local authorities were given responsibility for encouraging and facilitating agencies working together to improve children's well-being as defined by the five outcomes identified. The Act also introduced a Children's Commissioner to champion the interests of children and young people.

The Government's key ambition behind the new policy strategy is to 'make England the best place for children to grow up' by 2020 (Department of Health, 2009, p. 3). The first ever *Children's Plan*, introduced in 2007, was initiated within the Department for Children, Schools and Families, and is based on five guiding principles:

1 Government does not bring up children, parents do – so government needs to do more to back parents and families.

2 All children have the potential to succeed and should go as far as their talents can take them.

3 Children and young people should enjoy their childhood as well as growing up prepared for adult life.

4 Services should be shaped by and responsive to children, young people and families, not designed around professional boundaries.

5 It is always better to prevent failure than tackle a crisis later.

(Department of Health, 2009, p. 20)

The outcomes framework of the Children's Plan was revised in 2008 to include goals for 2020. In terms of enhancing the health of children at key transition points in childhood and adolescence, a major goal is to reduce the proportion of obese and overweight children to the levels found in 2000. As for children achieving economic well-being, the primary aim is to reduce by one half the number of children in poverty by 2010 and eradicate child poverty by 2020.

While the Children's Plan and the Child Health Strategy are intended to improve outcomes for all children and young people, the Government wishes to focus particular attention on children with special educational needs and children in public care. The policy strategy is also aimed at reducing the incidence of teenage pregnancy and reducing the proportion of 16- to 18-year-olds not in education, employment or training. By improving the five listed outcomes it is hoped that the gap between socially and materially disadvantaged children and their more comfortably off peers will be reduced.

Summary

- Developmental theories use the concept of the life cycle in describing human growth and development as an orderly and predictable passage through clearly demarcated stages marked by chronological age.

- Critics of the life cycle approach claim that it is unrealistic to assume that there is uniformity in the way people pass through life. They propose the life course as an alternative concept, which allows for individual differences, cultural diversity and historical variation in the ageing process.

- Childhood can be defined as more than a biologically determined stage in the transition to adulthood. From a sociological perspective childhood is viewed as a social construct. There is no one universal definition of childhood. Its definition can vary from one society to another and from one period in history to another. The notion of childhood with which we are familiar today is very much a twentieth century invention.

- Traditional approaches, such as the functionalist perspective, view childhood as a critical stage in the socialisation process. The child is portrayed as a pre-social being who plays a passive role in learning to embrace the norms and values of society. This is described as a crucial step, which serves to ensure that the individual becomes a conforming member of society. Whilst not denying the existence of child socialisation, critics maintain that functionalism tends to overlook the fact that children are active participants in primary socialisation. Until fairly recently, the process has been explored from the point of view of parenting and the needs of society, thus effectively ignoring the possibility of taking the child's view of the world as the focus of study.

- According to the new paradigm for the sociological study of childhood, children are not 'passive socialisation vessels' but active social participants. In the context of health care, children are depicted as 'embodied actors, seeking to maintain their health' (Mayall, 1998a, p. 276).

- Children's claims to the sick role are subject to evaluation by adults. Mothers are the primary carers of sick children and research shows that they are aware that how they deal with claims to sickness is interpreted as a measure of their maternal competence.

- Like childhood, adolescence can be seen as a social construct. However, some social scientists prefer to use the term 'young people' instead of 'adolescents' or 'adolescence', on the grounds that the latter 'tend to have a somewhat derogatory meaning – that the essence of being a young person is not in *being* but in *becoming*' (Brannen *et al.*, 1994, p. 1).

- Research suggests that young people negotiate rules with their parents with respect to a wide range of health-related issues. The nature and extent of this negotiation process is largely determined by the normative views parents have of adolescence. Whereas some parents see the status transition to adulthood as normatively ascribed, others view it as individually achieved. In the case of the former, parents are seen to exercise control overtly by way of the enforcement of normatively prescribed rules. As for the latter, parental control takes a less direct and more covert form through the use of maternal communication strategies. There is some suggestion that social class affects parental views of adolescence.

- There is no single lifestyle characteristic of childhood and adolescence. The lifestyles of children and young people are influenced by social and cultural factors. The development and expansion of the electronic media environment has led to the emergence of 'digital lifestyles'. Research into the harmful or beneficial effects of the electronic media has not produced any conclusive results either way.

- The *risk* factors and *protective* factors associated with mental health in childhood relate to the characteristics of the child, the circumstances of the family and the social and economic features of the community.

- The first decade of this century has witnessed much activity in the field of child welfare and child health policy including the *Every Child Matters* policy initiative, the introduction of a *Children's Plan* and the passing of the Children Act 2004.

Questions for discussion

1 Compare and contrast the concepts of 'life course' and 'life cycle'.
2 On what grounds is it possible to challenge the functionalist approach to primary socialisation?

3 What implications does the viewing of childhood as a social construct have for the sociological study of children?

4 How does knowledge of the 'focal concerns' of adolescence help us to understand this period of the life course?

5 How might children be seen as active participants in healthcare work and what implications does this have for those professionals engaged in the planning and delivery of healthcare services?

6 What part do adults play in assessing children's claims to the sick role?

7 Do children and young people lead healthier lifestyles today than they did fifty years ago?

8 Are internal or external factors more important when considering childhood resilience?

9 Is the electronic media damaging to children's health and well-being?

10 What constitutes a 'good childhood' and what policies can help to bring it about?

Further reading

Brannen, J., Dodd, K., Oakley, A. and Storey, P. (1994) *Young People, Health and Family Life*, Buckingham: Open University Press.

British Medical Association (2006) *Child and Adolescent Mental Health: A Guide for Healthcare Professionals*, London: BMA. Available at: http://www.bma.org.uk/images/ChildAdolescentMentalHealth_tcm41-20748.pdf (accessed 20 March 2009).

Coleman, J. and Hagnell, A. (eds) (2007) *Adolescence, Risk and Resilience: Against the Odds*, Chichester: John Wiley and Sons Ltd.

Corsaro, W. A. (2004) *The Sociology of Childhood*, 2nd edn, Thousand Oaks, CA: Pine Forge Press.

Hendry, L., Shucksmith, J., Love, J. and Glendinning, A. (1993) *Young People's Leisure and Lifestyles*, London: Routledge.

James, A. and Prout, A. (eds) (1997) *Constructing and Reconstructing Childhood: Contemporary Issues in the Sociological Study of Childhood*, 2nd edn, London: Falmer Press.

Kehily, M. J. (2008) *Childhood Studies: An Introduction*, 2nd edn, Maidenhead: Open University Press.

Mayall, B. (1996) *Children, Health and the Social Order*, Buckingham: Open University Press.

Wyness, M. (2006) *Childhood and Society: An Introduction to the Sociology of Childhood*, Basingstoke: Palgrave Macmillan.

Useful websites

Barnardo's: http://www.barnardos.org.uk/
ChildWise: http://www.childwise.co.uk/index.htm
Department of Health: Children's National Service Framework: http://www.dh.gov.uk/en/Healthcare/NationalServiceFrameworks/Children/DH_4089111
Department for Children, Schools and Families: http://www.dcsf.gov.uk/

Every Child Matters: Change For Children: http://www.everychildmatters.gov.uk/
Office for National Statistics, National Statistics Online: http://www.statistics.gov.uk/default.asp
NHS Information Centre: http://www.ic.nhs.uk/
The Children's Society: http://www.childrenssociety.org.uk
UNICEF, Convention on the Rights of the Child: http://www.unicef.org/crc/

CHAPTER 6

Later life

An ageing population

The population of the United Kingdom is ageing. In 2001, for the first time in the United Kingdom, there were more people aged over 60 than under 16. By 2051, an estimated one in four people will be aged over 65. Much debate on the ageing population has focused on the challenges it presents. We believe that, just as society has adjusted to accommodate the demographic changes that have been experienced so far, so too will it adjust to accommodate the challenges of the future.

(Select Committee on Economic Affairs, 2003, p. 5)

Changing age structure of the UK population

During the course of the last century the population of the UK saw a marked growth in the proportion of elderly people. Between 1911 and 2005 the percentage of people over 65 years of age increased over threefold, from 5.2 per cent to 16 per cent. The UK population as a whole is ageing. In recent decades in particular there has been an increase in the number of people aged 65 years and over and a decrease in the younger age groups. For example, in 1971 a quarter of the population (14.3 million) were under 16 years of age and 13 per cent of the population (7.4 million) were aged 65 years or over. By 2005 the number of people in the younger age group had *fallen* by 2.7 million, while the older age group had *risen* by 2.2 million. It is estimated that by 2014, for the first time ever, the population of the UK will contain more people aged 65 and over than aged 16 years and under. This trend is likely to continue into the third decade of this century (Office for National Statistics, 2007b, p. 3).

The population pyramids in Figure 6.1 illustrate how the age profile and sex structure of the population of Great Britain changed between 1821 and 2005. In 1821 there was a marked decline in the population with increasing age; each successive ten-year age band contained fewer people than the previous one. The

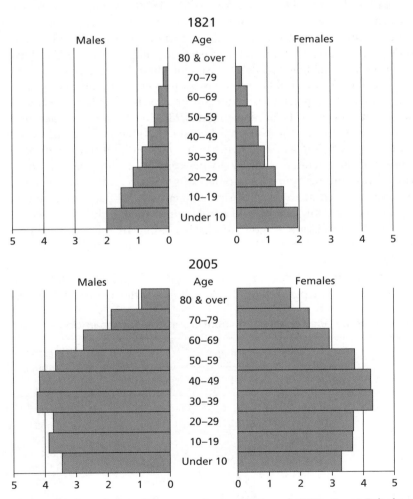

Figure 6.1 Population: by sex and age, 1821 and 2005, Great Britain, millions
Source: Office for National Statistics, 2007b, p. 3

age profile in 2005 displays a much more gradual and less regimented decline. In fact, there are increases in population numbers for people in their thirties and forties.

Two explanations can be advanced for this increase in the relative size of the older age groups. The first and most significant factor is the falling fertility rate, which has reduced the numbers in the younger age groups. The fertility rate has been below replacement level since 1973 (Smallwood and Chamberlain, 2005). The impact of fluctuations in the birth rate on the age structure of the population is illustrated in Figure 6.1. The low birth rate experienced in the late 1970s is represented by the indentation in the 20–29-year-old age group, while the bulge in the age profile, at 30 to 48 years, is a consequence of the 'baby boom' of the mid-1950s to the end of the 1960s. Population ageing will continue over the next few decades as those born in the 'baby boom' of the 1960s reach retirement age and are replaced by smaller numbers in the working population (Bray, 2008).

The second explanation relates to the fall in mortality rates in the older age groups and the overall improvement in life expectancy. Figures for the UK show that at the mid-point of the first decade of the twenty-first century, given current mortality rates, at age 65 men could expect to live a further 16.9 years and women a further 19.7 years. This represents a significant improvement in life expectancy among older adults since the beginning of the 1980s of 4 years for men and 2.8 years for women (Office for National Statistics, 2008c). More and more people are surviving 'early old age' and living to be 'very old'. Of those men born at the *beginning* of the twentieth century 15 per cent lived until their eightieth birthday; the corresponding figure for women was 35 per cent. It is estimated that of those people born at the *end* of the last century, 75 per cent of males and just over 80 per cent of females will survive until their eightieth birthday. Furthermore, of those individuals born at the beginning of this century, it is estimated that 30 per cent of those who reach 80 years of age will live to be 100 (Dini and Goldring, 2008).

Falls in both birth rates and death rates have produced ageing populations in many modern societies (Harper, 2006). Table 6.1 shows the age breakdown of

Table 6.1 Population by age for selected countries in the European Union, 2005

	Percentages			Total (=100%) Thousands
	Under 15	15–64	65 and over	
France	18.7	65.1	16.2	62,371
Germany	14.5	66.9	18.6	82,501
Ireland	20.7	68.1	11.2	4,109
Italy	14.1	66.4	19.5	58,462
Spain	14.5	68.7	16.8	43,038
UK	18.1	65.9	16.0	60,060
All EU countries	16.2	67.1	16.7	461,331

Source: Adapted from Office for National Statistics, 2007b, Table 1.4, p. 4

the population for selected countries in Europe. Italy has the largest proportion of people aged 65 years and over and Ireland has the lowest percentage of people in this age group.

Old age: a public burden?

There is a tendency among demographers, policy-makers and economists to interpret the increase in the proportion of elderly people in the population as constituting an economic burden on society. However, simply measuring the proportion of the population aged 65 or over does not take into account changes in the relative size of the other age groups. Consequently, in an effort to find a more accurate indicator of population change and predict its implications for future public expenditure on health and welfare services, an old-age dependency ratio is constructed. This is based on the population aged 65 and over as a percentage of those in the working age group, i.e. 16 to 64 years of age. The ratio is used as an indicator of economic potential: a low dependency ratio implies that there are relatively more workers (i.e. taxpayers) to support the dependent population of pensioners.

The ratio of persons of working age to persons of pensionable age has declined from 8.6 to 1 in the 1920s to 3.3 to 1 in 2006 and is estimated to decline to 2.9 to 1 by 2031 (Coleman and Salt, 1992, p. 546; Office for National Statistics, 2007c, p. 3). In terms of the provision of pensions and healthcare it is argued that an increasing proportion of retired people are imposing a growing financial burden upon a shrinking working population. The situation is exacerbated by the relative increase in the numbers of very old people, as the costs of meeting the medical and social needs of the elderly rise exponentially with age. It is in the field of geriatric medicine that significant progress has been made in easing suffering and improving the chances of survival.

This idea that the elderly constitute a costly burden on the state has been a constant theme in the political debate surrounding public expenditure since the second half of the last century. Expenditure on social security accounts for nearly one-third of total government expenditure and almost 50 per cent of this is directed at the elderly (Walker, 1986a). Curbing public sector expenditure was seen as the key to Britain's economic difficulties by Conservative governments in the 1980s. The policy of community care was introduced as a way of reducing costs (Department of Health, 1989). The prevalence of a discourse of dependency has served to foster a negative image of old age as an inevitable time of declining physical and mental health, increasing service need and financial hardship. The very word 'dependency' is emotionally charged especially when used in reference to the care of the elderly. As observed by Fine and Glendinning '. . . while "care" is a heart-warming concept with a positive valance, dependency is cold and its connotations are almost entirely negative. Those identified as dependent are assumed actively to seek to reverse their status' (2005, p. 605). Such are the perceived costs of providing for an increasingly dependent ageing population that the elderly are sometimes viewed as a problem for society.

The focus placed on the negative features of old age and the interpretation of the elderly as representing a public burden can be challenged on a number of grounds:

- Thane (1989) argues that we need to separate fact from speculation when determining the social and economic costs of dependency resulting from a change in the age structure of the population. She asserts that there is evidence to suggest that throughout the 1960s and 1970s 'the share of national resources going to the elderly has *not* risen proportionately with their numbers' (Thane, 1989, p. 65, emphasis in original). Also the anticipated rise in the number of elderly dependants in the first quarter of the twenty-first century is to some extent offset by a projected fall in the number of young dependants. Furthermore she maintains that general improvements in health currently enjoyed by younger age groups will ensure that they will experience a healthier old age, thus predicting a fall in per capita expenditure on health and social services.

- The old-age dependency ratio is a particularly crude indicator of the economic costs incurred by an ageing population. For example, it excludes those people aged 15 years and under, who also constitute a dependent sector of the population. Furthermore, the ratio does not take into account actual economic activity. Not all of those people in the 16- to 64-year-old age group are in paid employment; included in this group are full-time informal carers, the unemployed, those unable to work because of poor health or disability and people who have chosen to take early retirement.

- The old-age dependency ratio also ignores the fact that some people over pensionable age remain in the labour force as full-time or part-time workers. Others engage in a variety of unpaid activities, such as looking after elderly relatives, caring for grandchildren whose parents are working, or working for a voluntary organisation. Although for the purpose of calculating the dependency ratio they are not considered economically active, they do constitute a significant resource in so far as they provide (unpaid) supportive services for those who are active in the labour force, and provide care for those who would otherwise be dependent on state provision.

- There is an assumption inherent in dependency ratio calculations that *all* paid employment is of equal economic and social worth. As one critic has commented: 'Is the making and selling of hard drugs, pornography or "stink bombs" to count equally with the production of wholesome food and nursing skill? And what about the work which is done and valued but not paid for (like informal care and domestic labour)? Not only are the dependency ratio calculations simplistic and inaccurate, they embody a set of values which leave much to be desired' (Johnson, 1990, p. 220).

Clearly, it is erroneous to conceive of the elderly as simply dependent upon others. The old-age dependency ratio is a fairly crude measure, which concentrates on some of the basic economic costs involved whilst ignoring the nature and extent of the contribution made by the elderly both before and after retirement.

Theoretical perspectives on old age

> Many theories of ageing and older age have focused on the negative aspects of growing
> older, such as ill health and poverty . . . While there is no doubt that certain groups of
> older people suffer from poor health and poor financial status or both, it is not true
> that all older people are poor and sick.
>
> (Hyde *et al.*, 2004, p. 280)

The study of the social aspects of ageing, often referred to as social gerontology,
is a multi-disciplinary enterprise, which rather than attempt to develop its own
body of theory has relied heavily on theoretical perspectives generated in sociology and psychology. As Fennell *et al.* (1988) remark, social gerontologists have
seemed to be preoccupied with describing the lifestyles and behaviour patterns
of older people, rather than investigating the relationship between ageing and
the economic, social and political aspects of the society in which they live. In this
section the emphasis will be on how sociological concepts and perspectives have
made a contribution to the study of ageing.

Disengagement theory

This was one of the first theoretical perspectives to influence thinking in social
gerontology. The theory was originally proposed by Cumming and Henry (1961)
in an attempt to understand the changes that take place in the life of individuals
as they become older. Old age, which is characterised by a gradual and inevitable
withdrawal or disengagement from the mainstream of social activity, is viewed as
a developmental stage in its own right. On one level the theory is psychological,
in that it refers to individuals becoming introspective and self-preoccupied in
later life. However, a sociological dimension to the theory is revealed when the
process of disengagement is placed within a wider social context. This clearly
places the theory within a functionalist frame of reference.

According to disengagement theorists, on reaching old age individuals find they
have fewer social roles to perform and they experience a reduction in the number
and variety of social contacts. This is largely a result of retirement from work and
their changing position in the life cycle of the family. Thus in one sense old age
is characterised as a time of loss: 'Disengagement is a triple withdrawal: a loss of
roles, a contraction of contact and a decline in commitment to norms and values'
(Cumming, 1963, quoted in Townsend, 1986, p. 18).

However, this social withdrawal is seen as having a positive side; it provides
a solution, at the level of both the individual and society, to some of the problems
of adjustment to old age. The individual and society are considered to withdraw
from each other in a mutually satisfying way. The elderly individual is released
from previously demanding social roles and relieved of the pressure produced
by attempting to compete with younger people in an increasingly competitive world.
Successful disengagement is beneficial to society in general in that it ensures that
the eventual death of the individual does nothing to disrupt the smooth running
of the social system. Thus by freeing individuals from certain social expectations

and obligations, and legitimating a form of social redundancy, the process of disengagement is seen as functional for both individuals and society.

The disengagement theory of ageing has attracted strong criticism on a number of counts.

1 There is a lack of empirical evidence to support the theory

In a survey of old age in the USA, Britain and Denmark, Shanas *et al.* (1968) were unable to find any evidence of a significant reduction in the number or range of social activities of those old people who were in good health and maintained a reasonable level of income. Any observed decrease in social interaction was attributable to increasing physical infirmity in the older age groups. There was nothing to suggest that social disengagement constituted a widespread phenomenon. Indeed they discovered examples of integrating forces at work, as indicated in the following:

> Bereavement is perhaps the most important isolating experience in old age and yet even this, as at other ages, draws a chain of 'reintegrating' responses from family and community.
>
> (Shanas *et al.* 1968, p. 286)

Similarly, early studies of retirement cast doubt on the assumption, inherent in disengagement theory, that social withdrawal is positively welcomed by the elderly and considered to be a natural and normal part of the life course. Townsend (1957) describes the sense of loss, feelings of worthlessness and disorientation experienced by men on entering retirement. More recent studies show how for some individuals, given the right circumstances, withdrawal from full-time employment can lead to continued engagement through the development of new social relationships and activities and permit more time to be devoted to existing leisure pursuits (Atchley, 1972; Phillipson, 1987). As observed by Barnes and Parry: 'Whereas retirement has previously been conceptualised in terms of the loss of a social role, it is now more widely recognised that it entails the opportunity to acquire new roles (such as volunteer or part-time worker), and to continue in other roles (such as parent or friend)' (2004, pp. 217–18).

2 The theory does not consider how social and economic factors affect adjustment to old age

Disengagement theory does not explore how access to financial resources or the nature of the social circumstances in which people live their lives influences how successfully they adjust to old age. Indeed according to the theory, disengagement is a feature of the normal ageing process that occurs irrespective of ill health or poverty. A view that has not gone unchallenged:

> It is not ageing *per se* which determines disengagement, but a combination of factors associated with ageing (e.g. poor health, widowhood) and other factors associated with the nature of society and one's location in it which together influence engagement or disengagement.
>
> (Hochschild, 1975, quoted in Fennell *et al.*, 1988, p. 48)

What is being suggested here is that how old people respond to old age is not the inevitable outcome of a natural process of ageing but is determined by a number of factors, one of which relates to the position of the elderly person in the social structure and the implications this has for their socio-economic status and lifestyle. This approach acknowledges that successful adjustment to old age will in part be determined by structural factors. For those individuals with adequate financial support, disengagement may be seen as an ideal opportunity for self-directed activity. Those who are less fortunate may experience forced retirement as a struggle to make ends meet. It is difficult to see how disengagement can fulfil an adaptive function for the individual when for some people retirement has negative consequences.

3 The theory is gender biased

In its original formulation the theory appears to be based on the experiences of men. The assumption is that men find it more difficult to cope with disengagement than women do because they suffer considerably more disruption to their lives when they retire. It is argued that because women are far less likely to have been engaged in full-time paid employment they do not experience the same level of role loss as men in old age. Whereas men are faced with finding new roles, women continue to perform many of their established roles as they enter later life. However, since the 1950s, when this theory was first developed, the pattern of women's working lives has changed and they now account for a larger percentage of the labour force. Therefore if disengagement does occur it can no longer simply be assumed that the experience is less disruptive for women.

4 The theory can be used to justify discrimination

The disengagement thesis centres on the presumed inevitability of the disengagement process, which along with the belief that the elderly welcome the opportunity to be relieved of their obligations to society, is used to justify the way the elderly are treated in society. A bio-medical model of ageing prevails, in which the problems of old age are attributed to the natural consequences of physical deterioration and declining mental ability or to the failure of individuals to make the necessary adjustments in later life. This seems to preclude any serious questioning of those discriminatory practices that exclude and effectively marginalise the elderly. Disengagement is presented as a natural phenomenon; a process that should not be prevented from running its course. On the basis of this logic policy-makers are exhorted to develop policies that facilitate the process of social withdrawal, as this is deemed to be in the interests of both the individual and society.

5 The belief that disengagement is desirable is questionable

Finally, the claim that disengagement is desirable for the individual appears to be questionable when one takes into account the ways in which the elderly compensate for losses of role and resist the opportunity to 'disengage'. Retirement may lead to a reduction in social contacts as workplace friendships are lost, but this does not necessarily lead to social withdrawal. Elderly people may develop new relationships or increase their level of contact with relatives and friends. As Townsend states, '*Extensive* social interaction may be gradually replaced by *intensive* local interaction, involving many fewer people' (Townsend, 1973, p. 230).

The weight of criticism that has been levelled against disengagement theory has led one critic to observe that it is more appropriate to refer to 'industrial disengagement and increased socio-economic dependence' rather than 'social disengagement' (Bromley, 1974, p. 143). This acknowledges the fact that retirement can produce both losses and gains as far as social relationships are concerned. Despite the criticisms, Fennell *et al.* (1988) are reluctant to dismiss the theory entirely. While they agree that there is little evidence to support the existence of disengagement as a universal phenomenon, they are of the opinion that there are aspects of the theory that are worthy of further consideration. For example, a more detailed investigation of the conditions precipitating disengagement may help us to understand how some people come to terms with growing old. However, this need not necessarily involve adopting a functionalist perspective.

Role changes in later life

The concept of role features widely in theorising about the social implications of old age, particularly in relation to how individuals adjust to the role changes encountered in later life. As seen from a functionalist perspective, it is the loss of the work role that causes men to experience uncertainty about their social identity. According to Parsons (1942), they are stranded in a 'functionless situation', not only are they no longer engaged in activity which is culturally defined as purposeful, but they also discover that the ties they have to the wider community are weakened. While disengagement theorists see this role loss as something to be positively welcomed by the elderly, as it reduces demands on their time and energy, other theoretical perspectives focus on *role stability* and *role continuity* as being necessary in order to ensure a successful transition into old age.

Activity theory (Havighurst, 1963) maintains that:

- the majority of elderly people have a natural inclination to continue to pursue an active social life and maintain their links with the wider community.
- role loss leads to a reduction in self-esteem and low morale.
- successful ageing depends on maintaining a high level of activity by ensuring that some roles are preserved and any which are lost are replaced.
- in the interests of psychological and social well-being, retired people should be encouraged to take up activities commensurate with their age, health and personality, which promote continued social involvement.

Whereas disengagement theory encourages older people to relinquish some of the roles characteristic of middle age, activity theory suggests that new roles need to be adopted to prevent disengagement from leading to social isolation. In policy terms, disengagement theory emphasises age segregation, whereas activity theory supports measures designed to achieve the social integration of the elderly.

Not all theoretical perspectives that employ the concept of role to understand the transition into old age emphasise the discontinuities that occur between the earlier and later stages in the life course; some approaches focus on continuities instead. Age stratification theory (Riley *et al.*, 1972) and continuity theory are two examples.

According to **age stratification theory**:

- society is viewed as a system of social roles, in which age is seen as an important determinant of the nature and type of role allocated by society to the individual.

- age forms an underlying dimension of social organisation, such that role transitions are not a matter of individual choice but are influenced by formal and informal age norms which reflect the mainstream social and cultural values of the society.

- it is through the process of socialisation that individuals learn the role expectations and obligations applicable to their age.

- continuities can be observed through membership of a particular age stratum. People at similar points in the life course can be expected to have undergone similar experiences and therefore it is assumed that they will identify with a common set of values. For example, those people who were born in the first decade of the twentieth century were in their twenties at the time of the economic depression in the 1930s; they experienced personal loss and deprivation during the Second World War; they were in middle age when the British economy entered a period of high consumer spending and were in their seventies during the economic recession of the 1980s. These experiences are seen as having an impact on how people evaluate their place in society relative to that of members of other age groups.

Continuity theory asserts that:

- throughout the life course there is considerable continuity from one stage to the next.

- this continuity is maintained by means of anticipatory socialisation, which serves to ensure that individuals are prepared for the social roles they are likely to assume in the future.

- during the course of their lives individuals make efforts to achieve a secure and stable lifestyle. However, this desire for continuity is undermined in later life when the individual encounters major role changes, such as those initiated by retirement and widowhood, for which there is little anticipatory socialisation.

Whereas disengagement theory sees the solution in terms of social withdrawal and activity theory suggests replacing the lost roles with new ones, continuity theory maintains that successful adjustment to the social circumstances of old age will depend on how the individual perceives the situation. In this context, '. . . the decision regarding which roles are to be disregarded and which maintained, will be determined by the individual's past and preferred lifestyle' (Victor, 1987, p. 40).

In continuity theory the individual is seen as exercising some choice as regards role adoption. This is in direct contrast to functionalist accounts, in which social roles are conceived as being rigid sets of normative expectations to which the individual is expected to conform. This move away from the idea of role-taking as a simple process involving the passive acceptance of a socially prescribed role is a fundamental feature of another theoretical tradition in sociology known as the interactionist perspective.

The **interactionist perspective** maintains that:

- it is overly simplistic to argue that individuals are socialised into performing social roles imposed upon them, over which they have no influence.
- formal social roles do exist, but during the process of social interaction with others individuals play an important part in negotiating the roles they perform.
- role behaviour is an outcome of a compromise between the role prescriptions as formalised at the level of the group or society and the negotiations which take place between individuals during the course of social interaction.

According to interactionists, individuals play an active part in the construction of social reality. In learning to play roles they develop a self-concept and a social identity; these are not permanently fixed but are subject to renegotiation and redefinition. Entering different phases of the life course prompts a redefinition of the self. This is particularly pertinent in the case of retirement, as the individual loses an occupational role, which throughout adult life provided a major source of identity.

Political economy perspective

This image of the elderly as creating a problem for society is challenged by the political economy perspective. 'Political economy is understood to be the study of the interrelationships between the polity, economy and society, or more specifically, the reciprocal influences among government . . . the economy, social classes, strata and status groups' (Walton, 1980, quoted in Estes *et al.*, 1982, p. 154). When applied to the study of old age this perspective succeeds in locating the elderly within a wider socio-economic context. Unlike conventional gerontology, with its emphasis on the biomedical model of ageing, the political economy approach sees old age as a socially, as opposed to biologically, constructed status. This is clearly illustrated by Walker in an early attempt at promoting a political economy perspective on ageing:

> Thus rather than concentrating on biologically based differences in ageing and individual adjustment to the ageing process, it would focus on the social creation of dependent status, the structural relationship between the elderly and younger adults and between different groups of the elderly, and the socially constructed relationship between age, the division of labour and the labour market.
>
> (Walker, 1981, p. 75)

This is a structural approach, which focuses on the implications of inequalities in the distribution of income, wealth and power for the experience of old age. According to Walker (1986a), the social construction of old age is a function of two sets of relations.

- Older people do not encounter inequalities for the first time when they enter retirement; on the contrary they carry into old age the inequalities experienced during the earlier stages of the life course.

- The process of retirement itself results in a decline in the social and economic status of many older people when compared with younger adults in full-time employment.

Walker claims that social gerontologists have tended to concentrate on the latter rather than the former when studying dependency in later life.

The political economy perspective has a number of important features.

1 It recognises the diversity within the elderly population

In contrast to functionalist accounts, it avoids treating elderly people as belonging to a distinct social group. The notion of the elderly as forming a homogenous group with special needs and shared interests is a common misconception held by policy-makers (Walker, 1980, 1981; Daatland and Biggs, 2006). There is ample evidence of the existence of social divisions among the elderly. For example, Minkler and Estes (1984) describe how in capitalist societies class remains a major factor in determining access to social resources for the elderly. Class is not the only dimension of stratification to be used to explain the differential experience of ageing among the elderly population. Arber and Ginn (1991a), writing from a feminist perspective, describe ageing as a gendered process, and draw attention to the fact that ageing has different social and economic consequences for men and women. Ethnic minority status is also an important aspect of social stratification. Blakemore (1989) asserts that studies of ethnic minority groups serve to confirm the continued cultural heterogeneity of ageing. There is no evidence to suggest that elderly Asians and African-Caribbean people adopt a common elderly role. Indeed he claims that '. . . as people age they remain ethnically different from each other, or perhaps become more different from each other' (Blakemore, 1989, p. 172). All in all, a political economy perspective helps us to realise that class, gender and ethnicity strongly influence the experience of old age.

2 Dependency is seen as being socially and artificially structured

The political economy perspective offers a radical interpretation of the needs of the elderly. Dependency is not seen as being the inevitable outcome of the ageing process, but is a product of the social structure. This is explained by the concept of 'structured' or 'structural dependency', which draws attention to the macro economic structure and the role society plays in creating dependency (Townsend, 1981, 1986 and Walker, 1982). In Townsend's view the degree of dependency experienced by old people is unnecessary and partly the product of specific economic and social policies pursued by governments:

In the everyday management of the economy and the administration and development of social institutions the position of the elderly is subtly shaped and changed. The policies which determine the conditions and welfare of the elderly are not just the reactive policies represented by the statutory social services but the much more generalised and institutionalised policies of the state which maintain or change social structure.

(Townsend, 1986, p. 22)

Policies promoting early retirement, and increased levels of unemployment, have resulted in elderly people being excluded from engaging in socially valued activities through which they can assert their independence. It is well documented that poverty and the dependent status of the elderly are related to restricted access to resources prior to retirement and the low level of state benefits available following retirement from full-time employment (Walker, 1981).

It is argued that a number of economic and welfare policies have succeeded in creating artificial forms of social dependency among the elderly. For example, Townsend refers to statutory agencies providing domiciliary services in ways that suggest that they see elderly people as passive recipients of welfare provision. Consequently the type of service provided is not always the most likely to meet the needs of the individual and allow scope for self-development. Townsend contends that although policies have aimed to tackle the effects of dependency, some measures have tended to reinforce the dependent status of the elderly and encourage age segregation by presenting a public image of elderly people as non-producers who are reliant on state support.

3 The pathological model of old age is rejected

The political economy perspective rejects what Johnson (1976) has termed the 'pathology model of old age'. This model is characteristic of traditional approaches in gerontology, in which the emphasis is on the needs of the elderly and the problems associated with growing old. Although this problem-oriented approach highlights issues such as role loss, social isolation and disability, and focuses on the extent to which the individual can successfully adjust to the physical, emotional and psychological changes encountered in later life, the problems are not viewed in a wider structural context. The model has a tendency to 'psychologise the problems of old age', whereas from a political economy stance emphasis is placed on inequality and other social factors which have an impact on the health and social well-being of the elderly (Kart, 1987, p. 80). This concentration on needs and the ability of individuals to cope with old age can lead to the 'welfarizing' of the elderly (Fennell et al., 1988, p. 6). Old people come to be defined as a social problem. Identifying and meeting need is given priority; the social processes giving rise to the need in the first place are not considered. The fact that the problems experienced by elderly people may be attributed to social structural factors and that society itself constitutes a problem for the elderly are overlooked. It is the political economy perspective that takes up these issues by maintaining that in order to understand the inequalities in health, wealth and income in old age, it is necessary to appreciate how social class position, gender and ethnic status determine power relations and control access to resources, not only in old age but throughout the life course.

In summary, although an ageing population has given rise to increasing concerns about the burden of ill health in later life, the image of old age as a time of physical decay and social withdrawal has been challenged. According to Laslett (1996), we should cease to view old age as a residual stage in the life course, but see it as the 'crown of life' in which people have the freedom and opportunity to pursue personal interests and engage in a wide variety of leisure activities. The increase in healthy life expectancy and the growth in occupational pensions are just two of the factors seen to be responsible for a newly emergent cultural phenomenon of the 'third age' (Gilleard and Higgs, 2002). Clearly, when theorising about ageing account needs to be taken of the fact that on average people are living longer and healthier lives, are financially better off than their predecessors and have the opportunity to take on new, constructive and rewarding roles in retirement. However, at the same time, it is important not to overlook the existence of inequalities in old age. An adequate theoretical perspective on ageing must recognise the ways in which structural constraints and material disadvantage can prevent some groups of older people from experiencing retirement as a positive and fulfilling time of life. The situation is neatly summarised by Bajekal *et al.* when they assert that, 'Theories of structured dependency and the Third Age can be reconciled by seeing them as ideal types, which are located at the extremes of a spectrum of quality of life at older ages' (2004, p. 710).

Experiencing old age

Retirement

> This end of life is better than the other end, in the sense that you don't have the responsibility for other people, your children and so on, so that's changed. It's a very relaxed time, in the sense of not having those responsibilities. I quite enjoy that, and this is just a new thing, so I'm getting a buzz from it, because my youngest child has just turned 21, and I can take control of my life again, I'm able to let go. So it's quite an enlightening time I think, the later years, certainly in terms of the responsibilities.
>
> (Female interviewee talking about retirement in Barnes and Parry, 2004, p. 228)

Retirement is a significant event in the life course and has attracted increasing attention from social scientists. Early research from a functionalist perspective concentrated on role changes and the process of disengagement in an effort to illustrate how retirement from full-time employment created problems of adjustment for the individual. On entering retirement individuals were seen as becoming socially isolated as they were no longer required to perform the work roles which provided them with access to a range of social relationships in the wider community. Parsons viewed retirement as leading to 'structural isolation from kinship, occupational and community ties' (Parsons, 1942, p. 616).

Some theorists have argued that society has no positive conception of a role for old age. The ambiguity surrounding the social position of those who have retired from work is neatly captured by the phrase 'roleless role' used by Burgess (1960) when describing the experience of retirement. Following retirement the elderly are seen as being unable to maintain essential social contacts as they find themselves cut off from a number of social institutions. Not only do they experience a reduction in the number of roles they are expected to perform but they also find that the formalised role prescriptions associated with old age reflect the loss of status resulting from retirement. Old age is characterised as a time of loss. Individuals experience loneliness and isolation and feel a lack of attachment to society. As Berger and Berger state, 'In Durkheim's sense . . . old age is full of the threat of anomie' (1976, p. 358).

The idea of retirement as a seriously disruptive life event responsible for destroying the social ties an individual develops with society over a lifetime of working is not confined to functionalist accounts. In an early study of the family life of old people Townsend (1957) notes how retired manual workers suffered from financial hardship, low status, a lack of companionship and a sense of worthlessness. It is during the 1950s that the 'retirement impact hypothesis' found favour and numerous articles appeared in the medical journals warning against the negative aspects of compulsory retirement (McMahon and Ford, 1955). Retirement was considered to be detrimental to the physical and mental health of older men. A report by the World Health Organisation (1959) suggested that enforced retirement of healthy elderly people who wished to remain in their jobs was a significant factor in explaining the increased suicide rate among the elderly.

The advantages for the aged worker of remaining in paid employment were also expressed in government reports and policy documents. Here the emphasis was not only on the needs of active individuals to preserve their health and continue to lead full and satisfying lives, but on the benefits to be gained by the economy. The Philips Report (1954) presented an economic argument for retaining older workers. By remaining in paid employment they would ease the problems caused by a shortage of labour, help to increase productivity and delay their reliance on state-funded services and benefits.

What is clearly illustrated here is that images of the elderly are socially constructed. Attitudes towards old age not only differ between societies, but they also differ within societies over time. As Phillipson (1982) states, it is necessary to examine the relationship between economic policies and ideologies concerning retirement. In the 1950s there was concern about the costs of having to provide for an ageing population and also cope with a shortage of labour. Given the economic climate there were incentives to encourage older workers to stay in the labour force. The elderly were viewed as a valuable resource with a positive role to play in the nation's economy. Compare this with the very different situation in more recent decades, with technological innovations having a considerable impact on the structure of employment. There is no longer the same level of demand for traditional labour skills; a younger and more flexible workforce is called for. In this new economic climate retirement is no longer seen as an unnecessary evil to be avoided for the benefit of both the individual and society. Instead the virtues of retirement are extolled. Indeed in some industries middle-aged workers are encouraged to take early retirement.

Retirement is no longer portrayed as a personal crisis experienced by the majority of people: a debilitating event to be delayed for as long as possible. Atchley (1976) maintains that although work provides some individuals with a sense of identity and purpose this is not necessarily the case for everyone. It is realistic to assume that not everyone who retires misses work; some may see retirement as a welcome release which provides an opportunity for self-development through leisure pursuits and hobbies. For some people retirement can mark the beginning of the 'third age' of life, a time of personal achievement when individual ambitions are realised (Laslett, 1987). Cribier (1981), in a study in France, noted how there was an increasing number of people viewing retirement with optimistic anticipation. Findings such as these suggest that the effects of retirement are not common to all, but that there are variations in the experience of retirement. Some people adapt more easily to a life without paid work than others. In order to explain why this should be so, researchers have examined the personal, economic and social circumstances of retired people.

Numerous research studies have commented on the relationship between health and retirement. Surveys in Britain (Parker, 1980) and France (Cribier, 1981) reveal how poor health can be a cause rather than a consequence of premature retirement. In reviewing a number of American studies Palmore *et al.* (1985) claim that when considering the health of individuals who retire at the normal age the proportion reporting a decline in health is roughly matched by the proportion reporting an improvement in health following retirement from full-time employment. Thus they conclude that, 'Retirement at the normal age has little or no adverse effects on health for the average retiree' (1985, p. 167). Whether poor health precedes or follows retirement it certainly influences how individuals cope with this stage of the life course. When compared with healthy retirees those in poor health have greater difficulty in dealing with the initial problems of adjustment (Shanas, 1970) and show little improvement in adjustment over time (Levy, 1979).

Surveys show that lack of income is a major source of concern for many people in retirement (Braithwaite and Gibson, 1987). It is not only the size of the pension received during retirement but also the amount of capital accumulated over the years that is significant in determining the quality of life to be enjoyed in old age. Indeed whether or not an individual has access to an occupational pension, in addition to a state pension, will be an important factor in influencing decisions about early retirement in the first place. However, despite the improvements in the economic circumstances of some groups of pensioners, financial deprivation is experienced by the majority at some time during retirement. An estimated 1.1 million pensioners live in poverty and 4.8 million have incomes equal to or just above the poverty line (Phillipson, 1990, p. 159).

In a study of men living in Aberdeen, Taylor and Ford (1983) discovered that differences in health and income in later life are class related. They found that elderly working-class men reported more health problems than their middle-class counterparts, and were also less likely to enjoy the same level of financial security. Given these differences it seems reasonable to assume that middle-class retirees are better placed to take advantage of the opportunities offered by retirement. According to Guillemard (1982), social withdrawal is a typical response to retirement among the French working class as they lack the resources necessary to pursue a leisure-oriented lifestyle. From a theoretical point of view the political economy perspective readily acknowledges how social and economic factors can determine how successfully individuals cope with retirement. As Phillipson asserts:

> ... it is in the retirement transition that the individual calls upon the resources he or she has developed during the early and middle phases of the life course. In this sense the transition is not a movement from an old to a completely new life (as the disengagement and role theories would suggest); rather it is the final resolution of the advantages and disadvantages attached to given social and class positions.
>
> (Phillipson, 1987, pp. 165–6)

Old age itself is not a cause of poverty. Inequalities established during the pre-retirement years are carried into retirement and may be exaggerated with increasing age. For example, Walker (1986a) predicts that as a result of unequal access to occupational pensions there will be increased stratification among the retired. Many middle-class retirees will have the resources to ensure that the standard of living enjoyed in middle age is maintained in later life. For those who have occupied a less privileged social class position retirement may prove to be a more problematic proposition.

Up to now retirement has been discussed as if it were a singular self-contained episode in the life course, which can be isolated from other life events in order to measure its impact on the lives of individuals. According to Maddox, 'Too often retirement is treated implicitly as a fact with a given social meaning, rather than as a sociological variable to be understood within the social life-space of an individual' (1966, p. 163). Retirement may be preceded or followed by a partner or close relative becoming chronically ill and requiring constant care and attention. Given that how individuals respond to retirement varies according to their personal circumstances, some researchers have studied the transition to retirement by focusing on biographical accounts of work histories and family life.

The effect that retirement has on domestic arrangements and family relationships have formed a central feature of this research. As noted earlier, studies undertaken in the 1950s presented a picture of retirement as a time when men experienced a loss of self-esteem; robbed of a routine imposed by the structure of the working day they expressed feelings of boredom and found themselves spending long periods of time at home with little to keep them occupied. Townsend (1957) describes the impact this had on the organisation of domestic life. There was no sharing of domestic roles and responsibilities; on the contrary, women found the husband being around the house for most of the day irksome. In this case retirement served to reinforce an existing sexual division of domestic labour. This picture is not confirmed by more recent studies.

Phillipson (1987) describes differing reactions to retirement among three occupational groups: miners, car workers and architects. He interviewed a small sample of men and their wives to ascertain how retirement had changed their lives. Generally among the miners there was a reorientation towards domestic life. This was in contrast to the highly segregated nature of conjugal role relationships prior to retirement. The miners and their wives saw retirement as bringing them closer together and reported sharing a number of domestic chores. In some cases men stated that they had retired when they did in order to look after their wives who were in poor health.

The situation was different among the car workers. Here two groups emerged. In one group there was no marked change in the domestic relationship; in the other group there was evidence of increased conflict. In this latter group the former car workers lived in neighbourhoods dominated by young families and people in work; this made them feel like outsiders and their reliance on the state pension produced feelings of social inadequacy. Conscious of the need to economise they abandoned many of the social activities they had enjoyed whilst in work. As Phillipson noted, 'People would find themselves driven back inside the home as external contacts and supports fell away. One immediate effect of this was an increase in conflict within the domestic sphere' (1987, p. 173).

Of the three occupational groups studied, the architects reported the least change in their domestic arrangements. They had sufficient resources following retirement to enable them to continue employing domestic help, pursue their hobbies and maintain a full and active social life. The pattern of marital life was not unduly disrupted; both husband and wife continued to enjoy the joint and independent activities characteristic of the pre-retirement years. The architects' wives had interests outside the home; many were engaged in voluntary work.

By and large, research into retirement has tended to be largely oriented to the experiences of men: Szinovacz (1982) claims that there are three reasons, all based on common misconceptions, why women have been largely ignored by researchers.

1 It has been assumed that because fewer women than men engage in regular paid work outside the home, retirement is not an important feature of the lives of the majority of women. This is not supported by labour force statistics, which reveal a substantial growth in the number of women employees (Dex, 1985).

2 It has been suggested that women, unlike men, do not see work as a central element in their lives. For men, work provides not only financial rewards but also a sense of social identity. This assumption that men and women have markedly differing attitudes to work is challenged by more recent research, which suggests that there are important similarities in the orientations of men and women to work (Dex, 1985). More recently, Barnes and Parry (2004) found that where individuals had strong occupational identities they found adjusting to retirement more difficult. This applied to both men and women. However, men appeared to be more concerned by the loss of status following retirement, whereas women missed the sociability of the workplace.

3 It has been argued that retirement is a less disruptive life event for women, as they have a ready-made role waiting for them, that of full-time housewife

and carer. However, there is evidence to suggest that women can approach retirement with feelings of pessimism and actually encounter more problems than men in adjusting to life without paid employment (Streib and Schneider, 1971; Atchley, 1976).

To understand women's experience of retirement it is necessary to consider their employment patterns and ideas about women's role in society. Income inequalities in old age are primarily a function of access to resources over the 'working years' of the life course. Those employed in well-paid jobs that offer additional benefits, such as, occupational pensions, are well placed to make financial provision for later life through savings and investment schemes. Research has repeatedly shown that retired manual workers are more likely to experience poverty in old age than their non-manual counterparts (Townsend, 1979). What this research also reveals is that there are significant inequalities in income between women and men. Elderly women, particularly those living alone, are more likely to be living in poverty than are elderly men (Townsend, 1979; Walker, 1987). This can be partly explained by taking a brief look at gender inequalities in the labour market.

By far the main source of income for the majority of retired people is the state pension. As women tend to be concentrated in low-paid occupations they make lower pension contributions than men, which ultimately affects their state pension entitlement. Given their childcare and homemaking roles many women have a discontinuous employment profile: taking time out of paid employment to bring up children or care for sick relatives reduces their contribution record even further. Clearly, caring carries a 'pension penalty'. According to the Family and Working Lives Survey, one-in-five middle-aged women who had had caring responsibilities had stopped work altogether when they first took up the caring role and a further one-in-five female carers reported that they had undertaken less paid employment since they had become carers (Evandrou and Glaser, 2003). By working part-time, many women are ineligible for some occupational pension schemes. Access to occupational pensions is not only differentiated by gender; social class, ethnicity and occupational position are also significant (Gilleard and Higgs, 2000; Ginn and Arber, 2001). Pension schemes and employment practices need to address the social and economic circumstances of women workers. Indeed, there is evidence of a growing recognition of the need to help both women and men who have caring responsibilities to maintain contact with the world of work (Department of Health, 1999b). Employment schemes provided for workers with childcare commitments need to be extended to individuals who care for elderly family members.

The sexual division of labour not only restricts women's participation in the labour market, thus reducing opportunities to acquire the income and assets necessary for future financial security, but also ensures that their retirement experience will be structured around providing care for others. In one sense, it could be said that women who undertake paid employment outside the home do not experience retirement in the same way that men do; they exchange the role of paid worker for that of unpaid carer. However, this does require a series of adjustments in daily routines and life expectations, which have implications for one's sense of social identity. While some women may adopt the role of carer without question, they may still experience a sense of loss in having to withdraw from the labour market, especially if they had been strongly attached to their jobs. This is illustrated by the following comment from a woman who had retired from her managerial job in order to care for her elderly parents:

> It took me a while to get used to not going to my work and not having something to do like that because I felt looking after them wasn't really a job, if you know what I mean, although it was taking up all of my time, it wasn't quite how I had planned things.
>
> (Female interviewee quoted in Barnes and Parry, 2004, p. 221)

In actual fact women are never really allowed to relinquish the caring role entirely, for it is with them throughout their lives. It tends to dominate during the child-rearing years and again in later life when they come to care for a sick or disabled husband or relative. In some cases the need to provide care may be a reason for giving up paid employment temporarily or taking early retirement.

The structure of inequality in old age is influenced by the pattern of social stratification; therefore attention needs to be given to the combined influence of class, gender and ethnicity in determining life chances. Inequalities in the distribution of income, wealth and health confirm that class is a stronger predictor of lifestyle than age. As Bond and Coleman (1990) assert, there are more similarities between people of different ages in the same social class than there are between people of similar ages in different social classes. It is not age alone that is the significant factor. This becomes clear when considering the position of elderly people in minority ethnic groups. It has been argued that they are particularly vulnerable and face what may be termed a double burden or 'double jeopardy'.

> Like other older people in industrial societies, they experience the devaluation of old age found in most modern societies . . . Unlike other older people, however, the minority aged must bear the additional economic, social and psychological burdens of living in a society in which racial equality remains . . . a myth.
>
> (Dowd and Bengston, 1978, p. 427)

Some observers have described the situation as one of 'triple jeopardy' (Norman, 1985). This is when older members of minority ethnic groups can be seen to:

- suffer the consequences of the negative stereotyping and discrimination encountered by the elderly, irrespective of race or ethnicity, in modern society.
- endure the same social and economic difficulties experienced by sections of the working class.
- face additional discrimination on the basis of their religious beliefs, cultural practices and physical appearance.

Thus triple jeopardy is the result of a combination of the impact of age, social class and race on the lives of disadvantaged people in minority ethnic groups.

What is clear from a political economy perspective is how economic, political and social factors contribute to the creation of structural dependency. Following this approach, Bornat *et al.* (1985) have advanced a 'Manifesto for Old Age', which among its recommendations urges that steps should be taken to:

- improve levels of financial support;
- provide more imaginative policies for retirement;
- tackle age discrimination in society;
- eradicate inequalities in health and promote positive attitudes to health in later life;
- initiate new policies to meet the needs of elderly people from minority ethnic groups;
- establish education as a right for older people;
- encourage more investment in housing and transport for the elderly;
- ensure that elderly people are given the opportunity to participate in the planning and delivery of the services they receive.

The need for social policy to address the plight of older women could be added to this list. Sheila Peace (1986) draws attention to the 'forgotten female' when she states, 'It would appear that in our society old women are all around us and yet invisible – invisible in that their existence is seldom acknowledged; their needs are seldom recognised and their voices seldom heard' (1986, p. 61). It is only in the last decade of the twentieth century that feminist sociologists began to focus on gender inequalities in old age (Arber and Ginn, 1991a, 1991b).

There have been major changes in the pathways into retirement and the experience of retirement for many people in the UK in recent times. There is ample evidence to suggest that '[r]etirement is no longer the mass, forced expulsion from working life, and today's retirees, especially the newly retired, are on average wealthier and healthier than their predecessors' (Hyde *et al.*, 2004, p. 280). However, how well individuals adjust to this stage in the life course and how successful they are at developing a rewarding lifestyle is not simply a question of individual motivation and personal character, but depends upon a complex combination of social, economic and psychological factors. For example, where individuals see the transition as a voluntary one, feel financially secure and are able to achieve a certain degree of continuity in their social activities and friendships before and after retirement, they are more likely to have a positive experience. The opportunity structures available to individuals will of course vary according to gender, ethnicity and social class position.

Dependence and independence

Mabel, aged 84, is one of the liveliest residents. She's carved out a position for herself mending the socks for the men who can't afford to pay the seamstress who comes in once a week. She plays the piano for the occasional singsong. Both her legs are paralysed and she's been advised to have one off. 'But my brains aren't what they used to be', she complains. 'They're not right, you see. I can't concentrate on much.' One of the nurses chucks her under the chin and behind the ears like a baby; and Mabel looks up into her eyes. 'We do treat them like children', the nurse admits. 'That's what they *are* really, isn't it?'

(Harrison, 1973, p. 266)

Old age is commonly portrayed as a time of increasing dependency, when due to failing health and increasing levels of infirmity individuals are forced to rely on the support of family, friends and state-funded services to enable them to continue to live in the community. In simplistic terms, dependency is presented as a natural outcome of the biological process of growing old. However, as Johnson (1990) asserts, the notion of dependency is more conceptually complex than this stereotyped view suggests. For example, with reference to welfare provision in general, Fraser and Gordon (1994) identify four major types of dependency: economic, socio-legal, political, and moral or psychological. As regards old age, Walker (1982) offers a typology of dependency that differentiates between physical, psychological, social, economic and political dimensions (Box 6.1).

In actual fact modern societies are characterised by interdependency, with individuals being dependent on each other to some extent. The labelling of a group of people as dependent is part of a social process of definition and not based entirely on objective criteria. Defining dependency involves value judgements and ideological beliefs. For example, working men who rely on their wives to organise the day-to-day running of the home and make sure that appropriate childcare arrangements are in place, would not normally consider themselves to be dependent upon their wives: whereas women who undertake these unpaid tasks are officially considered to be financially dependent upon their husbands. There is also evidence that the term 'dependence' can present a negative image, as when critics of state-funded welfare programmes describe the creation of a 'dependency culture' among claimants as being responsible for increasing the burden on the public purse.

Professionals engaged in the planning and provision of care tend to see dependence and independence as opposites. Independence is the ability of the individual to live in the community without the aid of any extra help from statutory

---

Box 6.1   Definition

Types of dependency

- Life-cycle dependency
- Physical and psychological dependency
- Economic and financial dependency
- Political dependency
- Structural dependency

Source: Walker, 1982

agencies or voluntary bodies. Sixsmith (1986) suggests that this is not the only way of approaching an understanding of independence. He claims that it is important to gain an insight into how independence is defined at the individual level, that is, by the elderly themselves. In a study of what 'home' means in the lives of elderly people he explored their views on independence. He found that while the majority of interviewees placed a high value on independence in old age, three modes of being independent were mentioned:

- not having to rely on other people for personal care or to cope with day-to-day domestic chores;
- having 'the capacity for self-direction' (i.e. the freedom to make choices for themselves);
- not having to rely on charity or feeling under an obligation to anyone.

Arber and Ginn (1991a) discuss the relationship between the availability of resources and the likelihood of dependency in later life. They identify three broad categories of resources (Box 6.2). These three sets of resources play a key role in determining whether or not elderly people will be able to remain living independently in the community. In outlining these three categories Arber and Ginn do not suggest that independence is undermined when only one type of resource is unavailable. They recognise the existence of interconnections between the different types of resources. In fact they see the sets of resources forming an 'interlocking resource triangle' (1991a, p. 68). For example, if elderly people are to achieve a quality of life that promotes autonomy and allows them to make realistic choices as to how to meet their physical and social needs, they require the necessary financial resources. A frail or disabled elderly person with sufficient money to purchase aids or appliances to assist mobility can reduce reliance on others and maintain a degree of independence. On the whole, the extent to which an individual has access to the three major resources (material, health and caring) will depend to some extent on gender, social class and ethnic status.

Resources can be viewed on four different levels: the individual, the household, the community and the state. Independence is likely to be at a maximum when the individual has sufficient personal resources not to have to rely on immediate

---

Box 6.2   Definition

Resources in later life

1 **Material and structural resources** (including level of income, amount of wealth, quality of housing and car ownership).

2 **Physical health** of the individual and their ability to care for themselves and, if required, care for others.

3 **Caring resources** (including the degree of access individuals have to informal and formal types of health and welfare provision).

Source: Arber and Ginn, 1991a

family members, other relatives, friends, neighbours or statutory agencies for care and support. Dependency can therefore be seen more as a product of social and economic structures than as a natural and inevitable consequence of biological ageing. As previously noted, when discussing the political economy perspective, the concept of structural dependency helps to explain the nature and severity of dependency as opposed to just describing its existence. As Walker claims, dependency '. . . is to a large, and certainly unappreciated extent, manufactured socially' (1982, p. 121).

Similarly, Hockey and James (1993) argue that dependency can be viewed as being created within the context of specific social, economic and political relationships. They maintain that although dependency is a feature of various stages in the life course it is neither a property of individuals nor a natural outcome of the process of biological maturation, but is in fact, 'a social relationship resting upon the exercise of power' (1993, p. 45). In order to understand the way in which dependency is defined within in a particular society it is necessary to understand the power relationships within that society.

Hockey and James use the concept of 'personhood' to describe the culturally constructed model of dependency found in Western society. They define personhood as:

> that identity which is socially constituted for an individual, not with respect to his or her own sense of uniqueness, but with respect to a particularized set of cultural ideas about what it means to be fully human.
>
> (Hockey and James, 1993, p. 48)

Thus, what it means to be a member of society is culturally defined. In Western cultures personhood is symbolised through such ideas as active choice, self-determination and individual autonomy: the very characteristics used to define dependency. For Hockey and James, it is through the use of the concept of personhood that we are able to appreciate how perceived dependency and power are linked. It is necessary to discover the conditions and circumstances under which personhood is attributed or withdrawn at various stages in the life course.

The authors claim that childhood, with its emphasis on vulnerability and dependency, has become the dominant model of dependency, to the extent that it has implications for the lives of those who are physically dependent but not children, such as the elderly and disabled adults. Both children and the elderly are categorised as dependent and therefore not granted the status of full personhood. What is more, the language and ideology of childhood is simply applied to other dependent groups. This is referred to as the 'process of infantilization'. As Hockey and James assert, 'Metaphors of childhood permeate the very language we use and images we draw on, providing implicit frames of reference for everyday social interactions and encounters' (1993, p. 10).

The language and ideology of childhood play a part in structuring ideas about dependency in old age and help to create and sustain a stereotype image of the elderly as 'childlike'. There is a tendency for carers to adopt 'infantilizing practices' when dealing with the elderly, as demonstrated by the words and actions of the nurse quoted at the beginning of this section. Hockey (1990) describes how staff in a residential home distinguished the frail elderly from the fitter elderly by referring to the former collectively as 'the little people' and addressing them by nicknames. Similarly, Knowles (1987), himself a nurse, provides an account of how some nurses use terms of endearment, such as poppet, when caring for elderly patients. More recently, in a study of nurses' perceptions of dying and death on elderly care wards, one interviewee referred to a recently deceased patient thus: 'Oh, Little Elsie, she was a sweetie' (Costello, 2006, p. 596). Such responses to the physically dependent are not merely unfortunate occurrences but constitute a culturally acceptable way of understanding and coping with dependency. What is often overlooked is the humiliating consequences such practices can have for the individual recipient. Hockey and James see the tendency to attribute childlike qualities to the elderly as part of an ideological process that ensures that discrimination against the elderly is seen as natural. The metaphorical strategy places the elderly in a marginal social category, thus serving to sustain the ideological dominance of adulthood.

Quality of life in old age

> Quality of life is what you do yourself. You know, if you want to sit and watch television all day, well that's it, perhaps that's your equation of quality of life. . . . Mine is to get out and about and do things for myself, or see things that I would like to see or haven't seen, you know. I don't expect to sit back and expect quality of life to come through the door.
>
> (Interviewee quoted in Gabriel and Bowling, 2004, p. 684)

Social gerontology is not preoccupied with studying the impact and consequences of the negative aspects of ageing such as physical deterioration, functional loss, dependency, poverty and increasing service need. The discipline also embraces a more positive view of the experience of ageing, one in which old age is seen as a natural component of the life course and a period when life can still be satisfying (O'Boyle, 1997). In recent decades researchers have shown a growing interest in measuring social well-being and life satisfaction in old age, as witnessed by reference to such notions as 'ageing well' (Vaillant, 2002) and 'successful ageing' (Rowe and Kahn, 1997). Consequently, the 'quality of life' features as a key concept both in empirical research and policy debates. It is defined by the World Health Organisation as '. . . an individual's perception of their position in life in the context of the culture and value systems in which they live and in relation to their goals, expectations, standards, and concerns' (quoted in Smith, 2000, p. 422). However, despite this definition and the popularity of the concept it has proved to be difficult to measure. Although it has been the focus of a wealth of research activity, differences in methodological approach and research design have made it difficult to draw any firm conclusions about the actual mechanisms that influence quality of life or develop an understanding of how the different determining factors are interrelated. As Smith *et al.* have concluded in this context, the '. . . quality of life is best regarded as a multi-dimensional construct, the components of which may vary according to the nature of the sample studied, the contextual or environmental situation, and the methodology and design of the study' (2004, p. 797).

Research into life satisfaction and well-being in later life has identified several factors that contribute to an individual's quality of life. They can be roughly categorised under three broad headings:

1 personal characteristics (e.g. state of health, material standard of living and general psychological outlook);

2 social support (e.g. relationships with family members and relatives, friendship networks and social contacts with others);

3 local environment (e.g. perceptions of neighbourhood safety, local amenities and residential surroundings).

The concept of the quality of life is not always clearly defined in the literature and there 'is debate about whether these domains are predictors of (the quality of life) or constituents of the concept itself' (Bowling and Gabriel, 2007, p. 828). Given the multi-dimensionality of the concept, feelings of life satisfaction are likely to be the product of both the direct and indirect effects of the variables listed above. While research studies into the quality of life experienced by older people living in a variety of countries have produced equivocal results, the following findings are worth noting:

- In a study by Farquhar (1995), a majority of respondents aged 65 years or over stated that family relationships were the single most influential factor in determining their quality of life. In the 85 plus age group health and physical function were mentioned before material well-being as being significant determinants of life satisfaction.

- Older people living in poverty are twice as likely as those who are financially secure to describe their quality of life as 'very poor' (Scharf *et al.*, 2002).

- Surveys of older people's general satisfaction with the neighbourhoods in which they live show that physical characteristics (e.g. availability of local amenities and the general appearance of residential areas and public spaces) and social contacts with neighbours are important determinants of the quality of life (Richard *et al.*, 2005; Hanson and Emlet, 2006).

- The level of perceived loneliness is also an important determinant of the quality of life (Bramston *et al.*, 2002).

- While the factors which influence quality of life (e.g. feeling valued, having access to support networks and being independent) do not vary across ethnic groups, the ways in which they are played out in people's lives does show some variation according to ethnicity (Grewal *et al.*, 2004).

- Racism can have an indirect effect on quality of life, partly as a consequence of living in an area where racially motivated crime and racial harassment are in evidence, and partly as a result of discriminatory practices in the workplace leading to a reduced income in retirement (Moriarty and Butt, 2004).

As a multi-dimensional concept the quality of life is measured using both objective and subjective variables. The former refer to objective life conditions such as state of health, level of income and participation in social and community activities, while the latter reflect the subjective evaluations individuals make of these life conditions. There are a variety of standard measures of subjective well-being used in questionnaire surveys of life satisfaction, such as the World Health Organisation Quality of Life measure and the Satisfaction with Life Scale (Diener *et al.*, 1985). These measures consist of a collection of items or statements (e.g. 'In most ways my life is close to my ideal') to which the individual has to respond by indicating their level of agreement or disagreement on a Likert scale of one-to-five or one-to-seven. The individual item scores are aggregated and this figure is divided by the number of items in the scale to provide a single numeric measure of the quality of life for comparative purposes. In recent years there has been a growing debate over the relative significance of objective measures and subjective evaluations in this context. According to Bowling and Windsor (2001), subjective variables account for more of the variance in quality of life than do objective life conditions. Thus, more emphasis needs to be given to older people's views and perceived priorities if we are to develop a better understanding of life satisfaction in old age. As Gabriel and Bowling state quite categorically, 'A model of the quality of life and its associated measurement scales should be based on concepts derived from older people themselves' (2004, p. 689). From a study of old people living at home they demonstrate how the different domains of the quality of life are interrelated and there is a complex and dynamic interplay between personal characteristics and external social structures. What is important in terms of the quality of life from the perspective of older people themselves is outlined in Box 6.3.

Box 6.3   Research findings

Determinants of the quality of life in older age: a lay perspective

Quality of life is about having:

- good relationships, help and support;
- a home in a neighbourhood in which one feels safe;
- access to local facilities, services and transport;
- opportunities for engaging in hobbies and leisure pursuits;
- the ability to maintain social contacts and retain a role in society;
- a positive psychological outlook and accepting that some circumstances will not change;
- good health and physical mobility;
- enough money to meet basic needs and participate in community life;
- sufficient resources to maintain one's independence and control over life.

Source: Gabriel and Bowling, 2004, p. 689

Thus it can be seen that both objective and subjective variables play an important role in determining the quality of life in old age. However, it is difficult, if not impossible, to isolate the individual impact of any one variable. While some factors may exert a direct impact on quality of life, other variables may have an indirect effect or their influence may be mediated through other variables. Furthermore, there are considerable individual differences in people's assessments of their quality of life (Beaumont and Kenealy, 2004). Nevertheless, it is possible to identify broad overarching themes. One of these relates to issues of identity, belonging and participation in the local neighbourhood and community. The day-to-day behaviour of older people is to a certain extent shaped and influenced by the physical contexts and social surroundings in which they live. In essence these are 'socially constructed, socially filled out, and socially shaped physical environments' (Wahl and Lang, 2004, p. 17). Thus, not only do the physical features of an area have the potential to affect the collective well-being of older people but there is the possibility of links between physical features and social dynamics having implications for health and general well-being. In a study based in three diverse neighbourhoods in the Glasgow area, Day (2008) explored older people's understandings of the nature of the impact of the local environment on the health of the more elderly residents. The dimensions of the outdoor environment considered to be important for older people's health are outlined in Box 6.4. While the dimensions relating to facilitating physical exercise and supporting social interaction were considered to be the most important, all the dimensions were interlinked. For example, a physical environment that is clean, and in which residents feel safe and secure, will encourage people to exercise and socialise outdoors. In the final analysis, Day warns against adopting a position of environmental determinism and concludes that while the physical features of a local area may hinder or facilitate socialising, she found no evidence to suggest that these factors were capable of actually creating a community dynamic.

As regards the maintenance of identity and a sense of belonging in old age, research shows that for many older people their home and residential locale can

Box 6.4   Research findings

Dimensions of a healthy outdoor environment as defined by older people

A healthy outdoor environment is one that:

- is clean and free from pollution;
- is peaceful and quiet;
- facilitates physical exercise;
- supports social interaction;
- is emotionally uplifting.

Source: Day, 2008

be the source of a strong sense of emotional attachment (Phillipson *et al.*, 2001). The intensification and perpetuation of such attachments may constitute a strategy older people employ in order to attempt to maintain a sense of identity in a changing world (Rowles and Chaudhury, 2005). However, not all groups of older people enjoy the same level and degree of community attachment.

> What does seem clear is that while some groups of older people can actively re-shape communities which are meaningful to them in old age, others are relatively disempowered from the option of managing community and neighbourhood change. The key change over the past 50 years may lie precisely in the social division that has opened up between two groups: those that have expanding life styles and options, and those whose experiences of their neighbourhood are dominated by marginalisation and alienation.
>
> (Phillipson, 2007, p. 336)

Thus, when it comes to using community attachment as a measure of the quality of life, there is clear evidence of significant inequalities within the older population. While some groups of older people are free to choose where they live and can exercise some influence over their immediate physical and social environment, other groups do not have access to the economic and material resources necessary to make such decision-making a reality. Those in the latter group, especially those living in deprived communities, can experience social exclusion. Due to a lack of financial capital and possibly poor health, older people may find themselves excluded from full participation in socially valued activities. Also, living in a socially excluded neighbourhood may have implications for an older person's ability to acquire information and access public services.

Studies of people living in areas characterised by social exclusion illustrate that although not all inhabitants suffer financial deprivation, the quality of life for all residents can be adversely affected by problems encountered in the local environment. In a study of people aged 50 years and over living in a deprived neighbourhood in the north-east of England, researchers found that while the majority of respondents said they liked living there, they voiced concerns about specific problems and identified areas where they felt improvements could be made (see Box 6.5). The researchers compared the concerns and experiences of Beckfield residents with those reported by older people living in an affluent residential area in the south-east of England and found some differences. For example, fear of crime and worries over security featured as major issues only for those living in the deprived neighbourhood. Also, while residents from both areas raised the topics of transport and health, there was some variation in the nature of their respective concerns. In terms of transport, Beckfield residents relied on public transport and were concerned that services were not always available when they were needed. For their counterparts in the south-east, the main concern over transport was being fit and able to drive their own cars. Having control over their own mobility made it easier for them to visit friends and relatives, participate in social activities and access services both locally and in the surrounding area. In essence, those living in the materially disadvantaged neighbourhood lacked this level of personal control over their lives.

Box 6.5   Research findings

Major concerns expressed by local residents of Beckfield

- level of crime, fear of crime and worries about personal safety;
- need for the area to be better maintained and kept cleaner;
- need for public transport to be improved;
- need for the appearance and range of local shops to be enhanced;
- need for health services, including a GP, to be available locally;
- more opportunities for paid employment;
- improved local facilities;
- need for older people to be valued.

Source: Abbott and Sapsford, 2005, p. 42

The problems associated with living in an area of social exclusion have an impact on residents of all ages and old age can exacerbate some of these problems. However, we should be careful not to assume that people simply become passive dependants and recipients of informal care by family, friends and neighbours as they grow older. While some research has focused on the sense of a 'loss of community', particularly among older people (Charles and Davies, 2005), other studies have illustrated how older women actively participate in family and community health networks (Boneham and Sixsmith, 2006). The task facing environmental gerontology is to develop an understanding of the variety of ways in which older people form attachments to their communities and how this is influenced by their access to, and control over, economic and social resources. Any policies designed to support social integration, combat social exclusion and enhance the quality of life of older people need to be aware of the significant inequalities that exist within the older population.

Summary

- The UK has an ageing population. At the beginning of the last century one person in 20 was aged 65 years or over; this figure had reached just over one in six by the beginning of this century.
- It is inaccurate to view the elderly simply as recipients of services provided by others. Many people over retirement age make a significant contribution as unpaid, informal carers of sick or dependent relatives. By looking after their young grandchildren, grandparents provide an important support service for the families of their own adult children.
- Disengagement theory sees the gradual social withdrawal of elderly people as a natural and inevitable consequence of the ageing process. It ignores how the

adjustment to old age is influenced by socio-economic factors and structural forces, and encourages ageism.

- The political economy approach to the study of old age challenges the assumption that the elderly are a problem for society. Old age is viewed as a socially constructed status. This perspective avoids treating the elderly as if they constituted a homogenous social group.

- Economic, political and social factors all contribute to creating structural dependency in old age and influence how successfully individuals cope with retirement.

- Elderly people in minority ethnic groups can experience what has been termed 'triple jeopardy' in old age: they are subject to negative stereotyping, they experience financial problems and they have to contend with racial discrimination.

- When dealing with frail, elderly patients who are physically dependent, carers can sometimes treat them in a 'childlike' manner, thus denying them the full status of 'personhood'.

- Socio-demographic factors, health status, psychological outlook, access to social support networks and features of the residential environment collectively help to determine the quality of life experienced by older people.

Questions for discussion

1 What are the implications of an ageing population?

2 How has the way in which society treats old people changed over the years?

3 Does disengagement theory help us to understand how people adjust to retirement?

4 Identify and discuss three characteristic features of the political economy perspective on old age.

5 In what sense is old age a social construct?

6 Do men and women have different experiences of retirement?

7 What do you understand by the term the 'process of infantilization'?

8 What factors determine the quality of life in old age?

Further reading

Bengtson, V. L., Silverstein, M., Putney, N. M. and Gans, D. (eds) (2009) *Handbook of Theories of Aging*, 2nd edn, New York: Springer Publishing Company.

Biggs, S. (1993) *Understanding Ageing: Images, Attitudes and Professional Practices*, Buckingham: Open University Press.

Blakemore, K. and Boneham, M. (1994) *Age, Race and Ethnicity: A Comparative Approach*, Buckingham: Open University Press.

Bond, J., Coleman, P. and Pearce, S. (eds) (1993) *Ageing and Society: An Introduction to Social Gerontology*, 2nd edn, London: Sage.

Bytheway, B. (1995) *Ageism*, Buckingham: Open University Press.

Daatland, S. O. and Biggs, S. (eds) (2006) *Aging and Diversity: Multiple Pathways and Cultural Migrations*, Bristol: Policy Press.

Harper, S. (2006) *Ageing Societies*, New York: Hodder Arnold.

Hockey, J. and James, A. (1993) *Growing Up and Growing Old: Ageing, Dependency and the Life Course*, London: Sage.

Johnson, M. L., Bengtson, V. L. Coleman, P. G., and T. B. L. Kirkwood (2005) *The Cambridge Handbook of Age and Ageing*, Cambridge: Cambridge University Press.

Pilcher, J. (1995) *Age and Generation in Modern Britain*, Oxford: Oxford University Press.

Phillipson, C. (1998) *Reconstructing Old Age: New Agendas in Social Theory and Practice*, London: Sage.

Phillipson, C., Bernard, M., Phillips, J. and Ogg, J. (2001) *The Family and Community Life of Older People*, London: Routledge.

Sidell, M. (1995) *Health in Old Age: Myth, Mystery and Management*, Buckingham: Open University Press.

Useful websites

Age Concern: http://www.ageconcern.org.uk/
British Council for Ageing: http://www.bcageing.org.uk/index.htm
British Geriatrics Society: http://www.bgs.org.uk/index.htm
British Society of Gerontology: http://www.britishgerontology.org/
British Society for Research on Ageing: http://www.bsra.org.uk/
Centre for Policy on Ageing: http://www.cpa.org.uk/index.html
English Longitudinal Study of Ageing: http://www.natcen.ac.uk/elsa/
Help the Aged: http://www.ageing.org/ research/default.htm
The Oxford Institute of Ageing: http://www.ageing.ox.ac.uk/

CHAPTER 7

End of life

The end of the life course

> Dying and death are major categories of human experience that are culturally determined. Social science research documents the fact that defining someone as dying is a social process. Although critical medical conditions certainly have a physiological basis, disease states are given significance through interpretation.
>
> (Schulz *et al.*, 2006, p. 280)

The two preceding chapters explored aspects of the life course by focusing on three key stages: childhood, adolescence and later life. These stages represent distinctive biographical phases in the life of an individual and are socially defined. Sociologists use the term 'status passage' when referring to the transition from one social position to the next. Social and cultural rules govern the timing of a status passage and regularise the transition by sanctioning the behaviour of those involved. Ritual ceremonies, called 'rites of passage', often mark the change of status experienced by the individual. Rituals help people to make sense of the world in which they live, they represent a public reaffirmation of key social values and cultural norms and vary from society to society. According to the anthropologist Edmund Leach (1968), rituals are primarily invoked to deal with the transition from one status to another. Reaching adulthood, getting married, becoming a mother and retiring from work are all stages in the life course which involve a change in social identity for the individual and are marked by some form of public ritual or ceremony. For example, in most countries marriage ceremonies are imbued with ritual taboos and practices which have a sacred and/or secular significance.

Helman (1990) describes how biological events such as pregnancy and childbirth can also be viewed as social events, in so far as the ritual practices surrounding them can be seen not only to safeguard the pregnancy but to also mark the status transition from 'woman' to 'mother'. Anthropological accounts of traditional societies reveal that it is common for women to be subjected to culturally specific taboos regarding their dress, diet and interaction with others at some stage during pregnancy and in the early months following childbirth. This ritualisation of childbirth is not confined to traditional societies, but is also characteristic of modern societies where childbirth is under the influence of medical science.

Just as there are social mechanisms for dealing with birth, there are socially and culturally patterned ways of dealing with death. Death marks the final stage in the life course; it represents the final social transition whereby the individual relinquishes the status of a living person for that of a dead ancestor. What is unique about death as a 'stage' in the life course is that 'it is the only life event that can be anticipated with total certainty' (Finch and Wallis, 1993, p. 61). In all societies there are ritualistic practices surrounding the disposal of the corpse, taboos connected with physical contact with the deceased and culturally specific forms of behaviour expected of those relatives in mourning.

Attitudes to death and dying can vary not only between societies but also within one society over a period of time. In socially diverse and multi-cultural societies death, dying and grief are experienced in different ways in different social and ethnic groups. It is important that healthcare professionals recognise the existence of such diversity, as they will be involved in treating and caring for terminally ill patients and recently bereaved people from all walks of life. Given the life-sustaining impact of new technological developments and the emphasis placed on 'patient-centred medicine', individuals are increasingly more likely to be actively involved in making important decisions about their own care, or that of other family members, in cases of terminal illness (Box 7.1). This means that health professionals will need to develop the necessary skills for engaging in end-of-life conversations with patients and their relatives. In this context it has been observed that:

> **Box 7.1   Definition**
>
> ### Terminal illness
>
> Referring to people as being 'terminally ill' has become a shorthand way of describing a specific set of circumstances; that is, that any active therapy being received is not being offered with curative intent, physical deterioration has come to affect everyday functioning, the deterioration has become progressive and irreversible, and that survival is likely to be counted in weeks and months rather than years.
>
> *Source*: Robbins, 1998, p. 15

> Discussions about death are by nature disturbing and difficult for both clinicians and patients. Clinicians need better training in sharing information in a sensitive manner and both parties need support in dealing with the emotional impact of these conversations.
>
> (Zimmermann and Rodin, 2004, p. 127)

However, before health professionals embark on specialist training to help them to deal with the topic of death in the clinical setting, they need to appreciate the social and cultural diversity of attitudes towards death found in the wider society. This chapter will describe the changing approach to death and dying in Western societies and examine some of the major theoretical perspectives that contribute to providing a social understanding of mortality.

Death as a fact of life

> It may not be a coincidence that the two things we keep most secret from our children are birth and death. Somehow, we do not want them to be directly confronted with how they were created or how they will be extinguished. Perhaps the beginning and the end are linked in their common reference to the fact that there are boundaries to the state of being alive.
>
> (Fisher, 1973, p. 147)

Death is a natural life event, a universal human experience, which marks the end of the life course. Although death is a biological fact, an understanding of the human experience of death cannot be based solely on the biomedical model but needs to draw from a wide range of subject areas including philosophy, theology, history, social anthropology, psychology, sociology, literature and poetry. For example, from a sociological perspective the focus is primarily on exploring the ways in which attitudes, values, beliefs and behaviour concerning mortality reflect the social and cultural diversity that can exist both within a single society and between societies. Death from this perspective is viewed as a social issue. Sociologists concentrate on how societal responses to death, and institutional arrangements for managing death, vary according to a number of factors including the age of the deceased, the circumstances surrounding the death (e.g. its cause, nature and place of occurrence), and the prevailing social and cultural attitudes to mortality. It is within this wider socio-historical and socio-cultural context that individuals can be seen to make sense of their own mortality and encounter socially acceptable ways of expressing grief and coping with bereavement. Thus, although death may be perceived as an inevitable fact of life, the meaning attached to death and the rituals surrounding the disposal of the body vary according to the nature of prevailing social, religious and cultural beliefs.

In writing about death, grief and mourning in Britain in the middle years of the twentieth century, the anthropologist Geoffrey Gorer (1955, 1965) claimed that death had become 'unmentionable as a natural process' and had achieved the status of a taboo subject. He maintained that, 'While natural death became more and more smothered in prudery, violent death has played an ever-growing part in the fantasies offered to mass audiences' (Gorer, quoted in Peberdy *et al.*, 2004, p. 52). Death, it appeared, had become a legitimate topic for entertainment. According to Gorer, the fictional portrayal of violent death, through film, science fiction stories, detective novels and horror comics, gave a distorted picture of the reality of death and dying. In comparing attitudes to death with the Victorian approach to the subject of sex, he argued that 'natural' death had replaced sex as a taboo topic in the contemporary era. It is in this context that he coined the phrase 'pornography of death' when asserting that 'whereas copulation has become more and more mentionable, particularly in the Anglo-Saxon societies, death has become more and more "unmentionable" *as a natural process*' (Gorer, 1965, p. 193, emphasis in original). For Gorer, the social prudery surrounding the topic of natural death served to stifle any serious discussion about the end of life.

The use of the concept of 'natural death' suggests that there are some deaths that can be defined as 'unnatural'. First we need to understand what is meant by a natural death. This has been defined as 'a death which comes under medical care and finds us in good health and old age' (Illich, 1977, p. 180). As we will see later in the chapter, in historical terms this way of conceptionalising death is of fairly recent origin. In order to bring into sharp relief the differences between the two types of death, Prior (1989) utilises Goffman's (1974) conceptual distinction between natural and unnatural events. Natural events are seen as being the unintended or unmotivated product of purely physical processes. By contrast, unnatural events are the outcome of some form of human action or intervention. Consequently, natural death is that which results from an identifiable illness or disease that is located within the body; whereas unnatural death involves some form of human agency; this may be either intentional (as in premeditated murder) or unintentional (as in accidental death as a result of negligence).

We are offered a daily diet of stories of death from unnatural causes from the news media and the entertainment industry. Viewers of TV crime dramas encounter detailed depictions of crime scenes and witness graphic illustrations of victims' bodies being examined and dissected in an attempt to identify the nature and cause of death. Although these programmes are fictional, they expose the viewer to a scientific image of death when actors are seen to use the appropriate technical terms when estimating the time of death and describing and explaining the relevance of physical evidence such as damaged tissue and skin discolouration. Furthermore, such fictional dramas also show individuals coping with the sudden and unexpected death of a close family member. What impact this level of exposure has on the way in which individuals view death and dying is debatable. It could be argued that despite the access people have to such material, it is difficult to identify with the images presented on a personal level, as illustrated in the following comment.

> In a world full of instant mass media which can be 'beamed' to our homes 'live': dying, death and experiences of grief are all too common images on our television screens, in newspapers and on websites; to this extent death is ever-present in our lives. This, however, is the death and suffering of 'others' to be watched and observed, but something we often find difficult to relate to on a personal and individual level.
>
> (Exley, 2004, p. 111)

From an individual perspective, one's first experience of bereavement following the death (either natural or unnatural) of a close family member now tends to occur at a much later age than it did in previous centuries. Given the increase in life expectancy, death is primarily associated with old age and the majority of people do not experience the death of an immediate family member or near relative until they themselves are well in to mid-adulthood. This is in marked contrast to earlier times when death was a common occurrence in *all* age groups. For example, in reference to the Early Modern period (1500 to 1800), Stone notes how 'Death was at the centre of life, as the cemetery was at the centre of the village' (Stone, 1977, p. 54). Life expectation for infants and children was so poor in the medieval period that parents would give the same name to two living siblings as it was expected that both were unlikely to survive.

Returning to the contemporary era, Gorer's (1955) view that death has become a source of pornographic entertainment warrants careful reflection. Indeed, since he originally made the claim film scenes of violent death have become more graphic. Also, in 2002 the first public autopsy in Britain since the 1830s was broadcast on national network television. However, at the same time there has been a growing number of television programmes dealing with death and dying in less dramatic and visually explicit ways. For example, there have been documentaries on the end of life, coping with terminal illness and the question of euthanasia, which have addressed what may be termed the 'private' as opposed to the 'public' face of death. Although the media regularly report tragic deaths, deaths of celebrities are covered whatever the circumstances.

Natural death might not be the taboo subject it once was, but many people still find it difficult talking to someone who has recently been bereaved. We are quite happy to use words such as 'death' and 'dying' in everyday conversation when referring to highly emotive states or extreme experiences. For example, we may describe ourselves as being 'dead tired', 'dead drunk' or 'tickled to death'. We may begin an amusing anecdote or joke with the opening line, 'you'll die laughing when you hear this one'. However, when we actually talk about death and dying at a personal level we often deliberately choose not to use a direct vocabulary. Instead we resort to euphemisms and other linguistic devices to avoid any discomfort or embarrassment either on our part or on that of our listener. For example, we refer to someone as having 'passed away', 'gone to heaven' or being 'at rest' or 'at peace'. These are comforting words and phrases, which denote the end of life while conveying an image of death as representing a release from a state of suffering. It is possible that this reluctance to talk about death and dying owes a lot to the fact that people today have very little direct experience of death and bereavement. A view expressed by Walter when he asserts that:

> Death is not very much present today. If the bereaved person finds others embarrassed, crossing to the other side of the street, I suspect it is not so much because they dare not, cannot, confront death, but because they have had little practice at it, do not know what to do, are scared of saying the wrong thing.
>
> (Walter, 1990, p. 33)

Avoiding the use of certain words and phrases also applies when composing letters of condolence. We can experience difficulty in finding the appropriate form of words and there is an inclination to favour indirect phrases such as 'a sad loss'. The nature and type of written or spoken phrases employed, and the social etiquette surrounding interaction with the bereaved, will reflect the religious beliefs and socio-cultural attitudes towards death and dying of the particular group concerned.

Attitudes to death and dying

> The history of natural death is the history of the medicalization of the struggle against death.
>
> (Illich, 1977, p. 181)

The evolution of ideas regarding death

It would be wrong to assume that our views regarding the end of life, and the social practices and rituals surrounding the disposal of dead bodies, are similar to those found amongst people living in times and places different from our own. Indeed, there is a rich body of literature which charts the historical development of ideas about death and dying in different societies. The dominant image of death in any one society at a particular point in time is shaped by cultural values and social norms. Religion plays an important role in this context, as religious belief systems influence how people come to view life and death on a spiritual level. For example, some religions subscribe to a belief in an afterlife. However, there is a view that some modern Western societies have experienced a process of secularisation. In other words, spiritual ideas and religious beliefs have been undermined by advances in science and technology to such an extent that religion is no longer the dominant force that it once was. Commenting on the degree of secularisation witnessed in some European societies Walter observes that '[f]or many people today there is thus no afterlife to prepare for, on one's deathbed or at any other time' (Walter, 2003, p. 218).

A society's image of death changes over time. As noted in the previous section, the image of a 'natural' death in old age, following a good, healthy life, is an ideal of fairly recent origin. Illich (1977) argues that this view has evolved through a number of distinct stages over a period of some five hundred years. He identifies the main phases in the development of attitudes towards death and dying as follows:

1 The Devotional 'Dance of the Dead' – fifteenth century.

2 The Danse Macabre – sixteenth to seventeenth century.

3 Bourgeois Death – seventeenth to eighteenth century.

4 Clinical Death – nineteenth century.

5 Death under Compulsory Care – twentieth century.

6 Death under Intensive Care – late twentieth century.

Illich's depiction of stages in the evolution of images of natural death draws on a wide variety of sources including death ceremonies, rituals and customs, cultural and artistic representations of death, and a broad range of scholarly texts. The historical development of the changing views of natural death illustrates how the image of death has come to acquire an increasingly medical character.

In outlining the first of the six stages, Illich describes how Christian cemeteries were the scene of pagan practices, in which people danced on the tombs of the dead as a way of celebrating the joy of being alive. Towards the end of the fourteenth century the nature of these dances is seen to have changed as they came to reflect a more meditative response to the subject of death. Artistic works of the period show dancing partners as corpses, with each dancer representing a mirror image of the other. In this way, each individual is depicted as dancing through life with his or her own death. Throughout the Middle Ages, death was largely seen as the result of divine providence. However, the dance of the dead showed death as an inevitable part of human life rather than the consequence of a deliberate intervention by God. Illich suggests that this view of death as autonomous was illustrative of a readiness for the acceptance of a radical change in attitudes towards death: a change that would see death as a *natural* event or occurrence.

Illich's second stage in the changing image of natural death is labelled the 'The Danse Macabre' or 'Dance of Death'. Here the figure of death is symbolised by a skeleton and 'dance partners have shed their putrid flesh and turned into naked skeletons' (Illich, 1977, p. 186). In the dance of death of the sixteenth century, death was not presented simply in terms of a transition into the next world, but emphasis was placed on death as marking the end of this life. This suggests an acceptance of the finality of personal death. Death was perceived as a natural phenomenon and a force of nature, but it was a force with which to do battle.

The role of the physician was to engage in this battle by helping the healing process or assisting in achieving a comfortable death. However, any attempt to prolong life was viewed as interfering with the order of nature. The changing image of death had implications for the way in which the corpse was viewed. Whereas in the Middle Ages the human body had been regarded as sacred and the corpse had similar legal rights to those enjoyed by a living person, it was now reduced to an object. Towards the end of the seventeenth century public dissections were being performed at carnivals in Europe. If death is seen as becoming autonomous in stage one, in stage two it can be described as emerging as an 'independent figure' (Illich, 1977, p. 185).

The changing social and economic climate in Europe in the seventeenth and eighteenth centuries witnessed the emergence of what Illich terms 'Bourgeois Death'. This represents the third stage in his theory of the evolution of images of death. The Industrial Revolution led to a marked growth in trade and commerce, which provided new opportunities for the creation of wealth. The bourgeois class reaped the monetary benefits of this economic growth and could use their wealth to help to keep death at bay. Death now began to be perceived as an 'untimely event' when victim was not both elderly and healthy. There was no longer equality in death; a 'natural' death was the preserve of those who had the resources to die as patients. According to Illich:

> In an earlier epoch, death had carried the hourglass. In woodcuts, both skeleton and onlooker grin when the victim refuses death. Now the middle class seized the clock and employed doctors to tell death when to strike.
>
> (Illich, 1977, p. 198)

Illich contends that the dominant image of death in a society determines how health is defined and perceived. In the period in question a new concept of health had emerged, one that embraced the notion of a timely death.

'Clinical Death' marks the fourth stage in the evolution of images of death. According to Illich, this concept 'originated in the emerging professional consciousness of the new, scientifically trained doctor' (Illich, 1977, p. 200). The nineteenth-century physician was depicted as being engaged in a battle against a host of specific diseases. The hope and expectation that doctors would be able to identify and cure these diseases helped to create and perpetuate the myth that the clinician had power over death. Illich describes how in paintings and drawings of the period death is shown as taking the initiative, whereas by the early twentieth century the doctor is portrayed as having the upper hand and playing a more active role in the struggle against death. This constitutes Illich's fifth stage in the societal concept of death and he describes its emergence as follows:

> Only after clinical sickness and clinical death had developed considerably do we find the first pictures in which the doctor assumes the initiative and interposes himself between his patient and death.
>
> (Illich, 1977, p. 204)

In this era it is the doctor rather than the patient who is depicted as struggling with death. Health was perceived as a commodity and the 'good death' had 'become that of the standard consumer of medical care' (Illich, 1977, p. 202). Clinically trained doctors were deemed to be responsible for delivering the medical treatment necessary to prevent premature death. For the first time society was considered to have a duty to ensure that all citizens had the right to a natural death.

According to Illich death has become increasingly medicalised down the ages. In the contemporary era the doctor has replaced the priest at the final deathbed scene. Whereas the passing of life was once primarily explained in spiritual terms, in modern society it is seen as a scientific problem that is open to medical intervention. While the priest is concerned with preparing the dying person for death, the doctor focuses on relieving pain and prolonging life. Illich feels quite strongly that as a result of the medicalisation of society (i.e. the process by which aspects of social life have come to be viewed in biomedical terms and deemed appropriate for control by the medical profession) the patient is no longer able to set the scene for his or her own death. This is epitomised by the final stage of 'Death in Intensive Care', which Illich felt characterised the second half of the twentieth century. As he describes, the medicalisation of death ensures that doctors are in firm control of managing the dying process.

> Like all other major rituals of industrial society, medicine in practice takes the form of a game. The chief function of the physician becomes that of an umpire. He is the agent or representative of the social body, with the duty to make sure that everyone plays the game according to the rules. The rules, of course, forbid leaving the game and dying in any fashion that has not been specified by the umpire. Death no longer occurs except as the self-fulfilling prophecy of the medicine man.
>
> (Illich, 1977, p. 208)

One of the consequences of this arrangement is that when a patient dies medical staff can feel a sense of failure (Pietroni, 1991).

It is Illich's belief that the medicalisation of society, with its emphasis on health and living, has brought the era of natural death to an end and suppressed the development of a more enlightened attitude towards death. The medical profession has by its actions rendered patients 'pathetically dependent' (Illich, 1977, p. 111) and undermined their ability to express their own values. He does not offer any solution to the situation other than suggesting that intervention by professionals should be reduced to a minimum. However, it needs to be remembered that his medicalisation thesis was advanced in the mid-1970s, at a time when 'a much more unitary and optimistic view of medicine was in evidence than exists today' (Clark, 2002, p. 907). By comparison, doubt and scepticism feature in present-day medical practice. Furthermore, there is evidence of the emergence of a more holistic approach to understanding the meaning of life and death (Mellor, 1993). The growth in complementary therapies and alternative treatments suggests that the control of the medical profession over health issues is not absolute. There has also been recognition of the need to move towards the concept of a 'patient-centred death'. Traditionally debates about what constitutes a 'good death' have been dominated by health professionals, with relatively little attention devoted to the views of patients themselves. The need to readdress this balance by researching patients' perspectives on dying has been acknowledged (Clark, 2003). We return to the topic of a 'good death' in a later section.

The changing nature of death

In an effort to understand variations in the nature of morality and the handling of death in different societies, some social theorists draw a distinction between three broad societal types: *traditional* societies, *modern* societies and *postmodern* societies. The term traditional (or premodern) is generally used to refer to those societies that have not undergone a period of industrialisation. Included in this category are not only ancient societies, but the hunter-gatherer, nomadic and agrarian societies that have existed down the ages. Generally, traditional societies are characterised as having enduring extended family systems and a rudimentary form of community government. In the contemporary period, premodern societies tend to take the form of small, closely knit communities in relatively remote and inhospitable regions of the world.

In contrast, modern societies are those that have experienced major changes at the social, economic, cultural and political levels of activity. For historians the early modern era in Western civilisation began during the sixteenth century, while the first phase of modernity is associated with the increasing industrialisation of the nineteenth century. Giddens describes modernity as follows:

> At its simplest, modernity is a shorthand term for modern society or industrial civilization. Portrayed in more detail, it is associated with (1) a certain set of attitudes towards the world, the idea of the world as open to transformation by human intervention; (2) a complex of economic institutions, especially industrial production and a market economy; (3) a certain range of political institutions, including the nation-state and mass democracy. Largely as a result of these characteristics, modernity is vastly more dynamic than any previous type of social order. It is a society – more technically, a complex of institutions – which unlike any preceding culture lives in the future rather than the past.
>
> (Giddens, 1998, p. 94)

These features serve to set modern societies apart from their premodern counterparts. By comparison, on a structural level, modern societies are more complex and tend to have highly centralised and bureaucratised systems of production and government. Tradition and custom are no longer viewed as exercising the same degree of control over human behaviour and a high premium is placed on personal autonomy. Furthermore, the movement away from traditional social norms and moral constraints is reflected in the decline in the significance of religion. Under conditions of modernity, science and technology are seen as vehicles for human progress.

Social theorists maintain that during the late twentieth century Western societies began to undergo a transformation with the onset of what has been variously labelled as 'late modernity', 'high modernity' or 'postmodernity'. In essence, social values associated with modernity were beginning to be questioned and there was growing disillusionment with the idea that scientific knowledge and rational thinking were capable of making the world a better place. The move into the twenty-first century has seen a rapid growth in information and communications technology, a rise in the significance of the mass media and an expansion of popular culture. Consequently, it is argued that as a result of all this society underwent a fundamental transformation. Not only are people no longer tied to traditional norms and social conventions but *what* they think and *how* they think has undergone a profound change. In this context, some theorists refer to the process of globalisation. According to one such theorist, globalisation 'refers to the fact that we all increasingly live in one world, so that individuals, groups and nations become *interdependent*' (Giddens, 2006, p. 50, emphasis in original). On a macro-level we can see this process in terms of the expansion in world trade and the creation of transnational companies and commercial enterprises. However, this also has implications for the way in which people live their daily lives. Established social institutions are seen as being outmoded and economic and social life is considered to be in a constant state of flux. Within the context of highly diverse postmodern societies individuals have the freedom and opportunity to create and fashion their own self identities. Thus late modernity is characterised by a 'new individualism' (Giddens, 2006, p. 68), which encourages people to re-evaluate personal and intimate aspects of their lives. Whereas in earlier times traditional values determined the nature and content of the social roles people performed (for example, the man as the breadwinner and the woman as the homemaker), in the postmodern era people are much less constrained by normative expectations.

Walter (1996) uses the threefold typology of societies in exploring differences in social approaches to death (see Box 7.2). In premodern societies, to belong to a tribe or group is to share a common set of religious beliefs. As it is the belief system which gives meaning to life and death, religious leaders are in a particularly

Box 7.2   Definition

The changing nature of death in traditional, modern and postmodern societies

	Traditional death	*Modern death*	*Postmodern death*
Authority	Tradition	Professional expertise	Personal choice
Authority figure	Priest	Doctor	The self
Dominant discourse	Theology	Medicine	Psychology
Coping through	Prayer	Silence	Expressing feelings
The traveller	Soul	Body	Personality
Bodily context	Living with death	Death controlled	Living with dying
Social context	Community	Hospital	Family

Source: Walter, T. (1996) 'Facing death without tradition', in Glennys Howarth and Peter Jupp (eds), *Contemporary Issues in the Sociology of Death, Dying and Disposal*, p.195, published 1996, Palgrave Macmillan, reproduced with permission of Palgrave Macmillan influential position when it comes to organising how a community handles death and dying. In small, closely knit communities, the death of any one individual can undermine the family or communal group. Religious rites and ceremonies provide a way of dealing with death which serves to reaffirm existing social values and beliefs; religion is what binds societies together. In this sense, death rituals have considerable social significance and death is played out in the public arena with priests (or their equivalent) exercising their authority.

Ariès (1974) describes how in the period from the Middle Ages to the eighteenth century the actual event of dying was almost a public ceremony over which the dying person had some influence. From a study of historical evidence he suggests that during this period the majority of people died at home, and the bed chamber, in which the dying person lay, was regularly visited by family and friends. Indeed up until the eighteenth century, in portrayals of deathbed scenes in art and literature the presence of children was commonplace. In a sense the dying person was seen as playing an important role in the ritual practices surrounding the dying process and the community provided the social context in which death occurred.

In the modern period the doctor began to replace the priest as the principal authority figure at the scene of death. According to Howarth: 'During the twentieth century dying was no longer the preserve of the Church, but primarily the concern of medical science' (Howarth, 2007, p. 22). Death was now a medical event and doctors were the new authority figures. The doctor is assigned responsibility for pronouncing death, identifying the cause and issuing the death certificate. Whereas in premodern society death can be attributed to sorcery, witchcraft or an act of divine retribution, in modern society each death is officially classified according its physical cause. As described in the previous section, the medicalisation of death has meant that the hospital or hospice, and not the community, is where the majority of deaths take place. Thus, dying no longer constitutes a public ceremony involving the dying person. This transformation is aptly described by Illich: 'The medicalisation of society has brought the epoch of natural death to an end. Western man has lost the right to preside at his act of dying' (Illich, 1977, p. 210). The influence of the medical model is such that death is perceived as the enemy against whom the doctor must fight to prolong the life of the patient.

According to some social theorists, attitudes to death and dying have changed in the postmodern period. The fragmentation of social values and the growing emphasis placed on individualism in contemporary Western societies have brought about changes in the social understanding of mortality. As Walter (1996) claims, the authority for mortality under conditions of postmodernity is not tradition (as in premodern society) or professional expertise (as in modern society) but 'personal choice'; consequently the figure of authority is not the priest or doctor but 'the self'. Thus death is removed from the public sphere and in the process perceived as being more of a personal issue. This is referred to as the *sequestration* of death, which is described as 'the privatisation and subjectivisation of the experience of death, which in turn results in the increased presence of considerations of death for individuals' (Mellor, 1993, p. 12). Here privatised strategies and personalised rituals are emphasised when dealing with death and dying, in contrast to the public and communal death rituals favoured by traditional societies. There is a sense in which death has taken on new meanings for both the individual and society. The dominant discourse is no longer theology or medicine but psychology. Walter (1996) describes the contemporary situation as one in which the dying person negotiates their own passage through the various ways of dealing with the end of life. Given the importance attached to individualism (as opposed to collectivism), and the role of the family in the changing social context of death, counselling for individuals replaces collective ritual for society as the key mechanism for coping with death.

The typology of the changing nature of death outlined by Walter provides us with a broad overview of the different social approaches to death found in each of the three types of society. As an individual society develops, its view of death and people's beliefs concerning what happens after death may also change. However, at any one time there will be evidence of social and cultural diversity within an individual society. Therefore, it is more accurate to see Walter's framework as 'a tool for identifying *dominant* approaches surrounding death rather than as a portrait of attitudes within any one society' (Howarth, 2007, p. 19, emphasis added). Indeed, when commenting on Walter's description of postmodern death, Howarth comments that it might not actually be postmodern fragmentation that Walter is identifying but the existence of social and cultural diversity in approaches to mortality. This diversity has been forever present 'but has been pushed to the margins by dominant discourses that reflect the power of different social groups, for example, of those seeking only religious or medical understandings' (Howarth, 2007, p. 36). Thus while the broad typology provides a useful unified analytical construct that helps us to gain an insight into how different types of society handle death, we need to be aware that in contemporary Western societies there are a number of alternative discourses subscribed to by a variety of ethnic, cultural and religious minority groups.

The denial of death thesis

During the second half of the twentieth century the idea began to take hold that contemporary Western society was 'death-denying'. Fear of death was seen as a universal phenomenon that had to be dealt with in order for societies to function effectively. In premodern societies religion was the key institution that provided a framework for understanding the meaning of death and dying. Religious rites and mourning rituals governed the disposal of dead bodies and provided relatives and friends with a way of coming to terms with personal grief and the sense of loss. In the increasingly secular atmosphere found in modern societies the response at the societal level is best described as death-avoidance. Supporters of the denial of death thesis base their argument around three key themes already raised in this chapter: (1) the notion that conversation about death constitutes a taboo; (2) the medicalisation of death; (3) the segregation of the dying from the rest of society. The origin of these three themes will be discussed further in this section and the validity of the denial of death thesis will be explored. However, it needs to be borne in mind that these themes are clearly interrelated. For example, a consequence of the medicalisation of death is that dying has become more institutionalised, as more people are dying in hospitals and nursing homes rather than in their own homes.

From a psychological perspective individuals use denial as a defence mechanism when confronted with events of a potentially traumatising nature (Freud, 1940). Becker (1973) claims that such a response is not confined to individuals; a whole society can be characterised by denial. In fact he sees attempts to avoid the reality of mortality as a commonplace feature of modern society. The British social anthropologist Geoffrey Gorer and the French historian Philippe Ariès are recognised as early proponents of the idea of the existence of death-denying societies (Walter, 1991). Ariès (1974, 1981) provides an account of changing attitudes to death in Western Christian cultures from the Middle Ages to the twentieth century. He argues that death has gone from being public and familiar to being private and secret.

> The old attitude in which death was both familiar and near, evoking no great fear or awe, offers too marked a contrast to ours, where death is so frightful that we dare not utter its name . . . This is why I have called this household sort of death 'tamed death'. I do not mean that death had once been wild and that it had ceased to be so. I mean, on the contrary, that today it has become wild.
>
> (Ariès, 1974, p. 13)

According to Ariès, from the Middle Ages until the mid nineteenth century attitudes to death changed very slowly, but from that time on there occurred a 'brutal revolution' in traditional ideas and beliefs regarding death. In his opinion, death moved from being familiar to being 'shameful and forbidden' (Ariès, 1974, p. 85). This largely resulted from two developments in the management of death and dying. One was the emergence of a growing desire to spare the dying person knowledge of their impending fate and the other was the focusing on how the impact of death on society and the surviving relatives could be minimised. For Ariès this constituted 'the beginning of the lie', the 'hushing up' of death in modern Western society. While the initial intention had been to protect the terminally ill patient, by the early twentieth century any mention of death was avoided for the benefit of those people who were close to the dying person and for the sake of society in general. The idea was to avoid 'the disturbance and the overly strong and unbearable emotion caused by the ugliness of dying and by the very presence of death in the midst of a happy life' (Ariès, 1974, p. 87). Consequently, modern death (i.e. 'wild death') is depicted as taking place privately and secretly; shrouded in silence and denial.

There is no doubt that attitudes towards death have changed and that death is handled differently in modern-day society than it was in earlier times. However, the claim that in the modern era death is hidden away and not discussed is open to debate. Even Ariès himself acknowledges, when referring to the growing literature on death and dying in the early part of the second half of the twentieth century, that 'death is once again becoming something one can talk about'

(Ariès, 1974, p. 103). As previously mentioned, we are exposed to media images of death on a daily basis. The proliferation of news items and feature articles dealing with death and dying challenges the very idea that death is a taboo topic. In the case of celebrity figures, death is publicly announced and given extensive coverage on the radio, television and in newspapers. However, while the death of a celebrity generates talk about death and produces public displays of mourning, it is an impersonal experience for the vast majority of people. For example:

> . . . when Diana, Princess of Wales, died in 1997, there was an enormous outpouring of grief, not only in Britain but all over the world. Yet were people mourning a real person? . . . Princess Diana existed for most people only through the media. Diana's death was more like an event in a soap opera than a real event in the way in which people experienced it: . . .
>
> (Giddens, 2006, p. 115)

This highlights the significance of the media in the contemporary era as a vehicle for representing and transmitting social values surrounding mortality. Knowledge obtained via the media also provides important cues as to what constitutes appropriate behaviour when it comes to displays of grief (Walter *et al.*, 1995). It could be argued from this media coverage that the notion that death is a taboo subject has been grossly exaggerated and that there is in fact a public discourse around death and dying in our society.

Some critics of the denial of death thesis maintain that there has not been a silence surrounding death in more recent times; what has emerged is 'a new way of speaking about death' (Armstrong, 1987, p. 652). While Ariès claims a silence descended around the bed of the dying person, Armstrong maintains that changes in the nineteenth century resulted in death becoming subject to increased discussion and scrutiny by experts. The legal requirement that deaths should be officially recorded and a central register maintained meant that each death became public and the cause of death had to be identified in every case. Establishing the cause of death involved doctors, pathologists and coroners examining and interpreting a broad body of evidence. According to Armstrong talk about death was not silenced, it was more a case of a shift in focus. Legal and medical discourses emerged, in which the principal object was the dead body and not the dying patient.

When assessing the denial of death thesis it is important to distinguish between denial on the part of the individual (i.e. at the personal level) and denial as a feature of society (i.e. at the social level). Kellehear (1984) is critical of the way in which some sociologists have applied the label 'death-denying' to whole societies and accepted the fear of death as a universal phenomenon without exploring the conceptual distinction between personal fear and social fear. He notes that some studies have shown that fear of death is not universal and where individuals do express fear its nature varies. Furthermore, Kellehear maintains that supporters of the denial of death argument have been highly selective in their search for evidence to support their thesis. In short they have looked for examples and instances of denial and duly found them. Consequently, features of the handling of death and dying that illustrate social and cultural diversity, and have the potential to undermine the denial of death thesis, have been ignored.

Individuals may well refrain from discussing death in specific circumstances and social contexts. However, this may be a reflection of 'conversational propriety and emotional reserve', which discourages the talking about sensitive topics that are considered likely to make people feel uneasy and embarrassed in interpersonal encounters (Kellehear, 1984, p. 719). Given the intensity of the suffering associated with death and bereavement, discussing death can be extremely upsetting. Thus, while the practice of avoiding the topic of death in conversational exchanges may encourage an attitude of death denial, it does not necessarily follow that this avoidance is a reflection of the fact that the society as a whole is death-denying.

Proponents of the denial of death thesis draw on the medicalisation of death argument to support their case. They argue that not only is the dying process in modern culture firmly in the hands of the medical profession but curative medicine has embraced a death-denying ethos. Advances in medical science and healthcare technology have helped to create a death-avoiding attitude among physicians and other health professionals. As described above, when discussing the work of Illich, 'natural' death is seen as having been replaced by a form of technological dying. According to Illich, in modern Western society the individual no longer has control over the act of dying: 'Health, or the autonomous power to cope, has been expropriated down to the last breath. Technical death has won its victory over dying. Mechanical death has conquered and destroyed all other death' (Illich, 1977, p. 210). In other words, death has become largely a technical matter. In delivering the best care possible to the patient, doctors use every form of technology available to prolong life. The commitment to providing the best treatment that is technically possible is referred to as the 'technological imperative'. It is the operation of this imperative which is seen as encouraging an atmosphere of denial.

Not all sociologists subscribe to the view that the medicalisation of death is responsible for creating a death-denying attitude. Forms of treatment and clinical interventions to control premature death or relieve the pain and suffering of terminally ill patients can be seen as helping to produce a kind of 'natural' death. According to this view, the medical profession is not death-denying but actually accepts the scientific reality of death. The actions taken are designed to control the dying process until the inevitable finally happens. Thus, medical technology is not seen as being responsible for generating an attitude of denial (Parsons and Lidz, 1967; Parsons, 1978).

The idea of the medicalisation of dying is well established in the literature. Indeed, there have been major advances in medical technology, and historical research describes how the doctor has come to replace the priest at the bedside of the dying person. However, '[w]hat is less clear is whether or not this medicalisation indeed stems from or encourages a denial of death' (Zimmermann and Rodin, 2004, p. 125). The issue is confused by the fact that the concept of medicalised dying can be used when accounting for the existence of *either* 'death-denying' or 'death-accepting' attitudes. Consequently, Zimmermann and Rodin assert that it is too simplistic to categorise one society as 'death-denying' and another as 'death-accepting'. The way in which death is approached in a particular society will reflect elements of both denial and acceptance.

Modern medicalised death is described by Ariès (1974) as 'wild', 'savage' and 'dirty'; the very antithesis of the 'tamed death' characteristic of the premodern era. Along with Illich (1977), he sees death and dying as having been redefined in technical terms and managed by medical experts within the relative social isolation of the hospital. In essence, it is argued that the increasing use of medical technology has led to the physical segregation of the dying from the rest of society and the dehumanisation of death. This sequestration of death (i.e. its removal from the public sphere) has been referred to above as a characteristic of societies in the late modern or postmodern period. For the majority of people today the site of death is the hospital, hospice or nursing home. Death has become institutionalised: 'Never before have people died as noiselessly and hygienically as today . . . and never in social conditions so much fostering solitude' (Elias, 1985, p. 85). For those theorists who support the denial of death thesis, this social isolation of the dying is considered a direct consequence of the prevalence of a death-denying culture. Dying people are seen as being confined to hospitals and nursing homes as a way of protecting the living from having to face the full physical and emotional realities of death.

Although there is no doubt that in the contemporary period death has been sequestered and institutionalised, this does not necessarily constitute evidence in favour of the denial of death thesis. Indeed, it has been suggested that 'societies do not deny death but instead organise for it and around it' (Kellehear, 1984, p. 720). In other words, the growing tendency for people to die in an institution rather than at home, may be a reflection of the wider social and structural changes that have taken place in modern times. For example, families tend to be smaller than they used to be; the extended family has largely given way to the relatively isolated, nuclear family. Given that more people are now living alone or in smaller family units, it is no longer a realistic option for some families to provide continuous care for dying relatives. There is a greater likelihood of encountering a number of potential carers in large, cohesive extended families than there is in smaller nuclear families, where adult members are employed outside the home.

Sociologists who adopt a functionalist perspective argue that societies need to develop ways of handling and managing mortality in order to prevent it from disrupting the smooth running of society. Thus, the social arrangements that evolve to deal with death and dying are not a consequence of the existence of a death-denying culture but a reflection of a need to deal with mortality at the structural level. Blauner (1966) argues that as bureaucracy plays such an important role in organising people's lives, and is a fundamental feature of the social structure of modern societies, it is not surprising that it should have influenced the way in which death and dying are managed. The bureaucratisation and institutionalisation of death are seen as mechanisms for containing the potentially disruptive impact of mortality at the societal level. Thus, the segregation of the dying from the rest of society serves a particular purpose. As he asserts, the 'separation of the handling of illness and death from the family minimises the average person's exposure to death and its disruption of the social process' (Blauner, 1966, p. 384).

Proponents of the denial of death thesis maintain that the existence of a death-denying attitude has created a problematic situation when it comes to providing care for the dying. It is argued that dying is a natural process and needs to be recognised as such if better treatment is to be provided for the dying patient. However, as suggested above, the thesis is not without its critics. To describe contemporary Western society as death-denying has been described as 'simplistic if not altogether false' (Zimmermann and Rodin, 2004, p. 127). Ariès' historical analysis which exhorts a return to the natural, 'tamed' death of the past and a relinquishing of the medicalised, 'wild' death of the modern era has been criticised for underplaying the negative aspects of death in earlier times. While Elias (1985) accepts Ariès's general argument that there has been a major change in the way death is dealt with in the modern era, he draws attention to what he sees as an implicit romanticism in his interpretation of the historical evidence. Indeed, not all historians interpret the experience of death in the Middle Ages in a similar way to Ariès. For example, according to one account, 'Death was a grim business in the Middle Ages. With no alleviation of pain, no dulling of the horrors of surgery . . . the bitterness of death was very real' (Boase, 1972, p. 9). Ariès documents the fact that medical technology has succeeded in undermining the control individuals have over the final stage of the life course. However, whether this heralds the loss of what he terms 'tamed death' is another matter. Hospitals have become the convenient place to die, but this could reflect the fact that death has been 'tamed' by the medical profession who have, to a certain extent, taken over responsibility for dealing with the dying and play a major role in determining the nature and social context of death. This is not to deny the substance of Aries' original thesis, but merely to question his conceptualisation of 'tamed death'. Notwithstanding the medicalistion of death, the relationship between the dying patient and the medical profession is not always imbued with conflict. Great advances have been made in the control of pain and the treatment of terminal illnesses, which are capable of reducing physical suffering towards the end of life.

Theories of death and dying

> . . . although most conceptual models of the dying process and bereavement are dynamic, such as the stage theory of dying . . . most empirical studies still rely on single point-in-time evaluations that retrospectively recall the dying and bereavement process.
>
> (Carr, 2007, p. 975)

Since the sociology of death was first described as 'a neglected area of research' there has been a dramatic growth in studies of death and dying (Faunce and Fulton, 1958). Over the years a variety of theoretical models have been advanced as the focus of research attention has shifted. As Carr (2007) notes, although much empirical research has been conducted, a unifying theoretical perspective has not emerged. In the main, researchers have tended to work within their own areas of special interest and focused on death and dying accordingly. For example, those sociologists with an interest in ageing have limited their study to people aged 65 years and over, while medical sociologists have tended to concentrate on the social and ethical aspects of clinical decision-making towards the end of life and the interaction that takes place between healthcare professionals and dying patients and their families. What these various approaches have in common is that they are social in nature. In other words, they are primarily concerned with examining the social process and social organisation of death and dying in modern society. The context of awareness theory (Glaser and Strauss, 1965) discussed below is a good example of a sociologically oriented approach. However, not all theories focus on the social dimension to the same extent. For example, stage theory (Kübler-Ross, 1969) is interested in psychological responses to dying and how people approaching the end of life adapt to the institutional context in which they find themselves. The strengths and limitations of both context awareness theory and stage theories are discussed below.

Context of awareness theory

Much of the early research on death and dying took place in the USA in the 1960s and focused on the experiences of terminally patients and the management of death and dying in a hospital setting. Glaser and Strauss (1965) conducted a pioneering ethnographic study in three hospitals in San Francisco, using interviews and observations to collect data on the experience of dying in hospital. A key theme they explored was the nature of the interaction between hospital staff and terminally ill patients. In particular, they were interested in whether or not dying patients were aware of their terminal diagnosis. Analysing data collected during fieldwork on the wards they identified four contexts of awareness: closed awareness; suspicion awareness; mutual pretence awareness; open awareness (Box 7.3).

Closed awareness occurs when members of the healthcare team are aware that the patient is dying but do not share this information with the patient concerned. Essentially the patient's poor prognosis is hidden from them. According to Glaser and Strauss, hospital procedures and institutional arrangements are such that patients can easily be kept uninformed. As they point out:

> Records are kept out of reach. Staff are skilled at withholding information. Medical talk about patients generally occurs in far-removed places, and if it occurs nearby, it is couched in medical jargon. Staff members are trained to discuss with patients only the surface aspects of their illness and . . . they are accustomed to acting collusively around patients so as not to disclose medical secrets.
>
> (Glaser and Strauss, 1965, p. 31)

In observing interaction between hospital staff and patients, the researchers noted how nurses and doctors, when talking to patients, attempted to steer conversations away from discussing future events or tended to avoid certain topics

Box 7.3   Definition

Typology of awareness contexts

Closed awareness:

Health professionals and relatives are aware that the patient is dying but the patient is unaware.

Suspicion awareness:

The patient suspects a terminal illness but there is no confirmation of this from significant others.

Mutual pretence awareness:

Healthcare staff, the patient, family and friends have knowledge of the prognosis but refrain from discussing death.

Open awareness:

Everyone is aware of the terminal diagnosis and there is no pretence or hiding of the fact.

Source: Glaser and Strauss, 1965

altogether. In certain circumstances, maintaining such closed awareness can be particularly stressful, especially for those people who are in regular daily contact with someone who is terminally ill. It is an initial state, which may eventually give way either to suspicion awareness or full awareness. While some research suggests that closed awareness is less common today than it used to be (Field and Copp, 1999), there is evidence that non-disclosure policies operate on some wards (Costello, 2001).

Glaser and Strauss (1965) use the term suspicion awareness to describe the situation where the dying person suspects that they have a serious illness but keeps this suspicion to themselves. In the absence of any confirmation of a terminal diagnosis, the patient may adopt various direct or indirect tactics in an attempt to discover what she or he already suspects. This may involve confronting staff directly, which can be a potentially unsettling experience, especially for junior members of staff, as the following quotation suggests:

> The very first day that I came on to the ward I was very nervous. It was the first day in my foundation unit that I'd been up to the ward. The lady patient said, 'You can tell me that I am going to die, the others won't tell me, but I know. You can tell me that I'm going to die, aren't I?' I really didn't know what to say. I knew she was but I was really stuck for words. I just didn't know what to say. It was quite frightening.
> (A nurse quoted in Katz, 1989 and Katz, 2004, p. 57)

Glaser and Strauss (1965) describe this level of awareness as placing a 'fantastic psychological strain' on healthcare staff, the patient and the patient's family. In attempting to get at the truth the patient may initiate 'confirmation-seeking tactics' and indulge in behaviour designed to trap others into revealing the prognosis. Staff may respond by adopting counteractive strategies and being more circumspect when interacting with the patient in question. This may entail not only being careful as to what they say but also controlling aspects of their non-verbal behaviour (e.g. facial expressions) when dealing with the patient.

The interactional problems arising from the closed awareness and suspicion awareness contexts are absent from the state of mutual pretence. In this state of awareness, healthcare professionals, the patient and the patient's friends and family are informed about the prognosis but choose not to openly acknowledge the fact or discuss death. This ensures that any potentially embarrassing or emotionally difficult conversations and encounters are avoided. The main disadvantage associated with this response is that patients are not given the opportunity of discussing their concerns and fears about dying with people who are close to them.

The fourth awareness context is open awareness. This occurs when both staff and the patient are aware that death is imminent and choose to freely acknowledge this both in words and actions. There are no attempts at concealing the truth of the situation or avoiding discussing certain topics. This is not necessarily a tension-free state. For example, what the dying person considers to be an appropriate way of dying may not correspond with staff expectations.

Thus it can be seen that an understanding of awareness contexts can give us a better insight into the relationship between the dying patient and the professional practitioners and informal caregivers who provide care at the end of life. As Glaser and Strauss (1965) note, the problem of awareness has both a technical and moral dimension as far as medical and nursing personnel are concerned. In terms of the former, the focus is on whether the patient should be told he or she is dying and how to deal with patients displaying different states of awareness. From a moral perspective the problem is seen as involving professional ethics and personal values.

> Is it really proper, some people have asked, to deny a dying person the opportunity to make his [sic] peace with his conscience and with his God, to settle his affairs and provide for the future of his family, and to control his style of dying, much as he controlled his style of living? Does anyone, the physician included, have the right to withhold such information? Someone must decide whether to disclose, and when to disclose, but on whose shoulders should this responsibility fall – the physician, the family, or the patient?
>
> (Glaser and Strauss, 1965, p. 6)

The problem is compounded by the fact that dying people do not necessarily move in one direction from closed to open awareness. Depending on the length of time over which death occurs, patients may move between awareness contexts and may also reveal different states of awareness to different people.

Although Glaser and Strauss' research was published nearly forty-five years ago, their theory of awareness contexts is still seen as having relevance in the contemporary era. There is no doubt that their research has fundamentally changed the way we think about the management of dying and the nature of death itself. According to one observer, 'The most significant impact of their work by far, is their influence on healthcare professionals' approach to communication and interactions with the dying' (Copp, 1998, p. 385). In Western societies today there is a perceived preference for 'open awareness' among both patients and staff (Field, 1995). Doctors are now more likely to disclose a terminal diagnosis to patients. Indeed, given the emphasis placed on choice within the modern healthcare system, health professionals are expected to ascertain a patient's choice about preferred place of death (Department of Health, 2003b). Given the growing prevalence of open awareness, the concept has been refined in order to reflect more accurately the experiences of terminally ill patients and their carers. Timmermans (1994) distinguishes between three categories of open awareness:

Open suspended awareness: the dying person or informal carer 'blocks out' the information they have received regarding the terminal nature of the illness. They act as if the disclosure never occurred and live in a 'state of disbelief'.

Uncertain open awareness: where there is an element of uncertainty surrounding aspects of the diagnosis this opens the way for alternative explanations of symptoms. In this way patients and relatives can hold on to the hope of a recovery.

Active open awareness: there is no hope of a recovery. All those concerned accept that death is imminent and try to come to terms with the situation.

While acknowledging the significance of the general shift from closed awareness to open awareness, Field and Copp (1999) maintain that there has been a reversion to a state of 'conditional awareness'. They describe this as a more pragmatic approach, in which the right of the patient to be informed is fully accepted but at the same time it is recognised that not all patients are necessarily in favour of open awareness. Conditional disclosure can be a problem for healthcare professionals when they are attempting to provide patient-centred care and include patients and their relatives in end-of-life decision-making.

The degree of awareness that a particular patient has will depend upon a complex combination of professional, social, cultural and personal factors. For example, whether or not a terminally ill individual has a desire for open awareness may be influenced by cultural norms and values. There is evidence of cross-cultural variation both between societies (Seale *et al.*, 1997) and across ethnic groups within individual societies (Blackhall *et al.*, 1995). As Seale (1998) notes, cultural preferences for open awareness in dying are particularly marked when comparing Western societies with non-Western societies. He draws on research findings to illustrate how open awareness is culturally inappropriate in the Japanese context, which leads him to conclude that 'it appears that Japanese medicine and Japanese cultural expectations are characterised by the sort of "paternalism" and "denial" long decried in Anglo-American revivalist constructions of aware dying' (Seale, 1998, p. 111).

Glaser and Strauss' typology of states of awareness has proved to be a very important analytic device for understanding the management of dying in a hospital setting. What characterises this approach is its socio-environmental

---

Box 7.4   Definition

The dying trajectory

When the dying patient's hospital career begins – when he [sic] is admitted to the hospital and a specific service – the staff in solo and in concert make initial definitions of the patient's trajectory. They expect him to linger, to die quickly or to approach death at some pace between the extremes. They establish some degree of certainty about his impending death – for example, they may judge that there is 'nothing more to do' for the patient. They forecast that he will never leave the hospital again, or that he will leave and perhaps be admitted several times before his death. They may anticipate that he will have periods of relative health as well as severe physical hardship during the course of his illness. They predict the potential modes of his dying and how he will fare during the last days and hours of his life.

Source: Glaser and Strauss, 1968, p. 30

---

focus; it does not attempt to explore the inner psychological states of people who are facing death. Their research shows how the degree of awareness has implications for maintaining order and routine in the daily life of the hospital. The period of time over which death occurs is relevant and is one of the major factors influencing how staff respond to terminally ill patients and manage the dying process. In their book *Time for Dying* (1968) they use the concept of the 'dying trajectory' when exploring how an orderly ward routine is maintained despite the emotional sequence of events following the death of a patient (see Box 7.4). Individual dying trajectories vary in terms of time and shape. For example, in the case of the former, death may occur fairly quickly following a terminal diagnosis or the patient may experience a slow demise as a result of a long protracted illness. In terms of the shape of the dying trajectory, a person may experience a gradual, continual deterioration from the time of the initial diagnosis until death occurs. Alternatively, a trajectory may show signs of upward movement if a patient experiences a temporary relapse or brief episodes of remission. Glaser and Strauss describe how tension can be generated when there is an unexpected change in the predicted dying trajectory, such as when a patient dies unexpectedly or lingers when a quick death is anticipated. On the whole, hospital staff tend to find coping with sudden and unexpected deaths more difficult than dealing with deaths that are predictable and for which they have time to prepare.

Stage theories of dying

In the 1960s and 1970s several theories of dying were developed which focused on the needs of dying people and their families. These psychological theories presented dying in terms of a sequence of stages and became known as stage or phase theories. The most celebrated example is Kübler-Ross's (1969) five-stage

Box 7.5	Research findings

Kübler-Ross's five-stage theory

Denial:	'No, not me, it can't be true!'
Anger:	'Why me?' Initial shock gives way to rage.
Bargaining:	'What can I do to prevent this?'
Depression:	All hope is lost and thoughts and feelings are dominated by a sense of loss.
Acceptance:	The end of the struggle.

Source: Kübler-Ross, 1969

model of dying, which is based on interviews with over 200 patients who were dying in hospital. On one level, her study represents a critique of the medicalised and instutionalised way in which dying is controlled and managed in the modern era. She saw death in hospital as being far removed from the natural death that occurred in earlier times in more traditional community settings. As a result of modernist medical care, 'dying nowadays is more gruesome in many ways, namely, more lonely, mechanical and dehumanised . . .' (Kübler-Ross, 1969, p. 9). From her observational study of death in a hospital setting, she postulated that patients passed through five psychological or emotional stages in their response to dying: denial, anger, bargaining, depression and acceptance (Box 7.5).

At the core of this theoretical formulation lies the proposition that dying people pass through a series of identifiable stages as they approach death; each stage is characterised by specific observable behaviours and expressed emotions. According to this theory, when a patient receives the diagnosis of a life-limiting illness, the initial response to the shock is to refuse to believe the diagnosis. The patient is in a state of denial, which marks the first of Kübler-Ross's five stages. Once the patient accepts that there is no doubt concerning the accuracy of the diagnosis, denial eventually gives way to anger. During this second stage, the patient is seen as being full of rage and looking for someone or something to blame. The patient comes to view death as an undeserved punishment. The third stage identified in Kübler-Ross's research is one of bargaining. Here the dying person attempts to make a deal with fate or God in order to ensure that they do not die before a particular event, such as the birth of a grandchild. Depression represents the fourth stage in the model of dying. This occurs as the patient becomes weaker and shows signs of increasing physical deterioration. All hope of any recovery is lost as the progression of the disease can no longer be ignored. An acute and explicit fear of impending death may also be experienced. Feelings of anguish, despair and helplessness are not uncommon at this point in the dying process. Kübler-Ross also observed that patients in this stage may begin to withdraw from relationships with others and become less responsive to the world around them. The fifth and final stage is labelled 'acceptance'. This is when patients are ready to relinquish their hold on life. However, Kübler-Ross does not describe it as a necessarily happy state. Death with acceptance is the final stage wherein the emotional struggle to resist death is over and individuals have worked through their sense of grief and loss. This stage has been described as resembling Ariès's notion of 'tame death', 'where people have put their affairs in order, have made their farewells, and are ready to die peacefully' (Howarth, 2007, p. 136).

When it was first introduced, Kübler-Ross's theory was uncritically accepted by health workers and enthusiastically adopted to inform professional practice. Kastenbaum (1985) and Hart *et al.* (1998), among others, offer a number of reasons why the theory was originally so well received and widely used by professionals:

- The theory re-awakened interest in the subject of death and legitimised a once taboo topic.
- The focus of the theory was essentially on the dying person with the hospital context.
- The idea of an orderly sequence of unfolding stages of dying replaced an image of dying as a terrifying, lonely and dehumanising ordeal.
- The stage model provided professionals with a conceptual framework for making sense of the reactions of dying patients, thereby providing guidance for healthcare staff on how to respond to the emotional needs of individual patients.

In short, the 'model gained acceptance largely because it filled a void in health care theory' (Copp, 1998, p. 383). Also Kübler-Ross's status as a physician and psychiatrist gave the theory credibility among health professionals (Germain, 1980).

Kübler-Ross's stage theory was a pioneering work and succeeded in bringing attention to the emotional needs of dying people and their families. Nonetheless, the theory is not without its critics. From a methodological perspective it has been argued that the empirical study on which the theory is based is flawed because the focus is entirely on patients dying within a hospital setting. As such, the theory is limited in scope in that it reflects how dying patients adapt to a particular institutional context rather than describe the actual social process of dying (Charmaz, 1980). The emotional responses of dying patients may vary according to the situational context in which they are dying. Can we really assume that the five stages identified by Kübler-Ross apply equally to people dying in their own homes or in a hospice?

The theory is clearly useful in presenting the process of dying as a transition and providing a framework for identifying differences between people in terms of the way in which they respond to a terminal diagnosis. However, as Howarth notes, it was the 'wholesale adoption by professionals that led to the model being interpreted too rigidly, as a prescription for dying' (Howarth, 2007, p. 137). According to this interpretation, the dying person is seen as needing to progress through the universal five stages and experience the emotions and behaviours characteristic of each stage in order to achieve the goal of 'death with acceptance', which is defined as a 'good death'. Despite the fact Kübler-Ross never intended the model to be understood in such a prescriptive and mechanistic way, there is evidence to suggest that some health professionals have tried to apply the model in this manner (Rainey, 1988). This idea of an orderly linear progression is described as being contrary to the actual experience of people caring for individuals who are dying: dying patients are seen to 'oscillate between periods of calm, fear, hope, depression, anger, sadness and withdrawal' (Copp, 1998, p. 383). As Buckman (1998) notes, some emotions observed in clinical practice do not feature in Kübler-Ross's theory. Of those emotions omitted, fear is considered the most important.

Although Kübler-Ross's model of dying focuses on the needs of the individual at the end of life, the emphasis is firmly on the psychosocial dynamics of the situation, with scant attention being given to the relevance of the patient's physical condition or spiritual outlook. The five-stage schema is considered by some to fail to acknowledge the importance of individual differences. For example, it is claimed that, 'It is more useful to view the patient's emotions as a mosaic comprising different personal emotions often expressed simultaneously, but in a pattern that is a feature of that individual' (Buckman, 1998, p. 145). In other words, not only can individual patients experience multiple emotions at any one time but each patient will respond in a way that reflects her or his personal biography and individual characteristics. Where the five-stage model is used to identify what constitutes a 'good death' from the perspective of professional health workers, it can lead to a failure to appreciate the existence of individual diversity and the significance of cultural differences among patient groups.

Following a critique of Kübler-Ross's five-stage model, Buckman (1998) developed a more comprehensive three-stage model of the dying process, which he considered 'more accurately reflects the dying patient's progress and which will allow the professional greater power of analysis and prediction' (Buckman, 1998, p. 144). The model is informed by both clinical experience and findings from numerous research studies. At the core of the model are two primary principles:

- People who are facing death display a mixture of emotions and exhibit a variety of behavioural responses. These reflect the personality of the individuals concerned and are not seen as being characteristic of either the diagnosis or the stage the patient is at in the dying process.
- Each person goes through their own unique dying process. The individual's progress is marked by the extent to which the elements of those emotions that are relevant to them personally are resolved. Progress is not measured in terms of a change from one type of emotion to another.

As noted above, Buckman includes in his model emotions not featured in Kübler-Ross's five-stage approach and also sees individual emotions as forming a 'mosaic' or cluster rather than existing as part of a sequential process of transition from one state to the next.

For Buckman, the process of dying consists of three chronological stages: the initial stage, the chronic stage and the final stage (see Box 7.6). The emotional

---

> ### Box 7.6   Model
>
> ## Buckman's three-stage model of the dying process
>
> **Initial stage ('facing the threat')**
> A mixture of reactions characteristic of the individual including fear, anxiety, shock, disbelief, anger, denial, guilt, humour, hope/despair and bargaining.
>
> **Chronic stage ('being ill')**
> Resolution of elements of the initial response which are resolvable.
> Diminution of intensity of all emotions ('monochrome state').
> Depression is very common.
>
> **Final stage ('acceptance')**
> Defined by the patient's acceptance of death.
> Not an essential state provided that the patient is not distressed, is communicating normally, and is making decisions normally.
>
> *Source*: Adapted from Buckman, 1998, p. 146

states listed in the first stage are not experienced in any particular order and any one individual will not necessarily encounter all the emotions listed. When elements of the experienced emotions have been resolved the individual is seen as entering the chronic stage. If there is no such resolution then the chronic stage is not entered. In these cases the patient will require help and support in order to deal with their initial emotions. The final stage is characterised by a reduction in emotional intensity. Acceptance of death is a feature of this stage but not considered to be absolutely essential. What is of primary importance is that the patient is not distressed and is seen to be communicating normally with others.

Knowledge of the different stages may be of help to those people providing end of life care. It is important not only to understand particular psychological reactions to impending death (e.g. denial, anger, anxiety) but also to have an awareness of how these responses have a tendency to occur at particular times during the dying trajectory. Some emotional reactions will be characteristic of some stages more than others, and some may recur at different phases in the dying process. Not every person experiences all the emotional responses identified. For example, denial can be described as 'a subconscious defence mechanism' (Buckman, 1992, p. 101), a normal response to dealing with unwelcome news. However, some people diagnosed with a terminal illness may never admit that they are dying, while others may exhibit denial in the early stages but then eventually come to accept imminent death. In a guide for healthcare professionals, Buckman advises that:

> The way to respond to denial . . . is to respect the protective nature of it, and to realize that denial is a normal response to overwhelming threat. Further, you should demonstrate that you are allowing the patient the freedom to deny the bad news, until she or he is psychologically ready to deal with it head on.
>
> (Buckman, 1992, p. 101)

Thus, if denial is being used as a coping mechanism and appears to be working effectively, the patient should not be encouraged to accept the reality of the situation and move on to the next stage. Patients should only be encouraged to talk about their impending death when they show signs of no longer being in denial.

While Buckman's general model overcomes a number of limitations of the Kübler-Ross stage approach, it has not been exempt from criticism. Buckman's theoretical model is still stage-based and is therefore subject to the criticisms generally levelled at such approaches and 'falls into the trap of appearing "mechanistic"' (Copp, 1998, p. 384). Stage models are popular with health professionals, largely because they offer a framework for understanding psychological responses during dying. Consequently, they are seen as being particularly informative when it comes to the care and management of terminally ill patients. However, adherence to a stage-based perspective should not lead to individual differences being overlooked. A comprehensive theory of dying needs to incorporate an understanding of dying from the individual's own perspective. This is not necessarily captured by the stage theory approach.

Task-based approach

In exploring the process of dying from an individual's perspective some theorists refer to the notions of 'tasks' and 'coping with dying' as key concepts (Corr, 1992). Basically, the dying person is seen as being faced with having to perform a number of tasks as part of coping with the fact that death is near at hand. These coping tasks are identified by Corr (1992, p. 85) as falling into four broad categories:

1 **Physical:** There is a need to ensure that bodily needs are satisfied and physical distress is kept to a minimum. This needs to be achieved in accordance with the personal values espoused by the individual concerned.

2 **Psychological:** Here the key tasks relate to preserving and maximising psychological security and personal autonomy.

3 **Social:** The primary objectives are dealing with the social implications of dying and preserving and enhancing social networks and interpersonal contacts with significant others.

4 **Spiritual:** This involves developing or reaffirming spiritual beliefs, which can help to engender a sense of hope or cope with the realisation that death is imminent.

These tasks involve a wide variety of actions and behaviours on the part of the individual. Some tasks are primarily focused on the self, such as actions taken by the individual to cope with the increasing physical deterioration and frailty towards the end of life. Other tasks represent actions taken in the interests of others, such as making arrangements for the future financial security of one's family.

At the core of this approach is the view that the emphasis should not be placed solely on dying individuals and their coping tasks, but account should be taken of the actions and responses of those people involved in helping the dying person. Thus it differs from earlier approaches by bringing into the frame the relationships dying individuals have with their carers. Also, by including four broad areas of task work it represents a challenge to unidimensional perspectives such as Kübler-Ross's five-stage model. As a consequence, the task-based approach can be seen to acknowledge the multi-faceted nature of death and dying. However, much more empirical research needs to be undertaken before we can develop a theoretical framework for understanding fully the relationship between dying and tasks and how the tasks themselves are related to coping (Weisman, 1992).

As far as the different models and theoretical perspectives are concerned, concepts of awareness contexts, psychological states and coping tasks only apply in contexts where patients know or suspect that they are dying. This is clearly not always the case, as for example with patients who have dementia or have suffered a stroke. Death in intensive care units provides another example; here 'opportunities are markedly absent for the facilitation of awareness of dying, for development of self-identity through the dying process, and for social and psychological preparation for death' (Seymour, 1999, p. 694). When death occurs under conditions of intensive care the patient is nearly always in a state of unconsciousness as a consequence of the severity of the illness and/or as a result of receiving pain-relieving medication.

Good death, bad death

> A good death has always been important in all cultures. To achieve your chosen afterlife you died either well (euthanatos) or nobly (kalosthanein). But what is a good death in a world that for many is post-religious and medicalised?
>
> (Clark, 2003, p. 174)

The ideology of the good death

As individuals we can make lifestyle choices which have implications for our health and general well-being. However, while we have *some* freedom in making choices as to how we live our lives, there is very little scope for making choices when it comes to when, how and where we die. As discussed in an earlier section, at one time people died in their own homes surrounded by members of their family (Ariès, 1981). Nowadays, although the majority of dying still takes place within the home (Field, 1996), official mortality statistics show that the majority of deaths actually occur within an institutional environment such as a hospital, hospice or care home. Recent decades have witnessed a continual fall in the proportion of deaths taking place in the domestic sphere. This is despite the fact that it is assumed that the majority of people would prefer to die at home. A number of studies reveal that if given a choice, the majority of people with a terminal illness would prefer to die at home rather than in hospital (Dunlop *et al.*, 1989; Townsend *et al.*, 1990). At a national level, current policy is directed at giving terminally ill patients the opportunity to choose a home death should that be their wish (Department of Health, 2006b). However, some commentators maintain that the enthusiasm for home deaths expressed by policymakers is based as much on perceived cost savings, as it is on meeting the stated preferences of dying patients (Holmes, 1995). This is a contentious area of debate. Despite an increase in community-based palliative care provision in the UK over the last 20 years there has been a decline in the home death rate (Munday et al., 2007).

Although we have a considerable amount of information about what people die of, we know relatively little about how people die. Research findings can tell us a great deal about the quality of life but much less about the quality of death. What we do know from research is that patients and health professionals view some forms of death as 'good' and others as 'bad'. Definitions may vary across historical periods and from one cultural setting to another. Notions of death as either good or bad are not particularly straightforward but the result of a complex interplay between patients' expectations, the ability of health professionals and caregivers to meet these expectations and the extent to which the process of dying is subject to social control (Lawton, 2000; Bradbury, 2000). There may be differences between patients and health professionals when it comes to defining good and bad deaths. However, drawing on Smith (2000), it has been noted how, 'There is a consensus that a "good death" is that which best suits the preferences of the dying person and their close family while also protecting the integrity and values of professional career' (Seymour et al., 2002, p. 287). The true complexity of the situation is revealed when we consider the following:

> Modern dying involves a struggle for control. Some doctors fear failure when they cannot keep their patients living. Families, filled with grief and sometimes guilt, often have their own strong views on how and where patients should die. This can lead to struggles with doctors, who may see such assertions as an affront to their authority. The 'needs' of the dying patient are defined and thus filtered through the views of family and healthcare professionals.
>
> (Clark, 2003, p. 174)

Clark (2003) goes on to argue that if the experiences of dying patients are to be improved it is essential that patients' notions as to what constitutes a good death are considered alongside the views of professional health workers.

Although there is considerable diversity in the way people view and respond to death and dying, many people share some basic ideas about the kinds of situations and circumstances that make for a more or less good or acceptable death. For example, when we hear that someone has died we often ask questions concerning the age of the deceased, the timing of the death and the nature and cause of the death. We then find ourselves responding accordingly. Where death occurs to someone who is very old we may refer to the deceased as having 'had a good (long) innings'. When death is premature we are less likely to see it as acceptable. If we hear of a death following a long and painful illness, we sometimes refer to it as being a release from suffering and in this sense acceptable.

> **Box 7.7   Definition**
>
> **Elements of a 'good death' in modern Western culture**
>
> - Pain-free death
> - Open acknowledgment of the imminence of death
> - Death at home, surrounded by family and friends
> - An 'aware' death – in which personal conflicts and unfinished business are resolved
> - Death as personal growth
> - Death according to personal preference and in a manner that resonates with the person's individuality
>
> *Source*: Clark, 2002, p. 907

We all have our own views concerning death. When people are asked how they would like to die, the common responses are 'suddenly', 'quietly', 'peacefully', 'painlessly', 'in my sleep'. Conversely, people often express the view that they do not want to die following a long, painful, debilitating and lingering illness. However, what is defined as a good or a bad death is not simply the result of an expression of personal values; deaths are defined according to wider social and cultural norms. The elements of a good death in modern Western society are outlined in Box 7.7.

As Walter (2003) describes, in any one society cultural norms about the good death largely depend on three factors: the extent to which secularisation has taken place; the extent of individualism (i.e. the degree to which individuals are granted personal autonomy to make their own choices as to how they should live and die); the length of the typical dying process. Other writers have recognised the role played by cultural norms in establishing what constitutes a good death. Bradbury (1999) refers to the existence of culturally prescribed ways of representing death, which can vary according to time, place and context. For example, from one perspective, the death of a soldier in battle can be presented as a heroic deed, a noble sacrifice (a good death). However, the same death may be interpreted differently by pacifists and others who do not support the war. From this perspective it may be viewed as a tragic waste of a life (a bad death).

The notion of a good death is highly contentious and many definitions can be found in the literature on death and dying (Seale, 1998; Hart *et al.*, 1998). Kellehear (1990) used the concept of the good death in his study of the experiences of 100 terminally ill people. None of his interviewees showed any signs of being in denial or openly displayed any distress concerning the terminal nature of their illness. Concentrating on the social life of the dying person he identified five main characteristics of the good death:

- awareness of dying;
- adjustments to death;

- preparations for death;
- relinquishing of roles, responsibilities and duties;
- bidding farewell.

According to Kellehear, the dying person plays an active part in the social management of dying by making arrangements and preparations for the end of their life. The social transition involved is accomplished by means of a set of established cultural norms and prescribed modes of behaviour that are features of the dying process. In this way the very act of dying is given meaning for everyone concerned. Thus, the concept of the good death serves a particular purpose for the individual and those people with whom he or she comes into contact. It ensures that the dying person has a script and responds in a socially acceptable manner. Similarly, those people engaged in providing care also have some idea what to expect in terms of the behaviour of the dying person. In essence, Kellehear maintains that there are two major aspects to understanding a good death. First, from the perspective of the individual, a death can be considered to be good, in a psychological sense, if the dying person is seen to have the opportunity to exercise some influence over events and participate in the social management of the dying process. Second, from a social perspective, a good death is one in which the social impact of death is managed and controlled in such a way as to avoid any social disruption or other negative consequences. For Kellehear, there is an ideological dimension to the concept of the good death for both the dying and others in society. In the case of the former, the idea of a good death is used to justify both the kinds of decisions taken by dying individuals and their behavioural responses to impending death. As regards the latter, the good death concept serves the ideological needs of others, such as those in the medical profession, by reinforcing a culturally sanctioned and socially approved form of dying. Kellehear is described as concluding that:

> . . . the ideology of the good death reveals a picture of social values and ideas that are aspired to by the dying, and it also reveals that these ideas often exist as social pressures derived from the social conditions and social interests of the time.
>
> (Hart *et al.*, 1998, p. 71)

Thus, the good death model may be seen as a social construct through which powerful professional groups may influence how dying people organise and shape the ending of their lives.

Hospice and palliative care

The ideology of the good death, which upholds dying with awareness, acceptance and dignity, is a core feature of the hospice movement, out of which palliative care developed. The modern hospice movement began at the beginning of the second half of the twentieth century. Although there is evidence of some hospice provision before this time, the modern-day movement dates from 1967 when Dame Cicely Saunders founded the St Christopher's Hospice in Sydenham, London. This hospice, founded outside the mainstream medical establishment, 'blazed the trail for the British and indeed international hospice movement' (Katz, 2004, p. 12). The model of care it provided was developed as a direct response to the criticisms levelled against the medicalisation of dying and the realities of hospital deaths, particularly the neglect of pain relief in the case of cancer patients (Clark, 1998). Since its inception the basic principles of hospice care have been introduced into a variety of settings including day units, residential units providing short-term care and home-care services.

The primary aim of hospice care is to provide a good death for dying people. In pursuing this aim the hospice model is guided by six basic tenets:

- that it provides *holistic* care;
- that it involves *interdisciplinary* teams;
- that it is *non-hierarchical*;
- that it is *not rule-bound*;
- that hospice work should be viewed as *vocational*;
- that it should be committed to *research and education*.

(Howarth, 2007, p. 140)

The emerging treatment philosophy was originally designed to offer an alternative to the dehumanised and undignified form of dying that was seen to be characteristic of medically controlled deaths in the hospital environment. As Seymour (1999) asserts, the persuasiveness of the hospice model of care is embedded in its promise of reclaiming the 'natural' course of dying from the power and control of medical technology. In this sense, the hospice movement can be seen as a response to the demise of the image of 'natural death', or to use Ariès' term, 'tame' death.

From the very beginning hospice care placed a strong emphasis on the importance of pain control. Given the holistic perspective, pain was understood on a broad front, which gave rise to the concept of 'total pain' (Saunders and Baines, 1983; Clark, 1999a). According to this conceptualisation, there are four levels of pain: physical, emotional, social and spiritual. There is an underlying belief that physical pain is capable of masking pain encountered on the other three levels. Furthermore, emotional and social pain have the potential to exacerbate physical pain. In pursuing a holistic approach and targeting total pain, the hospice model of care sees the reduction of physical pain as helping to reduce the suffering experienced in relation to the other levels of pain. Pain relief calls for multiple interventions. This 'holistic vision of patienthood' was extended to include a familial dimension (Seale, 1998, p. 114). Cicely Saunders was of the opinion that family members were also in need of care and felt that the hospice should actively involve patients and their families in all decision-making.

The ideology of the good death permeates thinking and practice in contemporary palliative care (Hopkinson *et al.*, 2003). In accounting for both the rise of the hospice movement and the emergence of palliative care, Clark (1999b;

2002) describes how around the mid-point of the twentieth century there was a growing climate of opinion that was conducive to promoting changes in the management of dying and death. He identifies four innovations that took place during the first two decades of the second half of the last century:

1 The literature on the care dying patients received began to be informed by findings from systematic empirical research studies, as opposed to being dominated by anecdotal accounts. Leading British medical journals were using the research evidence in focusing on the promotion of care for the terminally ill.

2 A new approach to dying was beginning to emerge which raised issues of awareness, meaning and dignity.

3 There was evidence of a change in the provision of care for dying people. The passive approach, characterised by the belief on the part of the doctor that nothing more could be done (i.e. fatalistic resignation), was replaced by a more active response, whereby doctors sought to identify new ways of providing care for terminally ill patients.

4 The interdependent relationship between physical and mental distress was increasingly being acknowledged and this influenced how personal suffering was conceptualised. This represented 'a profound challenge to the body–mind dualism on which so much medical practice of the period was predicated – brilliantly captured in Cicely Saunders' notion of "total pain"' (Clark, 2002, p. 905).

The word 'palliative' is derived from the Latin 'pallium', which means 'cloak' or 'cover'. In a symbolic sense, palliative care can be seen as a protective cloak that carers (both formal and informal) provide for terminally ill patients. The patient is comforted by the 'cloaking' of the symptoms. There are many formal definitions of palliative care. Indeed, the term 'means different things to different people, and modern definitions are rapidly evolving' (Hallenbeck, 2003, p. 5). One such example, from the European Association for Palliative Care, is presented in Box 7.8. Originally the term was used exclusively in relation to the care of patients who were terminally ill but it is now applied more broadly to encompass the provision of care for patients with chronic, life-limiting illnesses whether or not they are dying (Hallenbeck, 2003). A distinction is usually made between palliative *care* as a philosophy or an approach to healthcare provision and palliative *medicine*. The latter, although similar in meaning, has a 'more formal ring to it' (Hallenbeck, 2003, p. 6) and refers to the incorporation of social, psychological and spiritual aspects of care into the medical model.

Palliative care is administered long before the final stage of a terminal illness is reached. The primary aim is to ensure that the dying person receives pain relief and is allowed to die with dignity. The purpose of any treatment is not to prolong life but to make the patient as comfortable as possible. In essence, palliative care is designed to:

• control symptoms, provide pain relief and avoid inappropriate or unnecessary treatment;

Box 7.8   Definition

Palliative care

Palliative care is the active, total care of the patients whose disease is not responsive to curative treatment. Control of pain, of other symptoms, and of social, psychological and spiritual problems is paramount.

Palliative care is interdisciplinary in its approach and encompasses the patient, the family and the community in its scope. In a sense, palliative care is to offer the most basic concept of care – that of providing for the needs of the patient wherever he or she is cared for, either at home or in the hospital.

Palliative care affirms life and regards dying as a normal process; it neither hastens nor postpones death. It sets out to preserve the best possible quality of life until death.

Source: European Association for Palliative Care: http://www.eapcnet.org/about/definition.html (accessed 6 July 2009)

- provide a holistic approach to care by creating a system of support for dying people which addresses practical, emotional, social and spiritual needs in an individualised manner;
- enable dying people to assert their independence and exercise choice when it comes to making decisions about how their needs are to be managed;
- provide care and support for the dying person's family and friends during the course of the illness and after death;
- create an environment in which the dying person and his or her family are able to participate in decision-making;
- deliver care through a process of teamwork involving all those engaged in providing care for the dying person (e.g. general practitioner, social worker, dietician and voluntary support worker).

Palliative care is a recognised specialism within nursing and medicine for which staff receive expert training. However, the basic underlying principles on which palliative care is based may inform the professional practice of health and social care workers employed outside specialist units or palliative care services.

As described above, the modern hospice movement emerged partly as a response to what was seen as the medicalisation and bureaucratisation of death and dying by a healthcare system dominated by the philosophy of curative medicine. Consequently, it championed an alternative philosophy of care, which perceived death as a natural process and emphasised the importance of adopting a holistic approach to meeting the needs of dying patients. However, there is a view that in recent years the hospice model of care has undergone a number of changes as it has become increasingly incorporated into mainstream healthcare systems. As a result, it is argued that it is debatable as to whether a hospice death still constitutes a good death for dying patients. For example, Clark (1993) suggests that although the hospice developed as a reaction to the medicalisation of death, the emergence of specialist palliative care professionals and an increasing emphasis on the physical, as opposed to the psycho-social aspects of care, has created a situation in which dying has become subject to 'remedicalisation'. According to some observers, as a result of the increasing institutionalisation and bureaucratisation of hospice care, the original philosophy of treatment has been compromised and a good death is interpreted as one which meets the professional ideals of the carers. Research in Australia by McNamara *et al.* (1994, 1995) describes how hospice staff worked towards the good death ideal while accepting that it was difficult to achieve, given the organisational constraints under which they worked. A death was defined as 'good' by health professionals when they felt comfortable with the situation and how they had interacted with the dying person and her or his family and friends. In contrast, bad deaths were those where patients or their families did not accept that death was imminent and did not prepare accordingly. As Hart *et al.* note, in this study '. . . the hospice ideology of the good death was contrasted by caregivers with the medical model's perceived bad deaths; a good death was a victory to the hospice staff and for hospice ideology' (1998, p. 70).

Growing 'routinisation' and bureaucratisation are key themes identified by James and Field (1992) in their account of how hospice care has changed. They describe how initially the modern hospice originated outside the established healthcare system and was openly critical of the standards of care provided by the NHS for dying people. In contrast to established health service institutions the hospice did not have a formal, hierarchical authority structure. It was not a rule-governed institution but in fact supported a philosophy that involved the breaking of rules and orthodox medical routines in an effort to provide more appropriate care for terminally ill people. However, in the contemporary era the hospice has tended to become absorbed into mainstream healthcare and consequently professional standards of care have been laid down by local, regional and national health authorities. The Gold Standards Framework for community palliative care is part of the NHS's End of Life Care Programme. Under the Care Standards Act (2000), hospices in England that are part of the independent healthcare sector are subject to registration and inspection by the Healthcare Commission. In Scotland independent hospice care is monitored by the Care Commission. To some extent, this has resulted in a return to traditional hierarchical structures, which has given rise to the concern that palliative care has lost the radicalism it displayed in the early days (Corner and Dunlop, 1997).

Just as hospice care has been institutionalised, hospital care for the dying has been influenced by some of the principles and practices characteristic of the hospice movement. As Seale (1989) comments in a review of research findings, examples of hospice-type care can be found in hospital settings and the care of the dying in hospices is in some respects similar to that found in hospitals. The ideological boundaries are not what they used to be and the notion of a good death applies in both contexts. However, there is a sense in which the changes in hospice and palliative care have led to a new form of social control over dying people:

> In tandem, the institutionalization of dying and death has led to professionals acquiring and exerting increasing power over the lives of dying patients; there is a constant emergence of more efficient death technologies, more sophisticated and specialized forms of counselling, more control over the professional administration to dying people's identified needs, and professional power that seeks to shape the lives of others to the prevailing ideal.
>
> (Hart *et al.*, 1998, p. 72)

Dying people have choices but these are seen as very much being influenced and shaped by health professionals who are providing the care. Research suggests that hospice nurses see themselves as playing an instrumental role in enabling dying patients to achieve a good death (Taylor, 1993). In this context, as previously mentioned, a good death is perceived as a victory for hospice ideology.

As palliative care grew out of hospice care, and the latter came to be applied to a wider range of life-threatening illnesses, the focus of attention shifted from a good death to the quality of life experienced by the terminally ill. This led to '. . . the medicalisation of palliative care, a speciality that opens up a space somewhere between the hope of cure and the acceptance of death. In doing so, it makes a classic appeal to the desires of "patients" in a modern culture, where we dread not so much the *state of death* as the *process of dying*' (Clark, 2002, p. 907, emphasis added). Indeed, as result of advances in modern medicine many people now live the latter part of their lives knowing that they have a life-threatening illness. Hence, 'the question about how to die well today is how to live for months, or even years, knowing that we are dying' (Walter, 2003, p. 219).

Hospital death

The quality and effectiveness of hospital-based care for terminally ill patients has been questioned over the years. Indeed, as already noted, the instigators of the hospice model of care were originally motivated by what they saw as the negative features of the care received by patients dying in a hospital environment. Studies of terminal care in hospitals have highlighted issues such as poor symptom control and the neglect of patients' physical needs, a lack of individualised care for dying patients to enable them to die with dignity and poor communication about death and dying. Although palliative care is provided in hospital settings, there is evidence that standards, particularly in relation to symptom control, can vary between hospice and hospital (Eve *et al.*, 1997). There is a view that the provision of care for the dying in hospital is hampered by factors such as the lack of appropriate staff and insufficient resources (Rogers *et al.*, 2000). In a comparison of hospice and hospital care, it was concluded that: 'The busy public atmosphere of some hospital wards may not be conducive to the good care of dying people' (Seale and Kelly, 1997, p. 93).

In a study of older patients dying in hospital, Costello (2006) explored nurses' experiences of dying and death on three wards in two hospitals. One of the hospitals specialised in caring for older people and the other had a large unit for elderly patients. In-depth interviews were conducted with 29 registered nurses,

Box 7.9   Research findings

Determinants of good death

Control over death event including disposal of the body

High degree of predictability

Staff and (sometimes) patient awareness

The patient's death is desired by staff

Death takes place at an appropriate time, i.e. during the night, to minimize disruption to the ward

Source: Costello, 2006, p. 598

Box 7.10   Research findings

Determinants of bad death

Often sudden and unprepared, causing disruption to the sentimental order of the ward

Nurses unable to make preparations for death due to time/context constraints

Death takes place outside of the normal ward confines

Patient and family not aware of impending death, family conflict a feature

Insufficient time for nurses to get to know the family

Distinct lack or dignity and respect

Substantive diagnosis not made, climate of uncertainty about future prognosis

Death is traumatic, patient experiences pain or dies with unrelieved symptoms

Source: Costello, 2006, p. 599

who were asked to describe the circumstances surrounding the deaths of particular patients and reflect on how these deaths were reacted to both by themselves and their colleagues. In a thematic analysis of the interview data Costello constructed typologies based on the nurses' descriptions of their experiences. Collectively the data covered a total of 71 deaths that had occurred on the three wards over a period of 20 months. The majority of these deaths had been expected: in only 12 cases was the death described as 'sudden'. Costello describes how two major typologies emerged from the data, namely 'good death' and 'bad death'. The key determinants of both these types of death are summarised in Boxes 7.9 and 7.10.

Costello's study provides an insight into what constitutes a good hospital death from the ward nurses' perspective. Basically, in this context, good deaths are those that do not disrupt the 'sentimental order' of the ward (Glaser and Strauss, 1968) and over which nurses feel they have some control. Sudden unexpected deaths can be considered to be disorderly deaths given their potential to upset the daily routine of the ward. Where dying trajectories can be successfully managed in the interests of establishing and maintaining order, disruptive consequences are less likely to occur. Research suggests that ward staff are more comfortable with deaths where the patient is heavily sedated and unresponsive than they are in dealing with more natural deaths where the timing is unpredictable and the terminal phase is prolonged (Bradbury, 2000). Even when death is anticipated it can occur at the 'wrong' time from the point of view of nursing staff. Such a situation is described by one of the Staff Nurses interviewed by Costello, when she compares the deaths of two patients. Elsie's death was expected and happened quietly during the night; whereas Harold, who had been very ill for some time, 'died bang on 9.00 a.m.'.

> It couldn't have happened at a worse time – he had experienced another bad night and was very poorly, but he had been like that for ages. His relatives had a vigil at the bedside but became tired and went home. They were not there when he died, even though they wanted to be. It was chaos, the ward round was about to start, we were short-staffed and it was right in the middle of the morning routine. It was awful for him and a nightmare for us – we just closed the curtains and left him for a couple of hours.
>
> (Staff Nurse quoted in Costello, 2006, p. 597)

This death had many of the hallmarks of a bad death. Indeed, it was perceived as being a bad experience for all concerned: the patient, the family and the staff on the ward.

Clearly the timing of death is of central importance. When a death takes place suddenly and unexpectedly nurses do not have sufficient time to conduct an accurate assessment of the physical, emotional and spiritual needs of the patient and take the appropriate action. Furthermore, they are unable to establish a rapport with family members and prepare them for the impending death. In this context, Costello describes how a bad death was not simply determined by the nature and pattern of the dying trajectory but was largely a consequence of the circumstances surrounding the 'death event' itself. In other words, a bad death was one where nurses had limited control over the events leading up to, and including, the death. For example, if a patient died in pain and discomfort and did not respond to nursing care, nurses expressed feelings of guilt at being unable to relieve the suffering experienced by the patient. As Costello concludes: 'Hospital nurses' perceptions of death focus more on the death event and less on the dying process' (2006, p. 600).

Dying well

In the early fifteenth century, in European countries with a strong Christian tradition, there were well-established beliefs and practices relating to dying, death and the afterlife. A body of literature, the *Ars Moriendi* (or 'art of dying'), contained practical guidance on how the dying person should prepare for death and how both clergy and laypeople should administer to the dying. There was information on what attitudes, actions and responses would lead to a good death and secure ultimate salvation for the deceased. In the contemporary period, palliative care specialists provide information and support for carers involved in providing end-of-life care. Ideally, patients, informal carers and health professionals are envisaged as working together towards the common goal of a 'good death' in terminal cases. To a certain degree:

> . . . medical care during dying has become a 'sheltering canopy' (Seale, 1998, p. 4), which has largely replaced that of religion as a means of negotiating meaning during the transition from living to dying in terminal illness. Arguably, the negotiation of death through medical practices such as palliative care provides us with the elements of a new 'ars moriendi' (ten Have, 2001, p. 408) . . .
>
> (Seymour *et al.*, 2002, p. 299)

The is not to deny the relevance of a religious perspective: indeed in addressing the needs of dying people it is important that carers have an appreciation of the importance and significance of the various religious beliefs and rituals surrounding death. As Howarth (2007) describes, many hospice staff and specialist palliative care workers have access to such information, in the form of 'factfiles', relating to a range of religious and ethnic groups. Whilst this dissemination of information is to be generally welcomed, she points out, with reference to Gunaratnam (1997), that it should not be assumed that all individuals belonging to a particular religious/cultural group will necessarily subscribe to the values and beliefs of the group with the same level and degree of individual intensity. Furthermore, the experience of dying and the idea as to what constitutes a good death are also influenced by factors such as the age of the dying person, the nature of the social circumstances in which she or he lives and the level of personal dependency.

Over the last 40 years in modern democratic societies there has been a growing debate as to the steps people might take in order to gain more control over their dying and thus secure a good death. A major aspect of this debate has been whether or not terminally ill or severely disabled people should be allowed to request medical assistance to enable them to die a comfortable death at a time of their own choosing. The term euthanasia itself is derived from the Greek 'eu' meaning 'good or well' and 'thanatos' meaning death. The current focus on euthanasia is seen as a logical consequence of the social and cultural trends characteristic of many modern Western societies: namely the growth in individualism (with increasing emphasis being placed on personal autonomy) and increasing secularisation. As regards the former, the prevailing ethos is one in which individuals are seen as having rights and responsibilities and the ability to make choices as to how they live their lives. In this context, maintaining good health and managing illness is achieved with the help and support of healthcare professionals. While the onus is on the individual to maintain a healthy lifestyle by means of taking exercise and eating a well-balanced diet, there is an expectation that the healthcare system will provided appropriate care in times of illness. The emphasis placed on rights, personal autonomy and choice has created a sense in which people expect to be able to determine their own medical treatment, as well as exercise the right to refuse treatment even if this is likely to result in their death. Hence the growing popularity of 'living wills' and 'advance care directives' or 'advance statements', which are written statements made by individuals specifying the conditions under which they would withdraw support for life-supporting interventions. While an advance statement is fairly general and not legally binding, an advance directive or living will contains a more detailed set of instructions and has some legal authority. Although health professionals are not legally required to give treatment requested in advance if this is not deemed to be clinically appropriate according to their professional judgement, they are legally bound by an advance directive refusing treatment. Advance directives and living wills may contain statements referring to the extent of medical intervention in relation to such procedures as resuscitation, hydration and nutritional support. As such, they serve as a directive for the doctor providing end-of-life care. Living wills may also give the power to make decisions on behalf of a patient to a named individual such as a spouse or other close family member. However, there is some uncertainty surrounding the legal status of a Health Care Proxy.

The issue of advance directives and living wills is a complex legal area. These instruments only come into effect once the person concerned has lost the capacity to make a decision for themselves. The legal status of such a document or directive depends on the decision having been made when the person was in a fully competent state, was not subject to any pressure from another person, and there is no reason to think that the person changed his or her mind between making the statement and it being acted upon. Commenting on the impact of living wills on doctors' end-of-life decision-making, Howarth observes from research findings that: 'The efficacy of the living will is open to debate, particularly in respect of wills that name a close friend or relative as the surrogate decision-maker. Where documents are drawn up stating wishes regarding the specifics of medical treatment, these are more likely to be honoured' (Howarth, 2007, p. 149).

Living wills can thus be seen as offering an opportunity for people to acquire some control over the dying process. In making an advanced decision regarding future treatment, the individual is effectively guarding against the possibility of medical intervention leading to a lingering and distressing death. The emphasis is on the individual taking action, in the form of making a living will, to avoid a bad death in the future. In the case of euthanasia, there is an intention to hasten the ending of life and by so doing reduce pain and suffering and achieve death with dignity. However, there are many ethical, religious, social, legal and political issues surrounding the question of euthanasia. While for some people euthanasia may be an acceptable response to medicalised dying, for others it may be rejected as a type of 'bad death'.

As illustrated in Box 7.11, there are two important dimensions to the definition of euthanasia: voluntary/non-voluntary/involuntary and active/passive. The first of these concerns the degree to which the wishes of the person who is dying are known and respected. Euthanasia is described as voluntary in situations where the dying person is seen to be competent to make a decision and either makes the initial request or gives their consent should euthanasia be presented to them as an option. Non-voluntary euthanasia applies in cases where a patient does not

Box 7.11   Definition

Euthanasia and physician-assisted suicide

Voluntary active euthanasia: performed at the request of a patient.

Non-voluntary active euthanasia: performed on a patient who is unable to make a request.

Involuntary active euthanasia: performed against the wishes of a patient.

Passive euthanasia: deliberately withholding life-sustaining treatment.

Physician-assisted suicide: a doctor helps a patient to take his or her own life.

have the mental ability to make a request, such as in the case of severely con-genitally deformed newborn babies and patients in a persistent vegetative state. The term involuntary euthanasia is applied in circumstances where the act of euthanasia is actually against the expressed wishes of the dying person. The non-voluntary and involuntary types are sometimes subsumed under the single heading of 'involuntary' on the basis that there is an absence of a request from the patient.

The second dimension (active/passive) refers to the provision or non-provision of specific medical treatments. A doctor may perform a deliberate act to terminate a patient's life (e.g. by giving a lethal injection) or may intentionally terminate a life by an act of omission (e.g. by switching off a ventilator). While the former may be termed 'active euthanasia', the latter is usually referred to as 'passive euthanasia'. In short, active euthanasia means acting in such a way as to cause death, whereas passive euthanasia means not taking action to prevent death occurr-ing. An example of the latter is provided by the case of Tony Bland, who was seriously injured on 15 April 1989 in the Hillsborough Football Stadium disaster, which claimed the lives of 96 football fans. Trapped in a crush of spectators Tony's lungs were compressed and his brain deprived of oxygen. He never regained consciousness and was eventually diagnosed as being in a persistent vegetative state. He was kept alive by means of artificial hydration and feeding. In 1992 the hospital where he was being treated petitioned the High Court to discontinue the artificial feeding and hydration. The case went to the House of Lords where it was adjudged that artificial hydration and feeding constituted medical treatment and that it was lawful to withdraw this treatment on the grounds that it was of no benefit and consent had not been given. Expert medical opinion was of the view that the action would allow the patient to die from a pre-existing medical condition. As one of the Law Lords ruled:

> [T]he law draws a crucial distinction between cases in which a doctor decides not to provide, or to continue to provide, for his patient treatment or care which could or might prolong his life, and those in which he decides, for example by administering a lethal drug, actively to bring his patient's life to an end. As I have already indicated, the former may be lawful.

> (Lord Goof, quoted in Keown, 2002, p. 14)

Feeding via a nasogastric tube was discontinued and Tony died within days.

What the various definitions of euthanasia have in common is that they all refer to doctors making decisions and taking action which results in shortening the life of the patient. Euthanasia can be distinguished from physician-assisted suicide. In the case of the latter, the doctor provides the patient with the means to take his or her own life. The doctor has no direct involvement in performing the final act. As for euthanasia itself, this can only be said to have taken place where death is *intentionally* caused by what was done or not done by the doctor. Furthermore, the key feature which serves to conceptually differentiate euthanasia from murder is that the action of the doctor is based on the belief that the patient is better off dead. Thus, euthanasia is a way of bringing to an end a patient's prolonged suffering. The doctrine or principle of double effect is relevant here. This states that if an action that is morally good (e.g. relieving pain and suffering) has a morally bad side-effect (e.g. shortens the life of the patient) it is ethically acceptable to take the action as long as the side-effect is not the intended or desired outcome. Take, for example, the administration of morphine and terminal sedation to provide a quiet and comfortable death. It is impermissible for a doctor to inject a large dose of morphine if the intention is to hasten death. However, if the intention is to relieve pain and suffering, and the doctor merely foresees the possibility of the patient dying sooner as a result of the dosage given, this is permissible as there is no intention to cause death. The principle of double effect only applies under certain conditions. For example, the bad result must not be the means of achieving the good one. The principle cannot be used if the only way of controlling the pain is to kill the patient. The doctrine of double effect is well established in medical practice and enshrined in the criminal law.

Increasingly over the last two decades euthanasia has been debated in many countries. However, there are very few countries in which any form of euthanasia or physician-assisted dying is considered lawful. In Switzerland, physician-assisted suicide has been permissible since the early 1940s. In 1997, in the USA, the state of Oregon, following a second public referendum, enacted the Death with Dignity Act. This allows doctors to assist terminally ill patients who wish to end their life. The law permits physicians to issue patients with a prescription for a lethal dose of a medication which is then self-administered. The first death under this legislation took place the following year when a terminally ill woman in her mid-eighties took a lethal dose of prescribed barbiturates. More recently, in 2002 euthanasia was decriminalised in the Netherlands with the passing of legislation permitting voluntary euthanasia and physician-assisted suicide. In the same year, a similar piece of legislation was introduced in Belgium (Almagor, 2009). In legal jurisdictions where euthanasia has been decriminalised strict guidelines are imposed as to the conditions under which a life may be prematurely terminated. For example, in the case of Belgium, the doctor must be seen to be responding to the voluntary, written and well-considered request of the patient. The onus is on the doctor to provide the patient with information regarding the full extent of the illness, the patient's life expectancy and the nature and type of palliative care available.

In Australia in 1996 the Northern Territory passed the Rights of the Terminally Ill Act which gave individuals lawful access to euthanasia. However, this ruling was quickly overturned by the Australian Federal Parliament. During the short period the legislation was in force there was detailed and extensive media coverage given to the cases of five terminally ill people who had elected to die (McInerney, 2006). There have since been attempts to introduce pro-euthanasia legislation but these have been unsuccessful. In many other countries the debate continues and periodically attempts are made to introduce right-to-die legislation. There are interest groups on both sides of the debate and the ethical, social, legal, moral and medico-technical arguments advanced are similar from one country to another. In an analysis of support for active euthanasia in Britain and the USA, Emanuel (1994) points out how arguments in favour and against euthanasia are similar to those advanced in the nineteenth century when the topic first came to be widely debated.

Arguments in support of assisted dying tend to be based on a notion of patient autonomy and a belief in the idea that it should be a fundamental human right for individuals to be free to choose how and when they die if they are terminally ill and experiencing intolerable pain. Proponents maintain that in moral terms there is no real difference between hastening the death of a terminally ill patient by withholding life-sustaining treatment or by administering a lethal injection. They support the view that a person should have the right to take the decision to end their life not only to relieve chronic and unrelenting pain during the final stages of life but also to enable them to die with dignity. Opponents of euthanasia claim that with modern methods of pain control provided by hospice care many deaths are in fact pain free. Active and passive euthanasia are viewed as morally distinct categories and the former is likened to murder. Consequently, it is held that active euthanasia contravenes a fundamental ethical principle of medicine, namely the preservation of life. Furthermore, to legally permit a doctor to end the life of a patient will undermine the value placed on human life and not only have a negative impact on medical practice but also on society in general.

Critics of the legalisation of voluntary euthanasia often raise what is referred to as the 'slippery slope' argument. This maintains that one of the consequences of legalising euthanasia is that frail, sick, elderly people may find themselves in an increasingly vulnerable position. There is a potential for conflict between their needs and the needs of others. For example, there is a perceived danger that relatives may request involuntary euthanasia for an elderly relative for purely selfish motives. As Cicely Saunders has stated: 'I do not think any legalised "right to die" can fail to become, for many vulnerable people, a "duty to die" or at best the only option offered' (Saunders, 1992, p. 3). Thus, while the pro-euthanasia lobby stresses the importance of the individual having the right to take control over the dying process in order to ensure a dignified death, opponents of euthanasia draw attention to the potential for abuse and the threat this poses to the 'right to life'.

National opinion polls report considerable public support for euthanasia. Figures for the USA show over two-thirds of those interviewed in favour of euthanasia (Duncan and Parmelee, 2006). While there is evidence that the level of support may vary from one country to another, Cohen *et al.* (2006) describe how those European countries recording the highest level of support are also those in which individual autonomy and the right to self-determination are highly valued. However, views expressed by individuals in these types of sample surveys may not be an accurate predictor of the actual personal choices people might make when faced with a 'real life' situation. Research studies of dying people and their families provide a valuable insight into views regarding the best time to die and attitudes towards euthanasia. Seale and Addington-Hall (1995) compared the views of spouses and non-spouses (e.g. immediate family members, other relatives, friends and neighbours) and found a variation in views as to the perceived desirability of an earlier death. Spouses were less likely than non-spouses to express the view that it would have been better if the deceased had died earlier. They were also more likely than non-spouses to say that they felt that a later death would have been better; however, this did not apply in those instances where the deceased was described as having expressed a wish to die sooner. As regards the experience of providing care in the terminal stages, non-spouses found this more burdensome than spouses. Thus, the researchers concluded that, 'the very old were more likely to be cared for by people who, in retrospect, felt that it would have been better if the old person had died earlier' (Seale and Addington-Hall, 1995, p. 589). In addition, they noted that women were far more likely than men to be described as having taken on the view that they were 'too old' and also as having asked about euthanasia.

Studies of terminally ill patients making treatment decisions at the end of life provide an opportunity for researchers to explore issues around euthanasia. Unlike attitudinal surveys and opinion polls, these qualitative studies are based on relatively small samples of patients but allow for a more in-depth exploration and analysis of attitudes, feelings and beliefs. In one such study in Australia, 28 cancer patients were interviewed: all were in the final phase of their illness and were aware that they had only about three months to live (Eliott and Olver, 2008). All but four of the patients made positive comments regarding euthanasia and spoke of the importance of being able to exercise a personal choice. They referred to euthanasia as a way of putting an end to intolerable physical and emotional pain and preserving death with dignity. However, when they talked about euthanasia it tended to be with reference to a hypothetical future or a scenario involving a hypothetical other person. None of those interviewees who endorsed euthanasia considered it an option for them at the time of interview. These findings replicated those of an earlier study of cancer patients in Norway (Johansen *et al.*, 2005). Although the majority of patients in the Australian study voiced opinions in favour of euthanasia, a number expressed concern at the need for rigorous controls to prevent abuse. As one patient commented:

> If only they could surround it [euthanasia] in correct procedures, . . . I thoroughly agree with it. . . . [B]ut I don't know how you'd hold it within its boundaries. . . . But it's the other complications, . . . it being abused by professionals and people and, yes, and people are not all good holy souls . . .
>
>   (Vera, a terminally ill cancer patient quoted in Eliott and Olver, 2008, p. 652)

In this context, some interviewees referred to involuntary euthanasia and subscribed to the 'slippery slope' argument.

The debate about assisted dying and the right to die with dignity will continue for years to come as the various interest groups campaign for and against the legalisation of euthanasia. Empirical research can help to inform this debate by exploring the various social and moral meanings of euthanasia, as expressed by dying patients, family members, representatives of pressure groups and healthcare professionals.

Summary

- Attitudes to dying and death can vary from one society to another. In socially diverse and multi-cultural societies, death, dying and grief are experienced in different ways in different social and ethnic groups.

- A society's image of death changes over time. Social approaches to dying and death differ in traditional, modern and postmodern societies. According to Illich, the medicalisation of society has brought the era of natural death to an end and suppressed the development of a more enlightened attitude towards death. In contrast to the 'tamed death' of the pre-modern era, Ariès describes modern medicalised death as 'wild', 'savage' and 'dirty'.

- Supporters of the denial-of-death thesis base their argument around three key themes: the perceived existence of a taboo surrounding conversation about death, the medicalisation of death and the segregation of the dying from the rest of society. Critics of the thesis maintain that there has not been a silence surrounding death in recent times but a new way of speaking about death has emerged. When assessing the thesis it is important to distinguish between denial as a personal or individual response and denial as a collective or societal response.

- Glaser and Strauss' typology of states of awareness has proved to be a very important analytic device for understanding the management of dying in a hospital setting. They identify four contexts of awareness: closed awareness; suspicion awareness; mutual pretence awareness; open awareness.

- In her observational study of death in a hospital setting, Kübler-Ross describes patients as passing through five psychological or emotional stages in their response to dying: denial; anger; bargaining; depression; acceptance. Buckman describes the process of dying as consisting of three chronological stages: the initial stage, the chronic stage and the final stage.

- While stage theories are popular with health professionals, largely because they offer a framework for understanding psychological responses during dying, a comprehensive theory of dying needs to incorporate an understanding of dying from the perspective of the individual. Task-based theories see coping tasks as falling into four broad categories: physical, psychological, social and spiritual.

- Patients and health professionals view some forms of death as 'good' and others as 'bad'. However, what is defined as a good or a bad death is not simply the result of an expression of personal values; deaths are defined according to wider social and cultural norms. Social and cultural norms about the good death in any society largely depend on three factors: the extent to which secularisation has taken place, the degree to which individuals are granted personal autonomy to make their own choices (i.e. the degree of individualism) and the length of the dying trajectory.

- The ideology of the good death, which emphasises dying with awareness, acceptance and dignity, is a fundamental feature of the hospice movement, out of which palliative care emerged. Although the modern hospice movement was partly a response to the medicalisation and bureaucratisation of dying and death by a healthcare system dominated by the philosophy of curative medicine, some observers maintain that due to the increasing institutionalisation and bureaucratisation of hospice care, the original philosophy of treatment has been compromised and a good death is interpreted as one which meets the professional ideals of the carers.

- Research suggests that from the ward nurses' perspective good deaths are those that are anticipated, that do not disrupt the 'sentimental order' of the ward and over which nurses feel they have some control. Bad deaths are those that occur suddenly and where nurses have insufficient time to make an accurate assessment of the physical, emotional and spiritual needs of the patient and are unable to develop a relationship with family members in order to prepare them for the impending death.

- Living wills, advance care directives and advance statements can all be seen as offering an opportunity for people to acquire some control over the dying process.

- Euthanasia can be categorised as voluntary/non-voluntary/involuntary and active/passive. The first of these categories concerns the degree to which the wishes of the dying person are known and respected. The second category refers to the provision or non-provision of specific medical treatments.

Questions for discussion

1 What are the main characteristic features of sociological approaches to the study of death and dying?

2 Discuss the evidence both for and against modern societies being described as 'death denying'.

3 Of what use is the typology of awareness contexts?

4 What are the strengths and limitations of stage theories of dying?

5 What constitutes a 'good death' as far as dying patients, palliative care practitioners, ward nurses and doctors are concerned?

6 What are the main arguments for and against euthanasia?

Further reading

Bryant, C. D. (ed.) (2003) *Handbook of Death and Dying*, Thousand Oaks, CA: Sage.

Clark, D. (1993) *The Sociology of Death*, Oxford: Blackwell.

Currer, C. (2001) *Responding to Grief: Dying, Bereavement and Social Care*, Basingstoke, Hampshire: Palgrave.

Earle, S., Komaromy, C. and Bartholomew, C. (eds) (2009) *Death and Dying: A Reader*, London: Sage.

Howarth, G. (2007) *Death and Dying: A Sociological Introduction*, Cambridge: Polity.

Leming, M. R. and Dickinson, G. E. (2007) *Understanding Dying, Death and Bereavement*, 6th edn, Belmont, CA: Thomson Publishing.

McNamara, B. (2001) *Fragile Lives: Death, Dying and Care*, Buckingham: Open University Press.

Riches, G. and Dawson, P. (2000) *An Intimate Loneliness: Supporting Bereaved Parents and Siblings*, Buckingham: Open University Press.

Seymour, J. (2001) *Critical Moments – Death and Dying in Intensive Care*, Buckingham: Open University Press.

Warnock, M. and Macdonald, E. (2008) *Easeful Death: Is there a Case for Assisted Dying?*, Oxford: Oxford University Press.

Useful websites

BBC Religion & Ethics: Euthanasia: http://www.bbc.co.uk/ethics/euthanasia/

British Medical Association, End of life issues: http://www.bma.org.uk/ethics/end_life_issues/index.jsp

Help the Hospices: http://www.helpthehospices.org.uk/welcome/

NHS National End of Life Care Programme: http://www.endoflifecare.nhs.uk/eolc/

St Christopher's Hospice: http://www.stchristophers.org.uk/

The National Council for Palliative Care: http://www.ncpc.org.uk/

CHAPTER 8

Care, community and the family

The concept of 'care'

> The concept of care is framed by multifaceted argument and is subject to debate on a number of levels. Many of the current debates have a long history and evaluation and include philosophical, ideological, political and economic arguments concerning the definition of care, who provides it, how and where it is provided and who provides funding.
>
> (Phillips, 2007, p. 2)

When studying the nature and organisation of healthcare and social welfare provision a distinction is normally made between the formal and the informal sectors. The formal sector consists of the statutory agencies, voluntary groups and private organisations that make up the professional healthcare system and social care services. It is clearly distinguishable from the informal sector, which is best described as a lay support system of care provided by families, friends and neighbours. The majority of formal sector care is provided by paid workers, many of who are employees of large bureaucratic organisations. The arrangement is a formal one and the relationship between carer and client is characterised by affective neutrality. In contrast, informal care is unpaid. This type of care is less public and more private. It is usually characterised by a social tie or affective bond, based on kinship or friendship, between the carer and the recipient of care. It is this informal care that is the subject of this chapter.

Informal carers are at the forefront of community-based health and social care. Most healthcare takes place in the community or to be more precise within the home (Dalley, 1988; Stacey, 1988). It is estimated that in the case of child health, nearly 90 per cent of minor illnesses are diagnosed and treated at home, without any intervention from healthcare professionals (Spencer, 1984). Recent figures suggest there are 6.8 million informal carers in Great Britain providing care for sick, disabled or elderly people; this is equivalent to one in six people aged 16 years and over acting as caregivers (Maher and Green, 2002). There is a wealth of research evidence illustrating that it is within the private arena of the family that much is done to promote, maintain and restore health. The major providers of care in this context are women (Ungerson, 1983).

As regards the organisation and delivery of statutory healthcare and social welfare services, the emphasis for many years has been on a strategy of 'community care'. In order to understand the origins, development and impact of community care policies it is necessary to look closely at how the terms 'care' and 'community' are defined. Also, given the central role the family plays in the provision of care, knowledge of how the family, as a social institution, fits into the wider social structure is essential. Furthermore, we need to know something about the diversity of family arrangements and the changing social and economic circumstances of modern family life, if we are to understand the realities of family-based care.

All of us at some time in our lives experience a state of dependency, when we rely on others for help and support. This is particularly the case in infancy and early childhood when the care and protection of adults is essential for our survival. As we go through life we not only receive care, but we also provide care. In fact caring is seen as such an integral part of the daily routine of family life that its definition is almost taken for granted. All too often because informal care is unpaid work, done mainly by women in the privacy of the home, it is not seen as labour. However, caring involves both physical and mental effort and can be described as 'a kind of domestic labour performed on people' (Graham, 1983, p. 27).

Generally the term 'caring' is used to refer to the assistance and support given to those members of society who are unable to look after themselves. However, as Bulmer (1987) notes, such a broad definition tells us nothing about the different forms that help and support can take. In conceptualising care he claims:

'Care' . . . has three components: (1) physical tending, which is the most intimate kind; (2) material and psychological support which does not involve physical contact; and

(3) more generalized concern about the welfare of others, which may or may not lead to the other two types of help.

(Bulmer, 1987, p. 21)

Thus it is possible to distinguish 'caring for' from 'caring about'. As regards the former, Parker (1981) uses the word 'tending' to describe the various tasks undertaken by those engaged in caring work. 'Caring for' involves helping with daily activities such as feeding, washing and dressing; 'caring about' refers to feeling emotional concern for an individual. On the basis of this distinction it is possible to 'care for' someone without 'caring about' them. Hilary Graham (1983) identifies this dual aspect to caring when she distinguishes between caring as 'the transaction of goods and services' and 'caring-as-feelings'.

Clearly, there is a strong element of emotion in informal caring relationships. On a structural level, relationships are founded upon kinship ties and bonds of obligation: on an individual level a relationship may be experienced as being based on personal ties of love and affection. There is another sense in which emotion features in caring. As Twigg and Atkin assert, 'Carers do not simply do things for people, they can also support them with encouragement, personal attention and conversation that endorses their sense of identity and worth. Offering such support is part of the activity of caring' (1994, p. 8). Thus, the very act of caring itself can be seen as a form of emotional labour.

In raising this conceptual distinction the intention is not to suggest that the emotional aspects of caring are clearly and easily separable from the physical activity of providing personal care. For both professional and informal carers emotional ties can develop within the context of a caring relationship. Although healthcare workers are instructed to maintain an emotional detachment in their dealings with clients, it is inevitable, especially when providing long-term care, that some emotional ties are formed. As regards informal carers, in some cases emotional attachments predate the caring role, for example when a partner becomes a carer out of a long-established sense of love. Graham views informal care in terms of a labour of love when she states, 'Care – is experienced as a labour of love in which the labour must continue even where the love falters' (1983, p. 16). The reason for drawing a distinction between 'caring for' and 'caring about' is to obtain an insight into the different dimensions of the caring role in order to appreciate more fully what it means to be a carer.

According to Phillips, care is 'a nebulous and ambiguous concept and a part of everyday life which is taken for granted' (Phillips, 2007, p. 1). She maintains that it is helpful to adopt a life course perspective in order to understand the multi-dimensional nature of the concept and to appreciate the variety of meanings of care in a contemporary context. For Phillips, the giving and receiving of care takes place throughout all stages of the life course and is not a simple one-way process based on dependency but is more complex and involves an element of reciprocity. As she asserts:

Caregiving and receiving may be sequential or concurrent across the life course; a carer one day may be a care recipient the next. Care may also be reciprocal and interdependent rather than one way. Assumptions of dependency may mask more complex notions of interdependence: for example, children contribute to family life offering parents emotional support; young carers offer support to disabled parents, while parents provide emotional and financial support. The care parents give to their children may later be reciprocated when the children care for their parents in their old age.

(Phillips, 2007, p. 4)

Thus, care may be a normal part of everyday life and a feature of all human relationships but there is no objective universal definition of care. In recent years the term 'social care' has become increasingly popular. This focuses on viewing care-giving as a similar practice irrespective of where it takes place (in the home, community or institution) or whether the provider is a paid professional worker or unpaid informal carer. Whatever term is used, care or social care, it embraces a diverse set of activities, actions and behaviours and involves both physical and emotional labour. In any specific context the nature and degree of care required will depend upon the needs of the individuals concerned and the circumstances in which they find themselves. While the concept of social care helps to highlight the broad similarities between care-giving in different domains and contexts, '[o]ne of the most contested debates surrounding care is where medical care stops and social care begins' (Philips, 2007, p. 24). As Philips notes, the medical–social boundary is not always clearly distinguishable when considering the personal care received by an individual.

Community care: the policy context

Community care is hard to define. One broad understanding is the care of people in the community who have previously lived in long-stay institutions. A second element focuses on efforts to keep disabled people, older people and vulnerable people within the community rather than seeing them having to go into institutional care. A third key issue is the considerable unpaid support and help given by relatives, friends and neighbours.

(Sharkey, 2007, p. 1)

Although the promotion of community care has increasingly featured as a strategic objective in the formulation of healthcare and social welfare policies in the 1980s and 1990s the concept of community care is by no means new. The social origins of the term are difficult to trace (Titmuss, 1963). According to Hunter and MacAlpine (1974), the term was first officially used in 1930 when it appeared in the Annual Report of the Board of Control in reference to proposals for providing support for mentally handicapped people to live in the community.

In the contemporary era the idea of community care stems in part from a reaction against institutional care. However, this has not always been the case. Hunter and MacAlpine (1974) describe how some observers of the growing numbers of patients in lunatic asylums in the second half of the nineteenth century raised the question of the feasibility of home care for those suffering from incurable conditions. This did not constitute a call for an alternative approach to institutional treatment, but was recommended as a way of reducing inmate numbers, thus enabling hospitals to concentrate on those cases deemed likely to respond to treatment.

In the late 1950s there was a policy initiative to move away from a hospital-based system to a community-based approach for the care and treatment of the mentally ill. The Royal Commission on the Law Relating to Mental Illness and Mental Deficiency (1957) addressed the issue of community care, which they defined as consisting of 'all forms of care (including residential care) which it is appropriate for local health or welfare authorities to provide' (1957, p. 208). Many of the recommendations made by the Royal Commission were endorsed by the Government and incorporated in the 1959 Mental Health Act. Introducing the new policy the Minister of Health stated in the House of Commons that: 'One of the main principles we are seeking to pursue is the reorientation of the mental health services, away from institutional care towards care in the community' (Hansard, 1959, p. 598). In pursuing this community-centred policy the Government produced the Hospital Plan (Ministry of Health, 1962) which proposed a 50 per cent reduction in the total number of hospital beds for mental patients and recommended the creation of large district general hospitals which would concentrate on provision for short-stay patients.

Within this context the emphasis was clearly on care *in* the community. The notion of the community as the ideal locus of care attracted increasing support from many quarters as the dark side of institutional life was revealed. Research by social scientists described the mental hospital as a form of 'total institution' in which patients encountered degrading and oppressive regimes (Goffman, 1961; Perry, 1974). The dehumanising and damaging effects of institutional confinement were also commented upon by psychiatrists. Russell Barton (1965) referred to some of the behaviours observed among patients as being a response to the experience of hospitalisation, rather than symptomatic of the condition for which they had been confined. He coined the term 'institutional neurosis' to describe the adverse reactions to confinement. Not only was the therapeutic value of institutional treatment questioned, but allegations were also made about the neglect and ill treatment of patients. Robb (1967) drew attention to the plight of elderly patients on psychogeriatric wards and her allegations of ill treatment raised such concern that an official inquiry was set up by the Government (Ministry of Health, 1968). Mental hospitals were very much in the news and over the next few years press reports of cruelty and neglect were a regular occurrence (Martin, 1984).

It was not surprising that all the adverse publicity created a general climate of opinion that favoured the closing down of institutions for the mentally ill and mentally handicapped. As one observer has noted, the combination of research studies and newspaper reports had an important influence on policy.

> ... the chilling equation of the mental hospital and the concentration camp, originally the hyperbole of muckraking journalists, has now acquired the mantle of academic respectability. Ideologically this is a development of profound significance, for it has

effectively legitimized 'community treatment', not by a careful demonstration of its merits . . . but by rendering the alternative simply unthinkable.

(Scull, 1983, p. 329)

Thus support for a community-focused policy in the field of mental health was largely based on a critique of institutional provision, rather than a systematic appraisal of the benefits likely to accrue from a community-care model. The belief that any form of care was preferable to treatment in an institution was widely held.

Although the term 'care in the community' entered into policy rhetoric in the early 1960s it was some time before any attempt was made to provide a framework for community care. As Kathleen Jones recalls, a policy document entitled 'Health and Welfare: The Development of Community Care', published in 1963, 'gave no positive rationale for community care, and no positive lead' (1988, p. 34). It was not until towards the end of the decade that policy-makers and politicians began to address the administrative and organisational reforms necessary in order to secure a community-centred approach. Concern was expressed about the fragmentation of provision of social welfare services for families. In commenting on the role of local authorities in providing personal social services the Seebohm Committee proposed some major changes.

We recommend a new local authority department providing a community based and family oriented service which will be available to all. This new department will we believe reach far beyond the discovery and rescue of social casualties: it will enable the greatest possible number of individuals to act reciprocally giving and receiving service for the well being of the whole community.

(Seebohm Report, 1968, p. 11)

What is clear from the Report is that the provision of community care should not be the sole responsibility of the statutory services.

A whole chapter of the Seebohm Report is devoted to a discussion of the importance of the community. The term is used not only to define a physical location, but also to refer to the existence of a network of reciprocal social relationships. The community is envisaged as both a recipient and provider of social care. In this respect the increasing participation of individuals and voluntary groups is encouraged as a way of removing the distinction between 'givers' and 'takers' and establishing a partnership between the state and the client.

The idea that the community must bear more of the responsibility for providing care began to feature more prominently in policy documents from the late 1970s onwards. Not only was the policy of community care extended beyond the field of mental health but there was also evidence that the Government wished to see a change in the balance between formal and informal provision. The 1981 White Paper, entitled *Growing Older*, reflected the Government's intention to shift the burden of care:

Whatever level of public expenditure proves practicable, and however it is distributed, the primary sources of support and care for elderly people are informal and voluntary. These spring from the personal ties of kinship, friendship and neighbourhood. They are irreplaceable. It is the role of the public authorities to sustain and, where necessary, develop – but never to replace – such support and care. Care *in* the community must increasingly mean care *by* the community.

(DHSS, 1981a, p. 3)

The distinction between care in the community and care by the community is of particular significance (Bayley, 1973). Whereas the former term refers to the location of the caring services, whether provided by professional staff, volunteer workers or informal carers, the latter refers to the bulk of the support coming from the members of the community themselves.

In the early 1980s a number of initiatives were introduced with the aim of stimulating voluntary sector services. For example, *Care in the Community* (DHSS, 1981b) allowed for the transferring of funds from district health authorities to those voluntary organisations offering support in the community for former long-stay hospital patients. However, mid-way through the decade there was increasing evidence of dissatisfaction over the way in which the community care programme was operating. According to a House of Commons Social Services Select Committee (1985) the phrase 'community care' had become a meaningless slogan: there was too much rhetoric and not enough action. Insufficient resources were being made available to set up community support services for the increasing number of discharged mental patients. The Committee noted that, 'Any fool can close a long-stay hospital: it takes more time and trouble to do it properly and compassionately' (Social Services Select Committee, 1985, p. xxii). There was what amounted to a virtual 'crisis in the community'.

The Audit Commission (1986) also examined the community care programme and found it wanting. Local authorities were not receiving adequate funding to provide the kinds of community services recommended by Government policy. In short, resources were insufficient to meet needs. It was the opinion of the Commission that radical changes were needed to the funding arrangements in order to ensure that community care reached those people it was intended to help. A number of possible reforms were suggested. For example, the responsibility for organising care for the elderly could be placed in the hands of an 'independent community care manager', who would have the power to use funds provided by the NHS and local authorities to purchase the services required to provide community care. It was also suggested that local authorities could be made responsible for the long-term care of mentally and physically handicapped people living in the community. Funds could be transferred from the NHS to provide the necessary financial support. All in all the Commission felt that an independent review of community care policies was needed.

In response the Government appointed Sir Roy Griffiths, a member of the NHS Management Committee, to undertake an investigation into how community care policy is funded and make recommendations as to how these funds might be used to achieve a more effective community service. The Griffiths Report, published in 1988, remarked on the lack of a coherent and coordinated policy strategy. Indeed he commented that: '. . . in few areas can the gap between political rhetoric and policy on the one hand, or between policy and reality in the field on the other hand, have been so great' (Griffiths, 1988, para 9). Included among the main recommendations for change were the following:

- There should be a Minister of State responsible for community care.

- Local authority social service departments should, 'within the resources available' determine the community care needs in their areas and develop local action plans in consultation with health authorities and other public sector organisations and voluntary groups.

- Social service departments should act as 'the designers, organisers and purchasers of non-healthcare services'. Rather than provide care they should concentrate on coordinating 'packages of care' bought on the care 'market'.

- Health authorities should continue to have responsibility for the medical component of the community health services and where appropriate have an input into the assessment of needs and the delivery of 'packages of care'.

- General practitioners should ensure that social service authorities are aware of the social care needs of their patients.

The White Paper *Caring for People* (Department of Health, 1989), which set out the government's proposals for the provision of community care in the 1990s, endorsed many of Griffiths' recommendations. Furthermore it identified four essential features of community-based provision when it stated that services should:

1 be flexible and sensitive in their response to the needs of individuals and their carers;

2 intervene no more than is necessary to encourage and support independent living;

3 allow consumers to choose from a range of options;

4 ensure that services concentrate on those individuals in the greatest need.

Many of the policy reforms contained in the White Paper were formalised and given legislative status when the National Health Service and Community Care Act received the Royal Assent in June 1990.

The Act of 1990 marked the culmination of a process of policy reform, embarked upon in the early 1980s, designed to change the balance of welfare provision by reducing reliance on public sector involvement and promoting a mixed welfare economy. A strategy summed up in the following:

> The essence of the Thatcher and Major governments' approach towards community care . . . is that it is attempting, with some success, to reduce the role of local authorities as providers within the formal sector. Furthermore, it is intended to fill this artificially created care gap with a mixture of private, voluntary and informal care.
>
> (Walker, 1993, p. 216)

According to Walker, there was a deliberate policy of residualisation; new guidelines and initiatives ensured that social services authorities concentrated on the management of care rather than its actual provision. This was referred to as the 'purchaser–provider split'.

Shortcomings of the new policy soon began to be revealed. For example, there was no real recognition of the needs of carers and no consideration given to the protection of vulnerable adults from abuse. Some of the apparent shortcomings were addressed by legislation, such as the Carers (Recognition and Services) Act (1995). However, criticism has been levelled at the fact that legislation in this area has been all too piecemeal and that the time is now ripe for a complete overhaul in order to produce a clearer and more coherent legislative framework. According to Clements, 'Community care law remains a hotchpotch of conflicting statutes, which have been enacted over a period of 50 years; each statute reflects the different philosophical attitudes of its time' (Clements, 2004, p. 8).

The introduction of a New Labour Government did not produce any immediate major changes in community care policy. Emphasis was placed on improving existing facilities through a process of modernisation rather than making any structural changes to the administration and provision of services (Department of Health, 1998). Indeed, two key themes dominating Labour policy in terms of community care practice were modernisation and partnership working. In the case of the latter, this involved encouraging organisations to work together by breaking down the traditional distinctions between healthcare and social care. Promoting independence and focusing the system of provision on service users were two of Labour's key policy objectives; the early part of their administration witnessed a number of initiatives such as the introduction of a National Strategy for Carers and National Service Frameworks for a variety of user groups.

As this brief discussion of the concept of community care in a policy context has shown, it is a concept with a long history. Although it has been at the forefront of many health and welfare policy initiatives in recent years, there is some confusion as to what is actually meant by 'community'. It is to the definition of community that we now turn.

Making sense of 'community'

In short, 'community' stands for the kind of world which is not, regrettably, available to us but which we would dearly wish to inhabit and which we hope to repossess. . . . 'Community' is nowadays another name for paradise lost . . .

(Bauman, 2001, p. 3)

What is the 'community'?

Although the term 'community care' is widely used by policy-makers, professional practitioners and voluntary organisations alike, there is still some confusion surrounding its actual definition. This stems largely from the fact that what is meant by the prefix 'community' is never really precisely stated in policy documents. 'Policy pronouncements treat the term "community" in a glib fashion, when it in fact requires close scrutiny' (Bulmer, 1987, p. 26). However, defining 'community' is no easy task. Sociologists have been studying the concept of community for over two hundred years and have still to produce a satisfactory definition (Bell and Newby, 1971). Part of the problem lies in the very nature of the idea of community, with its 'many layers of emotional meaning' (Bender, 1978, p. 6). As Williams observes, community is a 'warmly pervasive word' that never seems to be used in a negative way (1976, p. 76). Some commentators have described it as a 'God word', in that 'when it is mentioned, we are expected to abase ourselves before it rather than attempt to define it' (Butterworth and Weir, 1984, p. 96). However, while the emotional connotations may have hampered critical analysis, this has not deterred social theorists from attempting to define the concept. In a review of the literature some years ago Hillery (1955) identified 94 different definitions. Indeed, a feature of the definitional problem is that there are too many definitions rather than too few (Lee and Newby, 1983).

Willmott (1987, 1989) describes 'community' as having three main meanings. First and foremost, the term community is used to denote an area or locality in which people live. This is often referred to as a 'territorial community' and can consist of a loose collection of streets, a housing estate, a town or a whole country. However, from a sociological perspective there is more to the idea of community than simply a collection of people sharing a common territory. 'Community' has a second meaning in the sense that individuals may form a community on the basis of shared interests. As Willmott describes, such communities are often referred to as 'interest communities', with '"interest" being broadly interpreted to cover shared characteristics as diverse as ethnic origin, religion, politics, occupation, leisure pursuit and sexual propensity' (1987, p. 52). Thus, we often hear reference to the black community, the business community, the scientific community, the Roman Catholic community and the gay community, to name but a few. The two broad types of community are not mutually exclusive. Although members of an interest community may be widely scattered geographically, interest communities can also be found in local areas. In other words, communities can exist within communities. For example, a multi-ethnic, inner-city, territorial community might contain a number of disparate groups that constitute individual interest communities.

Willmott maintains that these two definitions do not capture the full meaning of community. He suggests that there is a third meaning, which he labels 'community of attachment' or 'attachment community' (1989, p. 4). This refers to the patterns of social relationships which engender feelings of belonging and help to create a sense of shared identity (see Box 8.1).

The likelihood of a 'sense of community' emerging depends upon three factors:

1 the degree and extent of social interaction between people in a particular locality;

2 the extent to which values and interests are shared by neighbours and other residents;

3 the extent to which local people recognise that they live in an identifiable area and feel attached to it.

(Willmott, 1984, pp. 6–7)

According to this conceptualisation, a particular territorial community may be a community only in a geographical sense if local residents have little social

> ## Box 8.1   Research findings
>
> ### Conditions for attachment communities
>
> Research findings suggest that 'communities of attachment' are more likely to arise when the following conditions exist:
>
> - population stability with lengthy continuous residence in the area;
> - kin living in area;
> - many people work in local industry;
> - people are alike in social class and income;
> - people share membership of a particular minority;
> - numerous locally based organisations;
> - in response to an external threat residents form local campaign groups;
> - physical layout and building design create a sense of a separate physical identity and encourage casual neighbourly meetings;
> - the area is particularly isolated.
>
> *Source*: Willmott, 1989, p. 1

contact with one another, share no common interests and feel no sense of belonging.

Given the ambiguity surrounding the concept of community, some sociologists have suggested that rather than attempt to define the indefinable, the concept should be abandoned in sociological research. Stacey (1969) suggests replacing it with 'local social system'. In this way the researcher avoids the emotive overtones associated with the word 'community' and is thus able to focus on local social networks and patterns of social interaction which do not present the same definitional problems.

Is the community in decline?

When we hear people extolling the virtues of community life we often discover that they are mourning a contemporary 'loss of community' by referring to an earlier age when 'community spirit' produced cohesive, stable and harmonious communities. This idea of the decline of community is also found in the writings of those early sociologists who regarded the rise of urban industrial society as marking the beginning of the end of the traditional community. The work of Ferdinand Tönnies is a good example.

Writing in 1887, Tönnies (1957) argued that increasing industrialisation and the rise of commercial capitalism was changing the established social order and altering the form of human relationships. This constituted a threat to the quality of social life. In developing his thesis he introduced the two concepts of *gemeinschaft* and *gesellschaft* to describe two very different ways of life.

Gemeinschaft is best described as community. For Tönnies, it encompassed the essence of life in pre-industrial society. *Gemeinschaft* represented a traditional style of living, characteristic of rural society, in which social relationships were lasting, informal, affective and based on cooperation. Strong family bonds, clearly articulated kinship obligations and a sharing of values ensured that people experienced a strong sense of belonging to the community. The family and the Church were the two most important social institutions responsible for enforcing social rules and moral norms, thus ensuring that individuals subscribed to a common culture. According to Tönnies, *gemeinschaft*-type relationships were founded upon 'community of blood' (kinship), 'community of place' (territory) and 'community of mind' (friendship).

Gesellschaft is translated as 'society' or 'association' and is the very antithesis of *gemeinschaft* or community. It 'essentially means everything that community is not' (Bell and Newby, 1971, pp. 24–5). Tönnies used the term to describe the type of human relationships characteristic of the newly emergent urban industrial society. He saw *gesellschaft* relationships as impersonal, formal and rational, based more on calculated self-interest rather than cooperation. People associated with one another primarily for reasons of personal gain rather than as a result of shared experiences or a sense of duty.

Tönnies saw the growth of the *gesellschaft* at the expense of the *gemeinschaft* as the precursor of many social problems such as growing social isolation and increased levels of loneliness. However, as Lee and Newby note, this thesis was not just directed at urbanisation:

> ... Tönnies was referring to the dehumanizing consequences of contemporary social change in *any* geographical location ... [his] concern was not urbanization *per se* but the 'loss of community' in a much broader sense – the loss of a sense of identity, meaning and authenticity in the modern world.
>
> (Lee and Newby, 1983, p. 51)

For Tönnies, *gesellschaft*-type relationships were not natural but rational and artificial. Devoid of all sentiment and emotion they represented the hallmark of an immoral social system.

Tönnies' conceptual distinction between the two broad social forms is useful for highlighting the differences between traditional communities and modern societies. However, two points need to be made by way of evaluation. First, it needs to be remembered that the two concepts are presented in a pure form for analytical purposes and are not intended as empirical descriptions of the world as it is. In reality elements of both may be found together. As Gusfield (1975) maintains, it is difficult to conceive of a permanent human relationship that contains all the attributes of community and none of society and vice versa. Second, Tönnies was not an objective observer of social change. Influenced by the Romantic tradition in German social thought he was passionately opposed to the social transition he was describing. Consequently, he presented community and society as being in stark contrast to one another. In order to emphasise the dehumanising aspects of modern society he presents a glorified picture of the pre-industrial past.

The idea that industrialisation has led to the disintegration of traditional communities is not supported by a number of studies of working-class communities undertaken by sociologists in the 1950s and 1960s (Young and Willmott, 1957; Kerr, 1958; Tunstall, 1962). For example, in their study of family life in Bethnal Green in the East End of London, Young and Willmott found a close-knit, cohesive community, in which there was evidence of shared values and communal sociability. Local solidarity was fostered by a relatively stable population; half of the sample of people they interviewed were long-term residents who had been born in the area, educated there and then taken jobs there. As a result of this restricted geographical mobility, social relations revolved around strongly articulated friendship and kinship networks. Consequently, large numbers of residents knew each other and this familiarity was important in helping them to identify with the group and develop a sense of community.

This image of the traditional, tightly knit urban working-class community in which friends, workmates and neighbours live in close harmony and provide informal networks of mutual support is open to challenge on two broad grounds. First, there is a view that these communities have ceased to exist. It is argued that as a result of social and economic changes in the second half of the twentieth century these traditional communities can no longer be found. The old industrial areas have been redeveloped and many of the old-style neighbourhoods replaced by modern housing estates. There has also been an increase in geographical mobility. According to one estimate, only one in eight of the population lives near members of their extended family (Willmott, 1986). Family life has become more 'privatised' or home-centred, as the modern family has become more inward-looking and less community oriented. Many neighbourhoods now consist of independent families who have only superficial contacts with their neighbours and do not share a sense of belonging to a common group or locality.

Second, some observers question whether or not traditional working-class communities actually ever really existed in the shape and form depicted in the community studies of the 1950s and 1960s. These studies are criticised for portraying a romanticised picture of community life as a haven of mutual support and good neighbourliness. Cornwell (1984), in a more recent study of working-class life in Bethnal Green, describes how individual interviewees presented both 'public' and 'private' accounts of community life. In essence, public accounts contain what are considered to be socially acceptable responses, whereas private accounts offer a more accurate reflection of a respondent's personal opinion. Cornwell found that whereas in their public accounts respondents spoke of shared values and common interests, in their private accounts they commented on the diversity within their community. It is the uncritical acceptance of public accounts that serves to mask the reality of community life by perpetuating the myth of the close-knit, traditional working-class community. The idea of a golden age of community is a feature of many autobiographical accounts and oral histories of working-class life down the years. As Bourke maintains, these remembered communities are 'retrospective constructions' in which 'conflict is forgotten in favour of doors that were always open' (1994, p. 137).

The fact that conflict can be a feature of social relations within communities is all too often overlooked. Communities are not fixed entities but are constantly changing as they adapt to various internal pressures and external social forces. Newby (1980) describes how the gradual transformation of English rural villages into non-agricultural settlements led to the emergence of social divisions and conflicts between the local population and the middle-class newcomers. For the farmers and agricultural labourers the influx of commuters and second-home owners was perceived in terms of a 'loss of community'. Wary of intimate social contact with the newcomers the occupational community becomes a community within a community, or to use Newby's terminology, an 'encapsulated community'.

Sociological studies of the community have tended to ignore the existence of internal divisions and how these affect social relationships. This partly stems from the fact that 'community' is a word with strong emotive connotations that makes it difficult to define without making value judgements. This can be a problem for the sociologist. From a sociological perspective, Lee and Newby emphasise how it is important that the community is described as it actually *is* (empirical description) and not as it is felt it *should be* (normative prescription). However, as they acknowledge, 'normative prescription and empirical description are often closely intertwined in sociology' (1983, p. 57).

This confusion between empirical description and normative prescription carries over into the domain of social policy.

> The appeal to 'community' implicit in community care policies is an amalgam of elements from the image of the traditional village on the one hand and the historical features of these urban working-class neighbourhoods on the other. Not only do they sit rather uneasily together, but their social basis is frequently idealized and romanticized. At a popular level this occurs in stereotypes of the idyllic rural society, but it can be perpetuated also in sociological accounts of the solid, tightly-knit urban working class 'community'.
>
> (Bulmer, 1987, p. 51)

It is essential that those responsible for designing and delivering community-based health and social welfare services have a realistic understanding of the diversity and complexity of community life. Statutory agencies need to understand how social support networks are formed and maintained before they can establish and implement appropriate policies and support services to meet the needs of different sections of the community.

The twin processes of industrialisation and urbanisation have clearly had an important impact on local social relationships and neighbourhood ties but to what extent this has resulted in a 'loss of community' is open to debate. If we accept that the form a community takes owes much to the prevailing social, economic, historical and cultural conditions, then communities are products of their time. Any perceived decline in the level of involvement in the local community may be indicative of an adjustment to changing conditions, rather than evidence of an irreversible decline in the overall quality of life. For example, Willmott (1989) describes how modern transport and advances in communication technology have increased the scope for people to interact more with others outside of the immediate territorial community. This has given rise to what he calls 'dispersed communities', in which individuals are able to exercise greater choice as to whom they associate with.

The family

> What is a family? Is it just a genetic chain, parents and offspring, people like me? Or is it a social construct, an economic unit, optimal for child rearing and divisions of labour? Or is it something else entirely: a store of shared memories, say? An ambit of love? A reach across the void?
>
> (Obama, 2008, p. 327)

The term 'community care' is something of a misnomer when used to refer to the informal lay support systems of unpaid carers within the community. It is individual members of the community who shoulder the burden of caring for the sick and chronically ill living at home. The family plays such an important role in providing informal healthcare for its members that it has been described as being 'at the centre of the caring function' (Equal Opportunities Commission, 1982a, p. 1). Indeed, most healthcare takes place within the home. Much of the daily round of family life is concerned with meeting the physical and psychological needs of individual family members. It is within the general social context of the family that health is maintained and illness dealt with. According to Litman (1974) the family constitutes the basic unit as far as healthcare is concerned.

Under community care policy the family has been given an increasing role to play in the provision of care. In order to appreciate fully the impact of this policy it is necessary to understand something about the changing nature, structure and organisation of family life in modern Britain. We need to know how recent changes in family patterns are likely to affect the ability of the family to fulfil its caring function. However, before we discuss the impact of changes in the pattern of family life on the provision of informal care we need to be clear about what is meant by the term 'family'.

What is a family?

The family forms the basic unit of social organisation in our society; it is seen by many as a prerequisite of a stable social system. Indeed, some social commentators attribute many contemporary problems, such as teenage crime, to a perceived decline in the family as a social institution. They assert that the family has lost its moral authority and sense of responsibility and only a return to 'traditional family values' will halt the moral decline and bring about a recovery. For them the family is seen as a natural social grouping that has benefits for both the individual and society. However, they tend to subscribe to a particularly idealised image of the family: a heterosexual married couple comprising the biological parents of the children and forming a one-family household. The male breadwinner is the head of the household and his spouse is a full-time housewife. This standard stereotype constitutes what is for many people the 'normal' nuclear family or 'traditional' household.

Data relating to Great Britain reveal that there is greater diversity in household structure and family composition than the standard stereotype would appear to suggest. Figures reveal that the proportion of households consisting of a married couple with dependent children fell from 35 per cent in 1971 to 21 per cent in 2008. Currently around 29 per cent of all households consist of people living alone; the comparable figure for 1971 was 18 per cent. Over the 37-year period in question, one-person households formed by people *under* pensionable age more than doubled from 6 per cent to 15 per cent. Households comprising single individuals *over* pensionable age rose from 12 per cent to 16 per cent between 1971 and 1991 but has stabilised at around 15 per cent during the first decade of this century. Lone parents with dependent children now account for 7 per cent of all households, compared to 3 per cent in 1971. As regards multi-family households, whereas these formed 3 per cent of all households in 1961, this figure had declined to 1 per cent by 1971 and has remained at around this level ever since (Office for National Statistics, 1998a, p. 42 and 2009, p. 15).

Although the traditional family structure of married mother and father with child or children is the most common family type, the family is not a fixed entity but can take a number of different forms. During the first half of the 1990s there was a slight increase in the proportion of both cohabiting families and lone-parent families, and a corresponding reduction in the proportion of married couple families. In the period from 1996 to 2006, the number of families headed by a married couple fell by 4 per cent, while the number of lone-mother families showed an increase of over 11 per cent and cohabiting families increased by over 60 per cent (McConnell and Wilson, 2007). As regards dependent children, just over three-quarters of all such children live with both parents; this figure fell continually throughout the last quarter of the twentieth century. Currently, over one-fifth of families with children are lone-parent families. Between 1997 and 2008 the proportion of children living with lone mothers increased from 19 per cent to 22 per cent: the comparable figure for children living with lone fathers remained stable at 2 per cent. During the same period there was also an increase in the proportion of children living with cohabiting couples; this figure rose from 8 per cent to 13 per cent (Office for National Statistics, 2009). Although seven out of ten families with dependent children may be described as married-couple families, these do not all conform to the stereotype of the 'normal' family as some are step-families or reconstituted families. Step-families with dependent children account for 7 per cent of all families and there is evidence of an increase in the proportion of step-families in recent years (Allan and Crow, 2001). As illustrated in Table 8.1, the distribution of dependent children by family type varies across the different ethnic groups. All in all, given the existence of different family types, the use of the term 'the family' can be misleading. At an empirical level it makes more sense to refer to 'families' (Elliot, 1991).

Table 8.1 Dependent children:[1] by family type and ethnic group, 2008[2]

United Kingdom			Percentages
	Married couple[3]	Cohabiting couple[4]	Lone parent
White	63	14	23
Mixed	48	13	39
Asian or Asian British	87	1	13
Black or Black British	46	6	48
Chinese	79	*	21
Other ethnic group	72	4	24
Total	64	13	23

1 Children aged under 16 and those aged 16 to 18 who have never married and are in full-time education.
2 Data are at April–June.
3 Includes civil partnerships.
4 Includes same-sex couples.
Source: Adapted from Office for National Statistics, 2009, Table 2.5, p. 16

Social change and family life

In recent years there have been some significant changes in both family structure and the internal dynamics of family life; many of these changes have implications for the provision of informal health care.

Changes in family formation and structure

From a broad historical perspective the process of industrialisation is seen as having had an important impact on the family. It used to be thought that the growth of industrialism, which set in motion the transition to urban living, was directly responsible for the decline of the extended family and the rise of the nuclear family unit. According to this view, the traditional family in pre-industrial society consisted of a multi-generational collection of kin forming a single household unit. With agriculture providing the major source of livelihood, this type of family was self-supporting. The extended structure ensured that there were sufficient adult members to share the burden of caring for the young, the old and the sick. As industrialisation promoted a geographically mobile labour force this family structure was undermined, resulting in the disruption of rural communities, the attenuation of kinship ties and the emergence of smaller, nuclear family units.

This idea that the extended family was the predominant family type in pre-industrial society and suffered a decline following industrialisation has been challenged on a number of grounds. First, given the average life expectancy, the three-generation family, with grandparents contributing to the care of young children, was far from commonplace in the nineteenth century (Laslett and Wall, 1974). Second, evidence suggests that industrialisation did not lead to a reduction in family size but in fact encouraged the setting up of extended households (Anderson, 1971). For example, in order to take advantage of the opportunities for paid employment for women in the new factories, nuclear families brought in relatives to look after the young children so as to enable mothers to go out to work (Anderson, 1971). Third, research in the second half of the twentieth century reveals that the so-called 'isolated nuclear family' is part of a wider kinship group. Nuclear families exist as independent households but they still form part of a kinship network in which reciprocal support is an important feature. Kinship ties have been found to be intact among both working-class and middle-class groups, with the exchange of services between female members being of particular significance (Rosser and Harris, 1965). Grandparents, particularly grandmothers, are major providers of care within the extended family. In fact, maternal grandmothers are the most frequently cited source of childcare by mothers who are in full-time paid employment (Martin and Roberts, 1984). All in all, extended kin relationships are an important aspect of contemporary family life (McGlone *et al.*, 1998). The existence of a non-residential network of kin who provide help and support in times of need has led some sociologists to declare that the term 'isolated nuclear family' is somewhat misleading, as what we are in fact observing is a 'modified extended family' (Morgan, 1975, p. 65).

A core element in the modified extended family is the domestic unit composed of the conjugal couple and their dependent children. Changes in the patterns of cohabitation, marriage and divorce over the last four decades have had an important impact on family structure and relationships. Just over a quarter of people born between 1971 and 1975 were cohabiting between the ages of 25 and 29 (Office for National Statistics, 2009). Survey data reveal that not only has there been an increase in the incidence of cohabitation but there has also been an increase in the average length of time couples live together prior to marriage. In Great Britain, of those women who married for the first time in 1966 only 4 per cent had lived with their partner prior to marriage; by 1993 this figure had risen to 68 per cent (Office for National Statistics, 1997). Thus, while cohabitation may be seen as a substitute for marriage for some, for others it is a precursor to marriage. The rise in the number of cohabiting couples and the decline in the proportion of people getting married has been one of the major changes in family life in recent years. As Coleman and Salt assert, 'cohabitation is a common preliminary to marriage, especially to remarriage, and is to some extent a replacement for it' (1992, p. 175).

For many people marriage no longer marks the start of a new family. As Figure 8.1 shows, there has been a significant reduction in the number of first marriages in the United Kingdom since the peak year of 1970. In 1995 there were half as many first marriages as in 1970; this was the lowest recorded figure since 1926 (Office for National Statistics, 1998a). The increase in pre-marital cohabitation has led to an increase in the average age at first marriage, which is currently 31.8 years for men and 29.7 years for women (Office for National Statistics, 2009, p. 19). Despite these trends, the increase in the number of remarriages (i.e. marriages in which one or both partners have been married before) suggests that marriage remains a significant social institution and the basis for the formation of households. In approximately one-quarter of marriages that took

United Kingdom
Thousands

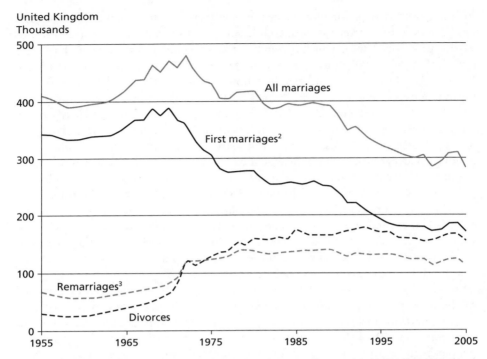

1 Divorce data from 1995 to 1970 are for Great Britain only. Divorce became legal in Northern Ireland
   from 1969. Includes annulments.
2 For both partners.
3 For one or both partners.

Figure 8.1 Marriages and divorces[1]

Source: Office for National Statistics, 2008, p. 20

place in 2006, one or both partners had been married or divorced at least once
before (Office for National Statistics, 2009, p. 19).

At the beginning of the 1960s there were just over 2 divorces per 1,000 married population in England and Wales. Following the implementation of the Divorce
Law Reform Act (1969) in 1971, the divorce rate rose to nearly 6 per 1,000 and
10 years later it had reached nearly 12 per 1,000 married population. Further
legislative changes were introduced by the Matrimonial and Family Proceedings
Act 1984, which allowed couples to file for a divorce after the first year of marriage instead of waiting for a period of three years. By the mid-1990s the divorce
rate had risen to 13.5 per 1,000 married people; however, there are signs that it
is beginning to level out, particularly among those in the younger age groups.
In 2007 the divorce rate for England and Wales stood at 11.9 per 1,000 married
population, its lowest level since 1981 (Office for National Statistics, 2008e).
One of the consequences of the rise in the divorce rate has been an increase in
the number of lone-parent families. Figures for Great Britain show that the proportion of all families with dependent children that are headed by a lone parent

Box 8.2 Research findings

Facts about marriage, divorce and the family

- About a quarter of men and women cohabit before their first marriage.
- Nearly 44 per cent of all live births occur outside of marriage.
- The average age for married women giving birth for the first time was 30 years in 2006.
- The average number of dependent children in a family is 1.8.
- Around one fifth of private households in Great Britain comprise two adults and dependent children.
- Twenty-two per cent of families with children are lone-parent families.
- One in 10 families contains a step-parent, usually a step-father.
- Around two-fifths of marriages are remarriages for one or both partners.
- Two in five marriages end in divorce.
- Nearly three-quarters of divorces are granted to wives.
- One-third of divorces in 2007 did not involve children.
- In 62 per cent of married couples with children both the husband and the wife work.
- Only 7 per cent of households comprise a male wage earner, a housewife and children.

Source: Office for National Statistics, 1997, 1998a, 2008d, 2009

rose from 7 per cent in 1972 to nearly 21 per cent in 1996. Approximately 90 per cent of lone-parent families are headed by a woman. Some basic facts about marriage, divorce and the family are presented in Box 8.2.

The fact that the family has undergone a number of major changes in recent years has prompted some social commentators to talk about the decline of the institution of marriage; thus suggesting that the traditional view of marriage no longer applies.

> Three old images of marriage have become obsolete in the twentieth century. The first is that marriage confers on a woman a secure, settled income and a status and a role based on children and housekeeping around which most of the rest of her life revolves. The second is that marriage lasts for the rest of an increasingly long life. The third is that marriage is the setting for almost all childbearing and sexual cohabitation.
>
> (Coleman and Salt, 1992, p. 175)

However, this does not herald the demise of marriage as a social institution but marks the fact that marriage is taking on a new meaning in response to the wider social, economic and cultural changes taking place in society. There may have been an increase in marriage breakdown but nine out of ten people still get married at some time in their lives. Many people who divorce remarry. In around

39 per cent of all marriages in 1994 one or both partners had previously been married; this was almost double the comparable figure for 1971 (Office for National Statistics, 1998a). Morgan (1994) describes this growing trend in remarriage as one of the most significant changes in family patterns in recent years.

The rise in the divorce rate, the growth in the number of remarriages and the increase in cohabitation, all point to the emergence of a new pattern of marriage. From a sociological perspective, marriage can be seen as an institutionalised social structure that provides a normative framework for regulating sexual relationships and raising children.

> Marriage itself can be regarded as a historically specific phenomenon, in that in many societies families have existed without it and that, as an institution, it appears to have evolved as a mechanism for controlling the inheritance of property and the legitimacy of sexual relations all with an eye to the reproduction of society.
>
> (Smelser, 1994, pp. 336–7)

Looked at in this way, it is easy to see why governments express concern when they feel that the status of marriage is losing some of its traditional significance. Legal marriage is viewed as a mechanism for establishing some form of social order and stability. For example, it is through the institution of marriage that parental responsibilities and obligations regarding the provision of primary childcare are formulated and formally endorsed. However, the traditional model of courtship, marriage and family formation is much less relevant than it once was. Cohabitation has become 'a prelude to marriage' for many couples (Morgan, 1994, p. 109), while for a growing minority of couples it has become an alternative to marriage. A third of all births now occur outside of marriage; however, in around 80 per cent of cases these births are jointly registered by both parents and in three out of four cases the parents live at the same address (Office for National Statistics, 1998a). Indeed, it has long been recognised that marriage now represents an incident in, rather than the start of, family life (Brayshaw, 1980).

The pattern of marriage characteristic of the contemporary era is sometimes referred to as 'serial monogamy'. In other words, the law may dictate that an individual can only be married to one person at any one time but during the course of a lifetime an individual may marry more than once. Consequently, as a result of the increase in the divorce rate and the rise in the number of remarriages, reconstituted families are 'an increasingly significant social phenomenon' (Abercrombie *et al.*, 1994, p. 298).

On account of these major changes in marriage and family life, some sociologists have suggested that the traditional concept of the family life cycle should be abandoned in favour of the notion of the 'family career' (Smelser, 1994, p. 337). At its simplest the traditional family life cycle approach constructs an image of the individual making a natural progression through a series of developmental stages. Following childhood and adolescence the young person embarks on a period of courtship, which culminates in marriage when they leave the family of origin to establish a new family of procreation. Smelser prefers the concept of 'career' because, like the notion of 'life course', 'it reflects the increased contingency in people's life patterns' (1994, p. 337), thus acknowledging the options and choices people have when it comes to the patterning of family life.

Marriage as a social institution is not so much in decline as changing. Individuals nowadays place a considerable emphasis on the quality of the relationship that exists between partners in a marriage. Expectations of marriage have never been higher. In this sense, the relatively high divorce rate may be interpreted as a reflection not of lower but of higher standards of marriage in our society (Fletcher, 1988). Furthermore, there is a greater flexibility about the arrangements surrounding family formation. As described above, cohabitation has grown in popularity to such an extent that it is 'virtually a majority practice to cohabit before marrying' (Kiernan and Wicks, 1990, p. 8).

How do these and other observed trends in family patterns affect the capacity of the family to provide care? The answer is that some family types are better able to cope than are others. One-parent families are in a particularly vulnerable position. To begin with, unlike two-parent families, there is no other adult with whom they can share the daily burden of childcare and the routine tasks associated with domestic life. Many of these families depend on Income Support and the links between poor health and poverty are well established. The economic hardship one-parent families have to endure can be a cause of considerable stress. By and large, lone parents provide care around the clock, which coupled with their limited financial resources means that they lead restricted social lives. Furthermore, women and men who are divorced or separated can experience social isolation as a result of the loss of contact with their former partner's family and the friends they shared when they lived together. The social stigma that still surrounds lone parenthood is also instrumental in producing feelings of isolation and exclusion. However, although lone-parent families face distinctive problems, the experiences of lone-parents are by no means uniform. For example, the unmarried teenage mother with very young children will experience a different set of circumstances than the older divorced or widowed mother with adolescent children.

Lone parenthood may be a temporary phase in a family career. Following remarriage a one-parent family becomes a reconstituted family. While this may go some way to easing financial problems it can give rise to new emotional difficulties as family bonds and kinship ties take on a new complexity. All this has implications for the future of the family as a major provider of care.

> Will members of stepfamilies, cohabiting couples or divorcees feel obligations to care for sick or aged relatives and ex-kin? As yet it is difficult to identify precisely what the impact will be on informal care. What we do know is that people are rethinking traditionally conceived family relationships and loyalties.
>
> (Taylor and Field, 1993, p. 184)

The changes in the patterning of family life over recent decades have given rise to a broad debate about moral responsibility and basic social values. While some observers take the view that any deviation from the traditional two-parent family structure is evidence of a disintegration of family life and a decline in moral standards, others see the changes as a reflection of how the modern family is adapting to changing social and economic circumstances. There is clearly a dilemma here for public policy. Should policy-makers strive to introduce legal reforms and social policies designed to prevent marital breakdown and promote the ideal of the traditional nuclear family, or should they concentrate on finding ways of helping individuals and families to adjust to the social changes that are taking place? In short, should the aim of policy be prevention or accommodation? However, this might not be an either/or question. The two policy responses are not necessarily alternatives (Kiernan and Wicks, 1990, p. 31) and the challenge facing policy-makers might be one of finding the right combination of policies that form a coherent strategy that incorporates elements of both.

Internal dynamics of family life

If we wish to understand how the responsibility for informal healthcare is distributed within co-resident nuclear families, we need to know something about both the nature of conjugal role relationships and the general division of labour within the home. Essentially this entails focusing on the differentiation of sex roles within the family. In discussing conjugal role differentiation, functionalist theorists in the 1950s and 1960s distinguished between masculine and feminine roles. They described the former as instrumental and the latter as expressive (Parsons, 1956). According to Parsons, the principal role of the husband and father was one of economic provider: it was the man who engaged in the external world of work in order to provide for his wife and children. In contrast, the role of the wife was conceived as more inward-looking, concentrating as it did on maintaining the affective side of family life. From a functionalist perspective, instrumental roles emphasise earning and are oriented towards the public world of paid employment, whereas expressive roles stress caring and are oriented towards the private sphere of the family. This role segregation or specialisation is deemed essential for ensuring the stability of the modern nuclear family as a social system. Indeed, it was Parsons' belief that it was through the clear delineation of the roles of mother and father that men and women were able to develop a sense of social identity, thus enabling the family to achieve one of its major functions, that is, the 'stabilisation of adult personalities'.

The existence of such rigidly segregated conjugal roles can be challenged on two broad counts. First, women's rate of participation in the labour force has increased significantly throughout the latter part of the twentieth century. In 1971 56 per cent of women aged between 16 and 59 were economically active, by 1997 this figure had risen to 71 per cent (Office for National Statistics, 1998a, p. 77). Data for married-couple families with dependent children reveal that the proportion of families where both parents are in employment rose from around 50 per cent in the early 1980s to over 60 per cent in the mid 1990s (Office for National Statistics, 1997, p. 30). Second, sociological research shows that in the second half of the twentieth century a home-centred family life style emerged, in which the family roles of men and women became less differentiated and more balanced. For example, Goldthorpe et al. (1969) describe how family life began to take on a new importance for affluent workers in the 1960s; this led to the emergence of what they call the 'privatised family'. It is suggested that one aspect of this development was that men began to participate in domestic tasks and activities that had once been traditionally defined as women's work, such as household chores and child-rearing. Young and Willmott (1973) also found evidence of a greater sharing of domestic work between husband and wife and claimed that this represented the beginnings of a new family form, which they labelled the 'symmetrical family'. In their view the roles of wives and husbands were becoming less differentiated and in due course would become identical. Consequently, the symmetrical family of the future would be a more democratic and egalitarian institution.

What implications do these changes have for the provision of informal healthcare within the modified extended family? To answer this question consideration needs to be given to the actual nature and extent of the changes in the division of labour within the home. While some studies show that in families where both partners are in paid employment there is a less traditional division of household labour, women's share of domestic work remains disproportionately large (Pahl, 1984). Research from a feminist perspective has done much to capture the realities of family life for wives and mothers and dispel the notion that male involvement in domestic labour heralds the arrival of an equal balance of power within marriage. As Abbott and Wallace assert:

> While it is evident that men are not sharing domestic work with their wives, even if their wives are in full-time employment, it is even more clear that they are not taking on responsibility for tasks. Men seem to be able to choose what domestic tasks they undertake and often take on those that women find more enjoyable, such as bathing children, rather than tidying up the toys or cooking the meal.
>
> (Abbott and Wallace, 1990a, p. 88)

Men may be playing a more active role in the domestic side of life but in the majority of cases the contribution they make falls well short of taking responsibility for the performance of any major routine household tasks. On an ideological level men are stereotyped as earners and women as carers. This, coupled with the fact that the domestic division of labour remains divided along gender lines, clearly has implications as far as the involvement of men in the provision of informal care is concerned.

Informal care

> The term 'informal carer' – or 'family carer' – is frequently used, but there is no consensus among researchers, policy-makers, service-providers, carers and cared-for persons as to what constitutes an 'informal carer' . . .
>
> (Dahlberg et al., 2007, p. 439)

Who cares?

Although families are the major source of informal healthcare, gender plays an important part in the organisation and delivery of this care. It has long been recognised that, 'Family care generally means care by women' (Equal Opportunities Commission, 1982a, p. 2). As Allan remarks, in reference to community care for the elderly, 'the caring is done not by communities or families as such but by female primary kin' (1985, p. 139). In general terms, Graham (1983) describes how the concept of caring is not only associated with home and family but is also presented as essentially 'women's work'. As she asserts, the caring role '. . . is constructed through a network of social and economic relations, within both the home and the workplace, in which women take responsibility for meeting the emotional and material needs not only of husbands and children, but of the elderly, the handicapped, the sick and the unhappy' (1983, p. 22). Gender stereotypes convey an image of women as the nurturing sex, for whom caring is essentially a natural function. Consequently, responsibility for maintaining the home and providing individual care for members of the immediate family are considered fundamental aspects of the role of a daughter, wife or mother. Furthermore, the caring role is not confined to the nuclear family and the raising and rearing of children.

> The caring role which is allocated to women moves from caring for her own children to caring for her parents (or her husband's parents) and back to her grandchildren. Even in her 60s and 70s, a woman may find her life predominantly shaped by the image of her as a caring and mothering figure.
>
> (Phillipson, 1981, p. 187)

Just as it is assumed 'natural' that mothers should carry the greater burden of housework and childcare, female kin are deemed the ones best suited to provide routine care for elderly dependent relatives. This is certainly the case where care involves attention to personal hygiene. The social taboos surrounding certain aspects of physical care ensure that some tasks are defined as essentially women's work (Ungerson, 1983).

Thus, abstract ideologies of kinship largely influence who becomes an unpaid, informal carer. For Ungerson, carers 'are selected, first and foremost, according to dominant, normative, and gendered rules of kinship' (1987, p. 61). Within families there is a recognisable hierarchy of obligations, which is gender related. By and large, female family members are more likely to be expected to take responsibility for the care of sick relatives than are their male counterparts (Parker, 1990). This is not only because gender-based stereotypes portray women as having the personal attributes and natural talents essential for caring. Gender inequalities in opportunities for paid employment and differences in the earning potential of men and women ensures that in many households women are the prime candidates to take on the responsibility of unpaid carer when the need arises.

Seeing caring in terms of kinship norms is not to imply that the social obligations associated with particular kinship roles are immutable or that caring is essentially a women's issue. As Finch (1989) argues, kinship rules can be the subject of negotiation in certain circumstances. It would be naïve to suggest that people simply recognise, accept and act upon a set of agreed social rules and moral norms governing the provision of informal care within kinship groups.

Consideration needs to be given to both the nature of the social context within which the need for care arises and the strength of existing kinship ties and family bonds.

To understand fully women's experience of caring it is necessary to appreciate the different dimensions of the informal health work undertaken by women. In the course of performing health work, female carers act as providers, negotiators and mediators (Graham, 1985). They are providers in the sense that they are expected to provide a home environment in which health can flourish. This involves a range of tasks from ensuring that the physical surroundings are secure and clean to purchasing and preparing food to meet the nutritional needs of individual family members. This is the most labour-intensive aspect of women's healthcare work and it is from this that their role as a negotiator stems. As Graham describes:

> In labouring for their families' health, women are also teaching it. In setting standards of diet and discipline, women not only facilitate health in a biological sense; they transmit a culture in which health and illness can be understood.
>
> (Graham, 1985, p. 26)

She contends that the bulk of the work that women do as informal carers is 'invisible' and 'privatised' (Graham, 1983, p. 27). In other words, it is carried out within the private domain of the family home. This clearly applies as far as the roles of provider and negotiator are concerned. When informal healthcare work becomes incorporated into the daily round of household chores it can be taken for granted and not appreciated as another aspect of the unequal division of domestic labour. However, not all women's healthcare work takes place within the private setting of the family. When women act as mediators they enter the public domain and engage with professional health workers such as general practitioners, health visitors and district nurses. In this context they function as 'go-betweens linking the informal health-care system with the formal apparatus of the welfare state' (Graham, 1985, p. 26).

Although women carry a heavy burden as informal carers, national estimates of the number of carers, based on data from the 2001 Census and 2000/2001 General Household Survey, reveal the contribution made by men. Of the estimated 5.5 million adult carers, 3.2 million are women and 2.3 million are men (Pickard, 2007, p. 21). Some of the findings from the two surveys are summarised in Box 8.3, which provides a useful insight into the major characteristics of informal carers.

The costs of caring

There is an established research literature focusing on the positive impact of informal care and family support on patient well-being. Also, informal caring activity is considered by some to enhance the fund of social capital in a community and this is considered to have a beneficial impact on the general health of the population (Cooper *et al.*, 1999). However, unpaid, informal caring also has its costs for the individual carers and other family members. Consequently,

---

Box 8.3   Research findings

A measure of informal care in Great Britain

- One in six people aged over 16 years provides informal care.
- Women (58 per cent) are more likely than men (42 per cent) to be the main carers.
- Women are more likely than men to be engaged in caring for someone living outside the household.
- Of those providing unpaid care for long hours over 60 per cent are women.
- Four per cent of the adult population provide unpaid care for 20 hours a week or more.
- Over one in five of the population between the ages of 51 and 59 provides unpaid care for one hour a week or more.
- Forty-nine per cent of carers are in full- or part-time work, 26 per cent are retired and 25 per cent are unemployed or economically inactive.
- Approximately one in three carers provides unpaid care for someone living in the same household.
- Nine out of ten carers care for someone to whom they are related.
- Eighteen per cent of carers look after more than one person.
- One in five carers have been looking after their dependant for at least 10 years.
- One half of all carers look after someone aged over 75 years.
- Over two-thirds of carers provide practical help such as preparing a meal, shopping and doing laundry.
- Every day 6,000 people take on new caring responsibilities.

Source: Department of Health, 1999b, 2008a; Maher and Green, 2002; Pickard, 2007

---

family support should not simply be viewed as a patient resource. The extra burden placed on individuals and families can have an adverse impact on health, the internal dynamics of family life and the way in which the family interacts with the wider community. According to one observer:

> . . . families are not merely static resource banks from which a seriously ill member withdraws desirable social supports. Families are also potential sources of stress, and negative social exchanges occur in all families. Most important, family systems collectively experience stresses associated with illness and engage in interdependent coping among members.
>
> (Ell, 1996, p. 174)

Thus, in order to understand fully carers' needs and interests we need to view the caring role within the wider context of both family and community. We also need to appreciate that the burden experienced by the carer has both an objective and subjective dimension. The objective aspect concerns what the carer actually does, for example the amount of time they devote to caring activities and the nature and type of caring they provide. In contrast, the subjective dimension refers to the personal experience of and feelings towards the caring role.

The costs to individuals and their families of providing care will depend to a large extent on the type and amount of caring tasks undertaken and the degree of help and support received from statutory agencies, voluntary organisations, extended kin and friends. It is only by understanding the nature and impact of these costs that we can begin to appreciate the problems carers face and identify ways in which professional workers in the health and social services sectors can help them in the work that they do. As Ungerson notes, 'the informal sector is the lynch pin of the community care reforms' contained in the National Health Service and Community Care Act of 1990. Therefore, 'policy has to be concerned with the maintenance of the sector, and research has to be funded to discover the conditions under which informal care works best' (Ungerson, 1998, p. 172).

There is a growing body of research documenting the impact of the caring role on informal carers and their families. Basically, the costs are physical, financial, emotional and social. These will of course vary according to the nature and severity of the disabling condition. Caring for children or adults with physical disabilities, severe learning difficulties, certain chronic illnesses or degenerative diseases can be extremely physically demanding. The recipient of care may need help with routine daily activities, such as getting out of bed, washing, dressing, eating and going to the toilet. There have been many studies over the past three decades describing the types of tasks performed by carers and the implications long-term caring can have for the physical, mental and social well-being of the primary carer. This literature suggests that carers are much more likely than non-carers to suffer from poor health (Nissel and Bonnerjea, 1982; Glendinning, 1992; Parker, 1993; Hirst, 2003). There is also some suggestion that caregivers who provide care within their own homes tend to have poorer health than informal carers who deliver care elsewhere (Barrow and Harrison, 2005).

In studying the difficulties experienced by carers, Twigg and Atkin (1994) divide physical care into four broad categories:

- personal care;
- the management of incontinence;
- medical and nursing care;
- household tasks.

From interviews with carers they describe how the intimate nature of some caring tasks can pose problems or difficulties for carers. As they explain, normative expectations and cultural rules influence what is interpreted as socially acceptable behaviour. The rules and expectations differ from one type of relationship to another. For example, what is considered acceptable for a parent to do for a young child of the opposite sex may not be deemed appropriate when that child reaches adulthood. Twigg and Atkin illustrate this with a quote from an interview with a father whose adult daughter, Dawn, suffered from muscular atrophy. Although he helped with looking after his daughter, he felt he had to leave the personal care to his wife.

Not with a girl of thirty-odd years old, let's be honest . . . If it had been a lad it would have been the other way round, wouldn't it? . . . It would be embarrassing for Dawn and embarrassing for me.

(Quoted in Twigg and Atkin, 1994, p. 32)

Cross-gender tending, involving personal care tasks, can also be problematic when adult children are caring for elderly parents.

The stresses and strains experienced by informal carers are well documented in the research literature. For example, in a detailed study of 44 primary carers of elderly dependants with senile dementia, Haley *et al.* (1987) report negative effects on both the physical and mental health of carers. Dealing with incontinence can be particularly stressful and a cause of much embarrassment (Levin *et al.*, 1989). Not only does the carer have to change and dispose of incontinence pads and colostomy bags but also has to cope with the problem of soiled clothes and bed linen. The extra work involved adds to the normal daily domestic chores and can be especially burdensome when the carer is elderly. Where the cared-for person displays behavioural difficulties, such as aggressive behaviour or an inability to communicate, the carer may experience emotional stress which may have a deleterious effect on their mental well-being and hence their ability to continue in the caring role (Pearlin *et al.*, 1990).

Providing long-term care for a chronically sick or disabled person also has its financial costs (Glendinning, 1992). In many cases there is an increase in daily living expenses as more money is spent on such items as laundry, heating and transport. In addition to this, where mobility is a problem, there is the cost of adapting the home environment. The financial situation of the family can also be adversely affected if the carer is forced to give up full-time paid employment in order to continue in the caring role. Where family members share the caring, or where the primary carer is not required to be in constant attendance, it may be possible for carers to continue to work part-time but this still means that they experience a loss of earnings. Furthermore, this forced change in employment status has implications for future career prospects and pension entitlement.

For many carers, especially those who live with the person they care for, employment outside the home is more than a source of income but also offers a temporary suspension of the caring role and provides an opportunity to connect with the outside world. As Pearlin *et al.* (1990) note, one of the stress-inducing aspects of caring is 'role captivity'; this occurs when the carer feels trapped in the caring role which is perceived as all-embracing. The identity and life of the carer comes to be so closely bound to that of the person being cared for that they experience a 'loss of self'. In this sense, work not only offers carers a means of temporary escape from a stressful and demanding situation but can also provide the resources to enable them to support a dependent relative. This is illustrated in Box 8.4 by the case of one informal carer reported in the study by Twigg and Atkin (1994).

Research shows that family caregivers also experience increased social isolation as the caring role impinges upon their general social activities (Jones and Vetter, 1984). Twigg and Atkin use the term 'restrictedness' to describe how being

> ## Box 8.4   Case study
>
> ### Combining caring and working
>
> The complex way in which employment could sustain caring was illustrated in the case of Mr Ensbury, a single man in his late sixties, who was caring for a mother with severe dementia. He used his income from his pharmacy to pay for private nurses to cover for him during the day. He would have liked to retire and sell the business, but this would have meant that he no longer had the income, nor the reason to pay for substitute care, and would be forced to stay at home twenty-four hours a day. He needed to work to generate the income to allow him to work and thus escape from the situation.
>
> *Source*: Twigg and Atkin, 1994, pp. 43–4

responsible for the care of someone else can lead to a reduction in the quality of life experienced by carers (1994, p. 37). They identify three dimensions to restrictedness. Firstly, there is the issue of the provision of physical care and attention. Severe constraints are placed on a carer's life when they are required to tend to the basic physical needs of the cared-for person and be on hand to provide for their personal safety. The carer may get little respite and be 'on call' 24 hours a day. The degree to which the carer's life is limited will depend on a number of factors, among which are the nature of the needs of the cared-for person, the extent to which the caring is shared among other family members and the amount and type of support received from statutory agencies and voluntary bodies. Secondly, in cases where constant attention is not called for, carers often admit to feeling anxious and uneasy about leaving a cared-for person alone. Some of the carers Twigg and Atkin interviewed talked about the uneasiness they felt when they were away from home, even for short periods of time. Although their fears were never realised, they nevertheless caused them to restrict their social activities and limit the amount of time they spent away from home. The third form of restrictedness is labelled 'shared or secondary restrictedness' (Twigg and Atkin, 1994, p. 38) and refers to instances where the limits placed on the cared-for person also affect the lives of the carer. This is particularly found in the case of partners who have enjoyed a joint social life prior to the onset of illness. As Twigg and Atkin comment, carers may feel both uneasy and guilty if they go out on their own.

As described in Box 8.5, Twigg and Atkin identified three modes of response to the caring role among the carers they studied: the engulfment mode; the balancing/boundary setting mode; the symbiotic mode. Engulfment occurs 'where the carer subordinates his or her life to that of the cared-for person' (1994, p. 122). This mode of response was particularly observable among those carers who faced a heavy physical burden and had strong emotional ties to the person they were looking after. The emotional closeness was often such that individual carers became distressed when seeing the person they cared about experiencing physical and mental anguish. Many of these carers structured their lives around providing care and support. This form of adaptation to the caring role was more

> ### Box 8.5   Definition
>
> #### Three modes of response to the caring role
>
> - *Engulfment*. Caring takes precedence; the informal carer is so immersed in the caring role that it becomes a core feature of her or his self-identity.
> - *Balancing/boundary setting*. The carer attempts to protect his or her autonomy by either making time to pursue individual interests or setting limits to the type of tasks and responsibilities he or she is willing to accept.
> - *Symbiosis*. The carer benefits from performing the caring role and has no desire to relinquish any of the responsibility.
>
> *Source*: Twigg and Atkin, 1994

prevalent among women than among men. In contrast, carers who fell into the balancing/boundary-setting category were not engulfed by the situation but attempted to find ways of fulfilling their responsibilities as primary carers while simultaneously maintaining a level of autonomy and emotional detachment. Although they acknowledged and accepted the role of carer, they identified what for them were the limits of their involvement. As was the case with engulfment, this response mode also displayed a gender bias, with male carers appearing better able to establish and maintain a sense of detachment than their female counterparts. According to Twigg and Atkin, this was particularly the case with husbands caring for wives who suffered from senile dementia or severe physical illness. Finally, the symbiotic response refers to 'situations where the carer derives positive benefits from their role, where they have no real wish for it to cease and where their and the cared-for person's needs are mutually reinforcing' (Twigg and Atkin, 1994, p. 126). This was characteristic of situations where the parent was the carer and the level of dependency was not particularly pronounced.

Twigg and Atkin argue that knowledge of these three broad categories of response is important for healthcare workers, as it gives some insight into how carers are likely to respond to the offer of help from outside agencies. For example, for those individuals for whom engulfment resulted in a total commitment to caring, asking for or accepting help was not an option they would entertain as it could be interpreted as an admission of failure on their part to provide the necessary support. By comparison, carers who adopted the balancing or boundary-setting mode tended not to view the offer of outside help as a sign of personal failure but saw such assistance as a valuable resource. Where a symbiotic mode of response prevailed carers were seen as being generally welcoming towards the involvement of the support services, provided that this did nothing to impinge on their own role as primary carer.

The individual circumstances of carers and the situational and familial contexts in which informal caring takes place vary widely. Carers do not represent a homogenous group and caring may take many different forms. The personal experiences of the carer and the person being cared for will be influenced by a

Box 8.6   Case study

Mutual caring

Elsie (88) lived at home with her daughter, Christine (60), who has a learning disability. They lived together all their life and they did everything together. Christine was declared 'uneducable' at the age of six and Elsie was told to 'take Christine home and keep her happy'. Christine did not use any services until she was 40 when her dad had a stroke and Elsie found herself suddenly caring for two people. However, Christine really enjoyed the new activities and the contacts that the services brought. As they both grew older, Christine did more and more things to help her mum, who found tasks like carrying the shopping increasingly difficult.

When Elsie was diagnosed with a terminal illness, both Elsie and Christine had full needs and carers' assessments as they were looking after each other. Services were offered to support Elsie when Christine was not at home, and to help Christine with things like cooking, cleaning and shopping for them both. Although Christine sometimes found it very difficult to care for her mum and watch her illness worsen, it was very important to both her and Elsie that they stayed together for as long as possible and she is proud of the care she provided while her mother was still alive. She says: *'Mum always looked after me and I'm glad I could look after her too because I know how she liked things done.'*

Source: Department of Health, 2008a, p. 22

complex pattern of individual personality factors, social circumstances and cultural expectations. The case studies presented in Boxes 8.6 and 8.7 describe two very different caring contexts, which illustrate examples of mutual and inter-generational caring.

From the above, it can be seen that the physical, psychological, social and economic costs associated with providing informal care can, either singularly or in combination, impair the quality of life enjoyed by the carer. It has been suggested that carer health and carer burden are related, in so far as the negative effects (costs) increase with the level of the burden borne by the carer and the patient's level of disability and/or distress (McKeown *et al.*, 2003). Where caring from the chronically ill is concerned, attention needs to be given to the transitional and dynamic nature of the caring role. For example, in cases of degenerative diseases, such as multiple sclerosis, the role of the carer takes on an ever-increasing burden as the cared-for person becomes more physically and functionally dependent. In circumstances such as these the role of the caregiver can be described as transitional. The caring role can also be seen to have a dynamic quality, in that the relationship between the carer and the recipient of care will at times be characterised by periods of relative calm and stability, while at other times it will be marked by distress and instability (Boeije *et al.*, 2003). Furthermore, where the provider and recipient of care are in a relationship the caring role has an interactive or dyadic dimension. As described by Forbes *et al.*,

> ## Box 8.7   Case study
>
> ### Intergenerational caring
>
> Ajmir (17) has cerebral palsy. He is unable to speak and uses British Sign language (BSL).
>
> His mother Kim is the main carer, and her husband Sarvjit helps when he can. Both parents work full-time, so three days a week, Ajmir attends a residential school. When at home, he has two daily visits from a local homecare provider, helping him to bathe and dress, and in the evening, get ready for bed. The homecare worker has learned signs in BSL, and some key words in Punjabi. She has learned about the Sikh religion and culture in order to show the family that she understands their culture.
>
> Sarvjit's frail and elderly parents live next door. Kim and Sarvjit care for them too, taking them to clinical appointments. However, the grandparents have a caring role with Ajmir too, supporting him when his parents go out. Ajmir is also able to reciprocate their help, assisting his grandparents by undertaking simple tasks for them such as putting the dishes away or closing windows.
>
> During the summer holidays, Ajmir, with support from his family, uses his direct payment to purchase care, which provides a break for Kim.
>
> *Source*: Department of Health, 2008a, p. 23

'A central element of this dyadic component is the collective health capacity of the patient and carer, considering the health of the patient and carer as a shared unit rather than each in isolation' (Forbes *et al.*, 2007, p. 564). In their study they found that although the level of patient-disease impact was the most important factor influencing the health status of the carer, the 'dyadic health' (i.e. shared health) of the patient and carer together also played a significant part in explaining carer burden and carer health problems. The specific health problems carers most commonly regarded as severe were tiredness, anxiety and depression.

Young carers

As the above discussion illustrates, we know a great deal about the circumstances, experiences and needs of informal carers from the findings of government-sponsored surveys and the growing body of academic research. However, in all this work there is very little mention of young carers, which has led some critics to refer to this as 'a literature of omission' (Aldridge and Becker, 1993a, p. 459). It is only relatively recently that researchers have begun to recognise young carers as an important subject group and attempted to estimate their numbers, identify their concerns and discover their needs (Walker, 1996). According to national data 1.4 per cent of all children in the UK provide informal care within the family (Doran and Whitehead, 2003).

It is not difficult to assume that children who provide primary care for a sick or disabled parent or relative living at home experience the same problems encountered by adult carers, especially if they are the sole provider of care. Where the cared-for person's mobility is impaired, providing personal care can be physically demanding. In certain situations the demands of the caring role may be so great that the child's social life is severely restricted. As Aldridge and Becker observe, children who care may experience 'a silent curfew' (1993a, p. 460). They may feel under pressure to limit the amount of time they spend away from home and feel unable to explain to friends the nature of their family circumstances. Whereas adult carers may experience a loss of employment opportunities, children may miss out on their education, which will have implications for their long-term career prospects.

These broad similarities aside, it is important to develop a child-centred perspective on informal care if we are to understand fully the experience and needs of children as carers. This approach requires research into the lives of young carers. One such example is provided by Aldridge and Becker (1993b) who carried out a small-scale qualitative study of young carers in Nottingham. They found that many of the children they interviewed associated the caring role with punishment in one way or another. This feeling of being punished was reinforced when the child was deemed to be the sole carer and received little or no support from other members of the household. The notion of punishment also featured in the way the child carers viewed their relationship with professional workers in the health and social welfare fields. Some young carers did not perceive such workers as necessarily supportive but saw them as a potential threat to the continuation of the caring role. For example, they feared that the involvement of social workers would eventually lead to them being taken into care, which they perceived as a form of punishment.

Child carers have been described as the 'unacceptable face of community care' (Meredith, 1991). Largely hidden from view their needs can go unrecognised and they can receive little support from statutory agencies. When young carers do come into contact with health professionals, such as general practitioners, community nurses and community care assistants (CCAs), their needs as carers may often be overlooked, as attention is focused on the recipient of care. In their study, Aldridge and Becker describe how some CCAs were of the opinion that where support services were provided these could be withdrawn once the child displayed an ability to cope and had reached 'a suitable age'. However, as the researchers note:

> The criteria of what constituted a 'suitable' age varied from 12 to 16, revealing a lack of consistency and resulting in uncertainty and confusion for the children themselves. Here again we can see how the young carers may believe themselves to be the subject of indirect punishment, in that outside support may be arbitrarily withdrawn leaving them inexplicably to cope alone when they, for example, reach their 12th birthday. This is particularly interesting considering that many adult carers have access to CCA and nursing support for the care receiver, regardless of their age or indeed their ability to care.
> (Aldridge and Becker, 1993b, p. 381)

A report by the Social Services Inspectorate (1995) entitled 'Something to Think About' summarised the research findings concerning the experiences of young carers: these are presented in Box 8.8.

Box 8.8   Research findings

Something to think about

Frequent effects for children and young people of providing care

- Problems at school with completing homework and gaining qualifications;
- Lack of time for playing, engaging in leisure activities and enjoying sports;
- Isolation from other children of the same age and from other family members;
- Conflict between the needs of the person they are helping and their own needs, leading to feelings of guilt and resentment;
- Feeling that there is nobody there for them, that professionals do not listen to them and only really engage with the adult receiving care;
- Lack of recognition, praise, or respect for their contribution;
- Feeling that they are different from other children and unable to be part of a group;
- Feeling that no one else understands their experience;
- Problems making the transition to adulthood, especially with regards to finding work, setting up a home of their own and establishing relationships.

Source: Adapted from Department of Health, 1999b, p. 76

Caring for the mentally ill within the family

Mental illness, like physical illness, has social and economic implications for the individual, the family and the wider society. Depending on the nature of the disorder, the prognosis and prescribed treatment, the patient may be temporarily indisposed, unable to fulfil his or her normal, customary social obligations. The concept of the 'sick role', as applied to the physically ill and discussed in the previous chapter, is in some respects relevant in this context. For example, the mentally ill person, like the physically ill individual, is granted exemption from some, if not all, his or her social role responsibilities during the period of the illness. However, the similarity ends here, on account of the different lay perceptions of physical and mental illness (Miles, 1981, p. 72).

The roles of the mentally ill patient and the patient suffering from an acute physical illness differ in a number of important respects. There is a general tendency for the physically sick to be absolved of responsibility for their condition, on the assumption that physical illness is the result of external factors over which an individual has little control. For example, we 'catch a cold' or accidentally 'pick up a bug'. In contrast, a mental disorder is perceived as being the result of a defect or weakness within the individual. Consequently, those so afflicted are considered to be in some way responsible for their condition. Furthermore, despite evidence to the contrary, the lay audience views mental illness as a long-term affliction, whereas acute physical illness is seen as being of a short-term duration. There is also a difference when it comes to laying claim to the sick role. Given the stigma associated with mental illness and the fact that an individual suffering from a psychiatric disorder might not recognise the symptoms, the mentally ill are less likely to embrace the sick role.

The policy towards 'care in the community', coupled with the closure of long-stay mental hospitals, has led to an increasing emphasis being placed upon the family as a caring institution. The demands made upon individual members of the family, and the degree to which the normal daily routine of family life is disrupted, will largely depend upon which member is mentally ill and the nature of their symptoms. It is not only in the early stages of mental illness, before professional help is sought, that the family is affected. Where a family member has an enduring psychiatric disorder and is receiving outpatient treatment, the consequences for the family can be both pronounced and long term. Consequently, it is important to have some understanding of the impact living with a mentally ill person has both on the family in general and its individual members in particular. This will enable health workers to appreciate and respond to the needs of the carers as well as the needs of the patient.

Researchers who have studied the impact of psychiatric illness on family functioning, describe how families often need to adjust their daily pattern of activities and household arrangements, in order to cope with the various practical problems that arise from caring for a sick relative at home (Creer and Wing, 1974; Wing, 1975). Where constant supervision is advised, ensuring that there is always someone on hand to help, may mean that shopping trips, visits to friends and other activities are curtailed or re-arranged. In some cases relatives may be forced to give up either full-time or part-time paid employment outside the home so as to be able to fulfil their caring role. This can have an adverse affect on the standard of living and jeopardise the future financial security of the family. The situation is exacerbated in cases where the mentally ill family member was formerly in paid work and contributed to the family finances.

Interestingly, as Miles (1981) observes, although relatives view the disruption of household routines and the loss of income as causing practical difficulties, they are not among what they consider to be the major problems of living with a mentally ill relative. What appears to be of paramount concern for relatives is the burden the patients' symptoms places upon the family, particularly in terms of the impact on the emotional climate of daily family life and the health of other family members. Miles quotes from Creer and Wing's (1974) study of families coping with schizophrenia to illustrate how symptoms such as bouts of incessant talking or prolonged silences can create an emotionally charged, stress-inducing atmosphere. The irrational behaviour of dementia suffers can be a source of distress for family carers (Haley *et al.*, 1987). Also the unpredictability of the behaviour of some psychiatric patients can be a source of insecurity for relatives, especially if the patients' behaviour at one time or another has been seen as physically threatening. Unlike professional mental health workers, the relatives of psychiatric patients are not trained for dealing with difficult and disruptive behaviour. Furthermore,

> ### Box 8.9   Case study
>
> ### An appeal for meaning
>
> You need somebody who will sit down and . . . you can say – 'How can we deal with this, how are we meant to react, what do you want us to do?' We can only be there for Donald, and you go through these stages where Donald thinks he hasn't got a family, he doesn't want to know you, he'll throw you out of the place, he'll scream at you, he'll shout at you . . . You need somebody when times like that happen, you know you're not immune to it all – it hurts. 'We know he's ill, can you explain to us what is going on in his brain that he is suddenly screaming and shouting at us, and abusing us and everything else, you know why? . . . what can be done about it and what do you want us to do about it, except make nuisances of ourselves, with both them and with him' . . . because that's what you feel like?
>
> *Source*: Caroline quoted in Jones, 1996, p. 98

their relationship to the patient makes it impossible for them to avoid becoming emotionally involved (Wing, 1982).

A number of research studies illustrate the complex feelings and emotional reactions faced by relatives: anger, grief, guilt and resentment are all commonplace. In a study of family members who have a close relative suffering from severe psychiatric problems, mainly involving symptoms of schizophrenia, Jones (1996) illustrates how anger, grief and a sense of loss predominate. Anger is sometimes directed at the professionals, particularly psychiatrists, for failing to provide a diagnosis and give relatives sufficient guidance. This is evident in the short extract above (Box 8.9), taken from an interview Jones conducted with the sister of a mentally ill patient. The interviewee is described as 'making an appeal for meaning' when she relates what questions she would like the professionals to answer (1996, p. 98). As Jones observes, Caroline is struggling with a number of mixed emotions. Despite the distressing circumstances in which she finds herself, she clearly cares for and wants to help her brother. Fadden *et al.* (1987) also refer to instances where relatives feel that psychiatrists have been unhelpful.

The uncertainty and unpredictability of patients' behaviour contributes to the heightened emotional climate found within families caring for mentally disturbed relatives. The extent to which family members experience the caring role as a stressful one is evident from the way they describe their situation. Phrases such as 'constantly on a knife edge, living on the edge of a volcano' (Creer and Wing, 1974, p. 30) and 'living on the edge of the world' (Jones, 1996, p. 100) occur frequently in interviews with family carers.

Relationships between family members can come under pressure when the family environment, or particular events in the history of individual families afflicted with mental illness, are reputed to be of aetiological significance. In the absence of a biogenetic explanation for the onset of a psychiatric disorder, there is an increasing likelihood that relatives may look for causes within the family. For example, parents may feel that the disturbed behaviour of a teenage child is in some way attributable to their failure to exercise adequate control as parents during the child's formative years. Attributing responsibility in this way generates feelings of guilt.

Caring for the mentally ill at home not only affects the quality of family life but also has adverse consequences for the individuals concerned. According to Gallagher and Mechanic (1996), many researchers have concentrated on the affective, social and economic consequences of caring for the mentally ill within the family and overlooked the impact on the physical health of household members. In those studies that have taken self-reported physical health into account, there is evidence that caring for mentally impaired relatives has negative health consequences. For example, following a comparison of family carers of Alzheimer suffers with a group of non-carers of a similar age, Haley *et al.* (1987) conclude that the carers reported more chronic illness and poorer subjective health.

Two factors that need to be taken into account when discussing the possible health effects of living with a mentally ill relative are the severity of the psychiatric disorder and the nature of the kin relationship between the patient and the carer. Where the symptoms are distressing, long lasting and severely disrupt family life, the physical and emotional strain placed on carers can be considerable. Studies of families caring for elderly relatives reveal that the burden of caring is perceived as being greater the more severe the illness (McCreadie *et al.*, 1987). As Gallagher and Mechanic conclude, 'This research on family burden suggests that disruptive or severe conditions may have greater negative health effects than do less severe conditions' (1996, p. 1693).

The notion of dependency features largely in any discussion of the importance of kinship networks in the provision of informal care. Given the relatively restricted nature of kinship connections in Western societies, the emphasis is on relationships between members of the immediate family. Within this context there are normative expectations and institutionalised practices surrounding the respective roles of mother, father, daughter and son. The obligations and responsibilities parents have towards their children, in terms of providing care and support during the formative years, are well established. Relations between kin are structured around normative expectations and culturally defined roles. In childcare it is the mothers who carry the major burden as primary carers. The general expectation is that children, as they grow older, become increasingly independent. Parental dependency in adulthood is not considered to be the norm. However, there are normative obligations concerning adult children caring for their elderly parents.

As Gallagher and Mechanic suggest, the type of kin relationship may be important when looking at the health effects of living with a relative who is mentally ill. It may be . . . that relationships in which dependency is more normative (e.g. one spouse being dependent on the other, or adult child caring for elderly parents) are less stressful, and therefore produce fewer negative health outcomes than do relationships in which dependency is less normative (e.g. parents caring for dependent adult children).

(Gallagher and Mechanic, 1996, p. 1692)

Indeed, they find some support for this assumption following their analysis of data from the National Health Interview Survey in the USA. Their findings reveal that respondents living with a mentally ill adult child reported poorer physical health than did respondents living with a mentally ill spouse.

Caregivers: the policy context

> Current policy and practice has fuelled an increasing focus on measuring the outcomes of health and social care over time, including the impact on carers.
>
> (Hirst, 2002, p. 579)

The unpaid activities undertaken by informal carers, whether young people or adults, prevent additional demands being placed on state-funded social care and community health services. Given the increasing number of older people, particular over 75 years of age, and the improvements in the life expectancy of severely disabled children, the demand for informal care is destined to increase in the years to come. Consequently, it is important that we have some idea as to the factors that are likely to influence the future provision of informal care. The population of potential carers will fluctuate in response to demographic, economic and social trends affecting the wider society. For example, the number of people who are willing and able to provide informal care, particularly of a long-term and intensive nature, will be influenced by changes in family structure and formation. Higher rates of cohabitation and the growing number of lone-parent and reconstituted families may affect the future patterning of informal care-giving.

As regards community-care policy and practice, supporting informal carers has emerged as a key issue over the last twenty years. In introducing the process of the market economy of welfare into the provision and delivery of health and social care, the 1989 White Paper, *Caring for People*, acknowledged that friends, families and neighbours were largely responsible for providing the 'great bulk' of community care (Department of Health, 1989). This was followed by a number of pieces of legislation which not only affirmed the role of carers but also provided support for them. The National Health Service and Community Care Act (1990) places a duty on local councils in England and Wales to carry out a care management needs assessment for anyone who might require community services. In undertaking such an assessment the Act stipulates that the views of carers have to be sought. Following the 1995 Carers (Recognition and Services) Act, when performing a community care assessment, social service departments have a duty to ascertain and assess the needs of those carers who are responsible for providing 'a substantial amount of care on a regular basis'. The rights of carers to assessment were also extended by the Carers and Disabled Children Act (2000), which places a duty on local councils to carry out a carer's assessment when requested to do so by a carer. Since the passing of the Carers (Equal Opportunities) Act (2004), local authorities are responsible for informing carers of their right to an assessment and in making such an assessment they need to take into account the needs of carers in relation to their current (or planned) leisure activities, education, training and work. In 2006 the government announced a New Deal for Carers in its White Paper on community services entitled *Our Health, Our Care, Our Say* (Department of Health, 2006b). Two features of this policy initiative were the provision of a comprehensive national information service to meet the diverse needs of carers and the establishment of a training programme for carers.

In recent years there is evidence that policy-makers and service providers have begun to consult carers and listen to what they feel would actually benefit them. Carers' expressed wishes for more information, better and flexible support services, and the provision of care for themselves are clearly reflected in the various policy documents. In 2008 the government announced its intention of moving towards a single community-based support system for carers in order to support independence and choice for those who use care and support services. (Department of Health, 2008b). It also renewed its National Strategy for Carers with the publication of a document entitled *Carers at the Heart of 21st-Century Families and Communities*. A major feature of this Strategy is a vision that in ten years' time 'carers will be universally recognised and valued as being fundamental to strong families and stable communities' (Department of Health, 2008a, p. 16). The aim is that by 2018 carers will:

- be treated with dignity and respect as 'expert care partners';
- will have access to the services they need to support them in their caring role;
- will be able to live a life of their own alongside their caring role;
- will not be forced into financial hardship by their caring role;
- will be supported in order to stay both mentally and physically well.

(Department of Health, 2008a, p. 16)

The Strategy also aims to ensure that children and young people are protected from inappropriate caring roles and given the opportunity to develop and learn and enjoy a 'positive childhood'.

The National Strategy for Carers outlines a comprehensive set of policy objectives based on an understanding of the relationships between the caring role and carers' employment situation, financial circumstances and physical and mental health. How effective the proposed policy measures will be remains to be seen. However, in order to increase the chances of success it is essential that support services meet the actual needs of carers. This means recognising the variation in needs between different groups of carers and avoiding making assumptions about the availability of informal care (and the need for external support) based on social or cultural stereotypes. Research has an important part to play here in providing the information necessary for policy-makers and service providers to make informed choices. From a research perspective we need to focus attention on 'subgroups of carers for their special needs and experiences rather than considering them undifferentiated members of a homogenous group of informal carers' (Navaie-Waliser *et al.*, 2001, p. 733). Carers constitute a diverse group of people and we need to understand the nature and rate of transition into care-giving. A dynamic perspective needs to be adopted, which sees the population of carers as constantly changing. For a substantial minority of carers the role is a short-term one; for others it can last for many years. By exploring how individuals come to be informal carers across the different phases of the life course we will begin to appreciate the diversity of carers' circumstances and how these impact upon the caring relationship.

Summary

- The concept of caring is a complex one. It is not just about physical tending (caring *for*) but also has an emotional dimension (caring *about*). The act of caring can be described as a form of emotional labour: a 'labour of love'.

- The idea of care in the community has a long history. The development of a policy of community-based treatment in the contemporary period gained momentum from the revelations of the deprivations suffered by patients in total institutions and the perceived financial savings that such a policy was expected to deliver.

- From a sociological perspective 'community' is a difficult concept to define. It can refer to a locality or territory, a system of social relationships that operate within a local area or a sense of shared identity or belonging experienced by individuals and groups, who may or may not live in close proximity. Some early sociological studies present a romantic or idealised view of community life by ignoring the conflict, divisions and diversity that characterise modern communities.

- Family care is the mainstay of community care. The majority of healthcare takes place within the home or family setting. When considering the ability of the family to provide informal care attention needs to be given to the diversity of family life. Whether care is provided within the nuclear family or within the modified extended family, women are not only the primary providers of that care but also play a major role in health promotion and general health maintenance. Men and children also provide care for chronically sick and disabled relatives.

- Policy-makers need to be aware of the fundamental changes that have taken place in family life in recent decades if they are to introduce the kind of public policies that will meet the needs of informal carers. The physical, financial, emotional and social burdens associated with the provision of informal care on a long-term basis are well documented in the research literature.

- The increasing incidence of cohabitation and the rising divorce rate are not necessarily symptomatic of a decline in the institution of marriage and a disintegration of family life. Marriage and the family are variable constructs that adapt to changing economic and social circumstances.

- Informal carers do not form a homogenous group, but constitute a diverse and changing population. Taking on the role of caregiver has its costs and research shows that carers are more likely than non-carers to suffer from poor health. In recent years legislation and policies have been introduced to give carers rights and provide them with information, support and care.

Questions for discussion

1 What is 'the community' and does it care?

2 Do women make more natural carers than men?

3 What factors influence how well carers adjust to the role of primary carer?

4 Is the family as a social institution in decline?

5 What have governments done in recent years to support families who care? What more could be done to help informal carers?

Further reading

Aldridge, J. and Becker, S. (2003) *Children Caring for Parents with Mental Illness: Perspectives of Young Carers, Parents and Professionals*, Bristol: The Polity Press.

Allan, G. and Crow, G. (eds) (2001) *Families, Households and Society*, Basingstoke: Palgrave Macmillan.

Jones, D. W. (2002) *Myths, Madness and the Family: The Impact of Mental Illness on Families*, Basingstoke: Palgrave.

Means, R., Richards, S. and Smith, R. (2008) *Community Care: Policy and Practice*, 4th edn, Basingstoke: Palgrave Macmillan.

Phillips, J. (2007) *Care*, Cambridge: Polity Press.

Scott, S., Treas, J. and Richards, M. (eds) (2004) *The Blackwell Companion to the Sociology of Families*, Oxford: Blackwell Publishing Ltd.

Sharkey, P. (2007) *Essentials of Community Care*, Basingstoke: Palgrave Macmillan.

Twigg, J. and Atkin, K. (1994) *Carers Perceived: Policy and Practice in Informal Care*, Buckingham: Open University Press.

Williams, F. (2004) *Rethinking Families*, London: Calouste Gulbenkian Foundation.

Useful websites

Community Care: http://www.communitycare.co.uk/Home/

Carers UK: http://www.carersuk.org/

Social Care Online: http://www.scie-socialcareonline.org.uk/

CHAPTER 9

Communication in healthcare settings

Communication in healthcare

> . . . a physician's communication style is an essential factor predicting patient satisfaction and compliance. . . . a good physician–patient relationship and high communication quality seem to be crucial elements fostering the activation of patients' self-healing powers.
> (Christen *et al.*, 2008, p. 1474)

Since the mid-1970s individuals have increasingly come to be seen as having a moral responsibility to look after their own health (DHSS, 1976). Health promotion programmes and health education initiatives have drawn attention to the role individuals play in maintaining good health and preventing illness. The World Health Organisation has defined health promotion as 'the process of enabling people to increase control over, and to improve their health' (WHO, 1984). Consequently, health promotion campaigns have urged individuals to take up immunisation, adopt healthier diets, reduce alcohol consumption and take regular exercise. Clearly the individual is seen to have an active rather than passive role to play in the production and maintenance of health. Health work has become 'everybody's business' (DHSS, 1976).

It is not only health promotion activities that have emphasised the potential for individuals to participate in the healthcare process. Nurses and other health professionals are often encouraged to involve patients in the caring process by promoting forms of self-care and encouraging patient participation. McCarthy (1985) asserts that positive health is more likely to be achieved by fostering a collaborative relationship between the patient and the nurse, whereby the patient is perceived as an active participant in, rather than a passive recipient of, healthcare. In this context the patient becomes a 'health worker' and 'can be said to be a producer as much as a consumer of that elusive and abstract good health' (Stacey, 1976, p. 194). This dual role of consumer–provider is well established in the health education literature (Kickbush, 1981).

Another change in healthcare provision since the early 1970s has been the growing emphasis placed on the concept of 'patient-centred medicine' in modern healthcare systems around the world. Patient-centred care is based on a holistic view of the patient as an individual with a unique set of life experiences and personal needs. Epstein *et al.* (2005) distinguish between *patient-centredness, patient-centred care* and *patient-centred communication*. With reference to McWhinney (1995), they describe patient-centredness as 'a moral philosophy with three core values':

1 considering patients' needs, wants, perspectives and individual experiences;

2 offering patients opportunities to provide input into and participate in their care;

3 enhancing partnership and understanding in the patient–physician relationship.

(Epstein *et al.*, 2005, p. 1517)

Patient-centred care refers to the actual actions, interventions and health system innovations that are guided by the underlying philosophy. Effective patient-centred communication is essential if health professionals are to provide care in accordance with the three core values stated above. The key elements of patient-centred

Box 9.1   Definition

Patient-centred communication

- Eliciting and understanding the patient's perspective – concerns, ideas, expectations, needs, feelings and functioning.
- Understanding the patient within his or her unique psychosocial context.
- Reaching a shared understanding of the problem and its treatment with the patient that is concordant with the patient's values.
- Helping patients to share power and responsibility by involving them in choices to the degree that they wish.

Source: Epstein *et al.*, 2005, p. 1517

communication are outlined in Box 9.1. A patient-centred approach involves not only health professionals and patients but also the family members of patients. It covers all aspects of healthcare delivery, including end-of-life care where there is evidence of a need to develop a greater understanding of patients' concepts of a 'good death' (Clark, 2003).

As a result of these changes increasing attention has been given to the nature of the relationship between patients and professionals involved in the provision of healthcare services. Sociological studies of this relationship have tended to focus primarily on patients' encounters with doctors. A possible explanation for this bias is that sociologists are interested in the distribution and exercise of power in society and doctors represent the most powerful profession within the health system. Although the majority of studies mentioned in this chapter relate to doctor–patient consultations the findings will be of interest to other health professionals for several reasons. Firstly, there are similarities between some of the tasks performed by doctors and other health workers. For example, nurses interview patients, collect personal health data and carry out a variety of nursing tasks that bring them into close physical contact with patients. Secondly, knowledge of how doctors perceive patients and what patients expect from their doctors can provide nurses with a better understanding of patient behaviour. Thirdly, an insight into how social class background, ethnicity and gender have an impact upon the doctor–patient relationship will encourage nurses to reflect on their own practice.

Perspectives on the doctor–patient relationship

> Where Parsons saw legitimate authority and trust, Freidson saw 'medical dominance' and suppressed conflict. And while Parsons saw the social control functions of medicine and the doctor–patient relationship as having positive outcomes, Freidson, in contrast, saw them as far from therapeutic.
>
> (Bury, 1997, p. 88)

In looking at sociological approaches to the study of the doctor–patient relationship a distinction can be made between those theoretical models which examine medical practice within the context of the wider social structure, and those which focus on the dynamics of the day-to-day encounters between doctors and patients. These approaches are sometimes labelled macro and micro perspectives respectively.

Talcott Parsons (1951) was one of the first macro social theorists to explore the social relationship between doctor and patient. Writing from a functionalist perspective he sees doctors and patients acting out socially prescribed roles. The role of the sick person is deemed to be undesirable, patients are expected to want to get better, to voluntarily seek professional medical advice and cooperate fully with the doctor. If they comply with these role expectations they are granted certain privileges, such as sick leave. The role of the doctor is also characterised by rights and expectations. Doctors are expected to use their skills and expertise for the benefit of their patients; to be objective and emotionally detached in their dealings with patients and to be guided, at all times, by a code of professional practice. In the performance of their duties they have the right to conduct physical examinations and ask patients questions about their physical health and personal circumstances. According to Parsons, the obligation on doctors to maintain a position of affective neutrality and ensure that they always behave in the best interests of the patient, serves to reduce the potential for conflict in doctor–patient encounters.

Clearly, Parsons presents a consensus model of the doctor–patient relationship. Although the relationship is seen as an unequal one, with the doctor having professional autonomy and exercising authority over the patient, the role of the doctor is portrayed as being complementary to the role of the patient. It is assumed that there is a shared value system to which both parties willingly subscribe. The patient accepts the doctor's authority in the belief that the doctor will always act in a manner that safeguards the health and well-being of the patient. The extent to which the Parsonian model is an accurate reflection of the doctor–patient relationship has been questioned, from within the functionalist perspective, by Szasz and Hollender (1956). They maintain that the relationship between doctors and patients varies according to the nature of the medical condition and where the encounter takes place. They identify three types of therapeutic relationship, as described in Box 9.2.

Szasz and Hollender's conceptualisation of the doctor–patient relationship is more elaborate than Parsons's original formulation. The cooperation/guidance model is the one that comes the closest to the role of the sick person as described by Parsons, whereas the activity/passivity and mutual participation models represent an attempt to modify the functionalist approach by taking into account different clinical conditions and a wider variety of medical settings. Szasz and Hollender also note the importance of wider socio-cultural factors. They acknowledge that the systematic differences in the therapeutic relationships between doctors and patients are influenced by wider social and cultural factors. For example, mutual participation is more likely to characterise doctor–patient interactions where both

---

Box 9.2   Definition

Three types of therapeutic relationship

1 *Activity/passivity*. Where the doctor plays the dominant role, as in the case of surgical procedures and medical emergencies.

2 *Co-operation/guidance*. Where the patient is compliant and co-operative and in accepting medical advice plays a passive role.

3 *Mutual participation*. Where there is equality between doctor and patient as in cases of chronic illness where a considerable amount of self-care is essential if the condition is to be managed successfully.

Source: Szasz and Hollender, 1956

parties have similar social origins, class locations and cultural backgrounds. Likewise, an active–passive relationship is more likely to be found when doctors and patients do not share similar socio-cultural profiles.

The idea that the relationship between doctor and patient is reciprocal and based on a shared value system has attracted considerable criticism. Consensus theorists have been challenged for failing to recognise the potential for conflict in the relationship. According to one critic:

> Common to functionalist accounts of medicine's role in society is an image of the sick person as a highly conditioned, passive social actor who has learned to respond obediently to the medical script of illness.
>
> (Hart, 1985, p. 620)

In other words, the functionalist description of the shared expectations of doctors and patients is nothing more than the medical profession's idealised view of the form the relationship should take. Studies of doctors and patients reveal that conflict is very much in evidence. Bloor and Horobin (1975) describe how conflict can stem from patients being subject to conflicting sets of expectations which places them in a 'double-bind' situation. This occurs in the following way. On the one hand, individuals are expected to be more knowledgeable about health matters so as to enable them to identify those symptoms which require expert medical attention. Indeed numerous studies reveal that general practitioners frequently complain about patients taking up valuable consultation time with trivial complaints which in their opinion do not warrant a medical consultation. They define the ideal patient as one who is capable of identifying which health problems justify a visit to the doctor (Fitton and Acheson, 1979; Jefferys and Sachs, 1982). On the other hand, doctors' role expectations of patients are such that they are expected to be deferential, accept the diagnosis and readily comply with the prescribed treatment. Herein lies the 'double-bind'.

Freidson (1970a) sees conflict, not consensus, as a fundamental feature of the doctor–patient relationship. For him the underlying assumption of mutual consensus, cooperation and sustained reciprocity is untenable. As he asserts, '. . . the separate worlds of experience and reference of the layman and the professional worker are always in potential conflict with each other' (Freidson, 1975, p. 286). Consequently, there occurs 'a clash of perspectives' in which the differences in interests, expectations and priorities between doctors and patients can give rise to conflict. In medical consultations individual patients are understandably pre-occupied with their own health problems, whereas the doctor has to bear in mind the health needs of a large number of patients. There is evidence to suggest that patients and doctors have different definitions of 'emergencies'. Calnan (1984), in a study of patients visiting a hospital accident and emergency department, found that in 59 per cent of cases patients considered their condition to constitute an emergency, whereas only 6 per cent of the cases presented were defined as emergencies by doctors.

A major potential for conflict in the doctor–patient relationship is the existence of a gulf between medical models of illness and lay explanations of ill health.

Doctors use a specialised language which patients do not always comprehend. This gives rise to what has been termed a 'competence gap', which is built into the very structure of professionalised medicine: the lay person does not share the highly specialised body of knowledge used by the doctor.

> The 'competence gap' is at least partly a consequence of the fact that the professional doctor has a social monopoly of expertise and knowledge which is the very basis of the professional claim to a privileged status in society.
>
> (Turner, 1987, p. 50)

This monopoly of knowledge ensures that the doctor has authority over the patient and thus accounts for the unequal nature of the doctor–patient relationship. Whereas traditional consensus theorists see patients as being passive and submissive, conflict theorists view them as active and critical (Freidson, 1970a). For Freidson, the image of mutual cooperation and reciprocity fostered by the consensus perspective assumes a correspondence of interest between doctors and patients which is not borne out by empirical studies which provide evidence of conflict in doctor–patient encounters.

Bury (1997) refers to a third model (the negotiation model) of the doctor–patient relationship, which acknowledges that while there is potential for both conflict and consensus, the doctor and the patient generally display a willingness to work together to achieve a desired outcome. Consequently, conflict and consensus in their ideal forms only come to dominate in certain situations. The negotiation model addresses the contingent nature of social interaction and operates at the micro-level. Bury sees this model as clearly exemplified in the work of Stimson and Webb (1975), which is referred to in the next section.

Medical consultations as social encounters

> Talk is a key ingredient in effective medical care. The talk that occurs in medical visits encompasses the manifest content of doctors' diagnoses and patients' questions as well as the deeper structure of patients' fears; physicians' unspoken, but viscerally communicated, assumptions; and the dynamic flow of nonverbal expressions – frowns, grimaces, smiles, and head nods. . . . It is no secret that in today's depersonalized medical system, talk between doctors and patients is characterized by physicians' interruptions, patients' failure to articulate their problems, and a depressing asymmetry between patient and physician needs.
>
> (Perloff *et al.*, 2006, p. 836)

Social theorists working at the micro-level of analysis are also concerned with aspects of conflict and consensus in encounters between doctors and patients. Research shows that the professional dominance of the doctor is not only maintained in these encounters but in certain circumstances it is in fact enhanced. There is ample evidence that doctors maintain a tight control over the consultation process. Their primary aim is to elicit from the patient the information necessary to reach an accurate medical diagnosis. In order to achieve this goal, many doctors are inclined to adopt what has been termed a 'bureaucratic, task-oriented' interviewing style. A characteristic feature of this style is the tendency for the doctor to concentrate on asking the patient a series of highly specific factual questions in such a way as to discourage the patient from playing a more active part in the encounter (Plaja and Cohen, 1968). In a study of nearly 2,500 tape-recorded general practitioner consultations Byrne and Long (1976) discovered that the majority of interviews followed a *doctor-centred* pattern, as opposed to a *patient-centred* approach. In the doctor-centred format the emphasis was on information gathering, to the extent that there was virtually no opportunity for patients to express their concerns. Doctors only tended to respond to information that was relevant from the point of view of reaching a diagnosis. As one doctor commented:

> The doctor's primary task is to manage his time. If he allows patients to rabbit on about their conditions then the doctor will lose control of time and will spend all his time sitting in a surgery listening to irrelevant rubbish. Effective doctoring is characterized by a 'quick, clean job'.
>
> (Byrne and Long, 1976, p. 93)

Not all general practitioners in the study saw their role in this way. In a quarter of the consultations a patient-centred approach to interviewing was employed with doctors displaying a willingness to listen to patients' fears and respond to their concerns. However, the researchers did notice a tendency for doctors to adopt the doctor-centred style of interviewing when faced with increasing demands on their time. Observational studies in other medical settings have produced similar findings. Strong (1979), in a study of consultations in paediatric clinics in the USA and Scotland, found the 'bureaucratic' or 'doctor-centred' interview format to be the most common.

The medical interview has been described as 'a constrained, pre-structured form of talk' (Freund and McGuire, 1991, p. 233). Its organisation and structure reflects the relative power positions of the principal parties. The verbal exchanges tend to be initiated and controlled by the doctor. Only a minority of questions in doctor–patient encounters are from patients (West, 1983). The doctors' control in these situations is also evident in that they are more likely to interrupt their patients than be interrupted by them. Heath (1981, 1984 and 1986) in a detailed analysis of the coordination of verbal and non-verbal behaviour by doctor and patient shows how a doctor may disrupt the talk of a patient by not looking at them while they are speaking. However, as he notes, '. . . patients are not without resources when wishing to encourage their co-participant (doctor) to display attention to their talk' (Heath, 1984, p. 329). From the analysis of video recordings of doctor–patient encounters he describes how patients use gesture, body movements and silence to regain the attention of the doctor. Thus patients are not entirely passive subjects in medical encounters.

Studies of medical consultations have revealed that only a small amount of time is taken up by the doctor giving information to the patient (Waitzkin, 1985). It is the access to knowledge and the ability to control the flow of information to the patient that highlights the inequality between doctor and patient. Surveys consistently reveal that this is a major source of patient dissatisfaction (Jefferys and Sachs, 1982). An early study of hospital patients by Cartwright (1964) reported that the lack of information was the most frequently heard complaint. In a study of general practice Cartwright and Anderson (1981) found nearly a quarter of patients unhappy with the information given to them by their doctors. Obviously many patients wish to know more about their medical condition. This raises two questions: is it important that patients are better informed and, if so, why is information not always forthcoming?

The answer to the first question must be a resounding 'yes' on three counts. Firstly, if individuals are to make choices, for example whether or not to consent to treatment, they need to be as fully informed as possible about the options available to them. Secondly, research suggests that patients who are satisfied with the amount of information provided by their general practitioner are more likely to follow the prescribed treatment (Kincey et al., 1975). Thirdly, new models of the professional–patient relationship have emerged in recent years. The concept of the passive patient has been replaced by that of the 'activated' (Sehnert and Eisenberg, 1975) or 'active' patient (Steele et al., 1987). If such patient involvement is to be encouraged then it is essential that there is a greater sharing of knowledge and information between professionals and patients. Why then is information not more readily available? There are a number of possible explanations for this. Doctors may underestimate the patient's desire for information or their ability to understand any information they receive. Medical staff may deliberately conceal knowledge in order to ensure patient compliance or avoid distressing scenes. Withholding information may be a strategy for dealing with medical uncertainty. Finally, health professionals may have difficulty in communicating information to certain types of patients.

The medical consultation is another form of social encounter and as such will be influenced by the class, gender and ethnic background of the participants. The amount of information given to the patient is not simply determined by the nature of the presenting symptoms, but depends on an array of factors including the expectations and attitudes of the parties involved, and the level of communication skills of the participants. Given what is known about patterns of social interaction it is reasonable to assume that doctors may find it easier to communicate with patients of a similar cultural and social background to themselves. Doctors are by definition middle class and research shows that middle-class patients, in comparison to their working-class counterparts, tend to be given more information either voluntarily or in response to direct questioning (Cartwright and O'Brien, 1976). The reluctance of working-class patients to ask questions may not be an indication of a lack of interest but a reflection of the status gap between doctor and patient which can constitute a barrier to communication (Pendleton and Brocher, 1980).

As regards gender, there is some evidence to suggest that doctors are less responsive to questions from female patients and are more readily inclined to offer their male patients a fuller and more technical explanation of their medical condition

(Wallen *et al.*, 1979). To some extent the interactional strategies observed in the consulting room reflect the cultural stereotypes of gender-appropriate behaviour which are prevalent in the wider society. Thus male doctors are more likely to expect female patients to adopt a passive role, not simply because they are patients and are expected to accept the authority of the doctor, but because they are women. Studies in the USA have found that female doctors spend more time than their male colleagues talking to patients (Langwell, 1982). Indeed, research suggests that the communication patterns of female and male doctors differ in a number of ways and that female doctors are more likely to adopt a patient-centred style of communication. Studies conducted in primary-care settings in the United States show that female doctors tend to conduct longer consultations, ask more questions and are more likely to discuss psychosocial issues than their male counter-parts (Roter *et al.*, 2002; Roter and Hall, 2004). In a study of gynaecological outpatient consultations Christen *et al.* (2008) found that although higher patient satisfaction levels were recorded when the doctor was female, the crucial factor was the gender-related specific communication skills (i.e. a patient-centred approach) and not simply the gender of the doctor.

Cultural factors can inhibit communication between health professionals and patients from minority ethnic backgrounds. Language barriers and differences in non-verbal behaviour are common causes of misunderstandings in medical encounters (Tuckett *et al.*, 1985). This is not surprising given that '[t]alk is certainly the fundamental instrument by which the doctor–patient relationship is crafted and by which therapeutic goals are achieved' (Roter and Hall, 2006, p. 4). In a study of people of Asian and African-Caribbean descent living in London it was described how both men and women experienced 'feelings of powerless-ness in the face of doctors' knowledge and attitudes' (Donovan, 1986, p. 255). Furthermore, a number of British Asian women were reported as stating a preference for Asian doctors as 'some of those who speak little English derive much comfort from being able to express their worries in their chosen language' (1986, p. 262). Clearly effective doctor–patient communication can be hampered if the participants are from different linguistic cultures. However, it is not simply a case of there being a language barrier; it is also a question of the expectations both parties bring to the medical consultation and how these influence what has been described as the 'dynamic dance of doctor–patient interaction' (Perloff *et al.*, 2006, p. 837). There is a suggestion in the American literature that inter-racial miscommunication may be a result of the fact that African Americans and Whites are accustomed to different interactional practices and conversational styles. Consequently, Black patients may experience the questions posed by White doctors as a form of interrogation (Perloff *et al.*, 2006).

Research reveals that when patients evaluate the healthcare they receive, they are seldom critical of the technical skills of the doctor (Cartwright and Anderson, 1981). Patient satisfaction is related to the amount and quality of information they are given about their condition and the extent to which the doctor appears to be willing to listen and take their worries and concerns seriously (Jefferys and Sachs, 1982). It is the personal qualities of the doctor which patients appear to value the most. Patients want their doctors to be considerate, understanding, willing listeners with good interpersonal skills. This applies irrespective of the social class background, gender or ethnic origin of the patient.

Comaroff (1976) in a study in South Wales found general practitioners adopted a variety of communication strategies. Some doctors withheld information from their patients in order to prevent them worrying, some gave as little information as possible and others saw the provision of information as an important aspect of their job. On the basis of the data Comaroff identified two broad communication strategies, the *unelaborated* and *elaborated*. The former was favoured by those doctors who felt the need to preserve their professional autonomy by ensuring that consultations were tightly controlled. They adopted a doctor-centred interview style, which was predicated upon the assumption of a competence gap between doctor and patient. In contrast, an elaborated strategy was discernible among those doctors who placed less emphasis on their professional status, acknowledged the limitations of their own knowledge, and recognised the importance of sharing information with patients. Comaroff concludes that the communication strategies are not determined by the need to preserve control over patients but by the image doctors have of their professional role and the type of relationship they wish to establish with their patients.

Some studies, particularly from an interactionist or ethnomethodological perspective, into the micro-politics and situated dynamics of the doctor–patient relationship reveal that not all patients adopt entirely passive and submissive roles in their encounters with medical personnel. The underlying theoretical assumption is that doctors and patients are social actors who have individual expectations as to what they want from a consultation and will therefore act in a way designed to achieve their objectives. Consequently conflict is depicted as a natural feature of these encounters. Stimson and Webb (1975), in a study of general practice provide data which supports this view. Following observations of 50 consultations they report instances of patients attempting to exert some control by means of negotiation. However, they acknowledge that despite this opportunity to negotiate conflict remains muted. Patients did not openly challenge their doctors when apparently dissatisfied with some aspect of their treatment. Their response was more likely to be non-confrontational and take the form of polite questioning. For example, the authors cite the case of a female patient who believed that her general practitioner had a tendency to over-prescribe and responded to a proffered prescription by saying: 'Are those tablets really necessary, doctor? Because, if they're not, I'd rather not take them, if it will clear up anyway.' While Stimson and Webb identify attempts by patients to influence the course of the consultation, they stress that opportunities for negotiation are limited and in the main the doctor retains the dominant role.

The asymmetry in the doctor–patient relationship is reflected in the clinical interview. The four phases of the interview have been identified as the opening, medical history, physical examination and closing phases (Fisher, 1984). From the doctor's perspective the consultation ideally should take the form of a highly structured interview. In the opening phase patients are encouraged to tell their story, explaining what led them to consult the doctor. The second and third phases are when the doctor gathers the information necessary to reach a diagnosis. This usually involves the doctor asking a sequence of questions that mainly require yes/no answers. The structure of the discourse between doctor and patient takes the form of a repetitive three-part pattern; the doctor asks a question, the patient responds and the doctor asks a further question. In the final phase of the interview the doctor offers a diagnosis and recommends an appropriate course of treatment. The doctor is clearly in control of the interview process.

Although patients are generally responsive to doctors' questions they do themselves ask questions and introduce topics into the interview, which the doctor might regard as irrelevant. This can result in:

> conflict between the 'voice of medicine', expressing a technical, biomedical frame of reference, and the 'voice of the life-world', reflecting the patient's personal, 'contextually-grounded experiences of events and problems', expressed in familiar terms.
>
> (Clark and Mishler, 1992, p. 346)

In a comparative analysis of two audio-taped consultations, Clark and Mishler (1992) reveal how whether or not patients are allowed to tell their story will influence how the clinical tasks of diagnosis, treatment and illness management are accomplished. In one case, by adopting the role of attentive listener and allowing the patient's story to unfold, the doctor acquires an understanding of the patient's 'life-world' and sees the illness and the patient's response to it in a wider social context. In the second case, the doctor asserts his medical authority by repeatedly interrupting the patient's narrative in order to elicit the medical facts. The doctor's frame of reference does not extend beyond the biomedical and he therefore fails to consider their experience of their illness. As Clark and Mishler state: '. . . the clinical significance of attending to a patient's story is that it changes the object of clinical intervention' (1992, p. 366).

When considering negotiation as an aspect of professional–patient encounters attention needs to be given to both the nature of the medical problem and the setting in which the interaction takes place. Patients suffering from chronic conditions will have prolonged contact with health professionals. In some cases they will be active participants in the treatment process, as is the situation with diabetic patients who monitor and control their condition by means of self-administered doses of insulin. The patient's knowledge of their condition and their regular visits to the clinic are likely to have some influence on the nature of their relationship with the health professionals they encounter.

Sociological studies of patients in long-stay hospitals reveal how negotiation and bargaining feature in the interaction process. According to Strauss (1978), negotiation is defined as 'getting things accomplished'. Roth (1963) describes how tuberculosis patients negotiated with staff in an effort to determine their date of discharge from the hospital. This involved them drawing upon the experiences of other patients in trying to convince doctors that they had reached a certain stage in the treatment programme. In discussing long-term treatment institutions in general, Roth (1984) describes how an informal bargaining process between inmates and staff can result in the establishment of 'working agreements' which have benefits for both groups. Strauss (1963) uses the concept of 'negotiated order' to describe how interactions between staff and patients are managed in general hospitals.

The majority of interactions between professional health workers and patients take place in hospitals, clinics and surgeries. The imbalance in power between professional and patient is markedly evident in these locations. In short, the professional is on home territory whereas the patient is on 'foreign' ground, faced with practices and procedures which are unfamiliar. In these circumstances it is understandable that many patients adopt a dependent and passive role. However, not all healthcare is delivered in institutional settings. District nurses, community midwives and health visitors all provide a service in the patient's own home. There is some evidence that home patients enjoy a stronger negotiating position than that experienced by patients in hospital. Not only do they not have to contend with the rules and regulations which operate in many institutional settings, but it has also been suggested that health workers are aware of the implications the change in treatment setting has for the professional–client relationship. In a study of home births Kirkham (1983) found that midwives described the relationships they developed with their patients as being 'colleague-like'. McIntosh (1981) describes how district nurses considered themselves to have the status of a guest when entering the homes of patients. They found themselves performing a kind of balancing act, trying to exercise some control in order to perform the required nursing tasks, while at the same time attempting to preserve a guest-like status.

Nurse–patient interaction

> Nurse–patient interaction refers to the dyadic reciprocal interactions that occur between nurses and patients in the context of providing and receiving nursing care.
>
> (Bottorff, 2005, p. 381)

Four types of mutual relationship

According to Armstrong (1983b), until relatively recently the relationship between nurse and patient depicted in the nursing literature could be described as being:

> . . . similar in its mechanistic passivity to that between customer and cashier. Certainly there was a relationship but it was extremely limited in the identity it provided for its participants. Patients had to obey and show respect, nurses had to follow sister's instructions and walk in a dignified way.
>
> (Armstrong, 1983b, p. 458)

Clearly the patient is presented as a passive object, a physical body to be observed, monitored and cared for. There is no room for a consideration of the psychological and emotional needs of patients. Armstrong remarks on how the role of the nurse changed radically during the 1960s and 1970s. With the introduction of the concept of the 'nursing process' and the growing acceptance of the ideology of individualised care, nurses were encouraged to adopt an active rather than a passive role. The newly emergent nursing process focused on the need for greater interaction between nurse and patient (Shetland, 1965; Kratz, 1979). The belief being that by achieving an insight into the social and personal worlds of their patients, nurses would be in a better position to determine health needs and implement appropriate care plans.

A central feature of the 'new models of nursing' is the emphasis placed upon the changing nature and quality of the nurse–patient relationship (Salvage and Kershaw, 1990). Many of the 'new models' challenge the traditional task-oriented role of the nurse and maintain that patients will benefit from more personalised care. Nurses are encouraged to view the patient as a subjective being with whom they need to establish a relationship. The role of the nurse is not simply to reconstitute the patient as a human being by establishing and maintaining a therapeutic environment (Johnson and Martin, 1965) but to become involved in the nurse–patient relationship to the extent of becoming the 'patient's advocate' (Watson, 1988). According to Watson, greater nurse involvement is an essential response to a biomedical model of medicine which, with its emphasis of technology, depersonalises patients, treats them as objects and denies them human dignity.

Morse (1991) illustrates how the relationship that is established between nurse and patient can be seen as '. . . the outcome of covert interactive negotiations or implicit interplay between the two persons' (1991, p. 456). On the basis of the results of a Canadian study she identifies four types of mutual relationship (Box 9.3). According to Morse the degree of involvement and level of intensity increases from one type to the next.

Involvement and intensity are at their lowest in the clinical relationship. This type of relationship occurs most frequently in situations where the patient is receiving treatment for a minor condition. The encounter is brief with the nurse carrying out the required procedures in an efficient and perfunctory manner. This is particularly characteristic of nurse–patient interaction in outpatient clinics. The therapeutic relationship is the one most commonly found. Again this applies to short-term cases where the patient has clearly identifiable needs which are not too great and can be quickly met. The role expectations of both parties are clear

---

Box 9.3   Definition

Four types of mutual relationship

- Clinical
  - Therapeutic
    - Connected
      - Over-involved

Source: Morse, 1991

and unambiguous. 'The nurse views the patient first within the patient role and second as a person with a life "outside"' (Morse, 1991, p. 458).

The third type of mutual relationship identified by Morse, and termed the connected relationship, develops when nurse and patient have been in prolonged contact with the result that 'the nurse views the patient first as a person and second as a patient' (1991, p. 458). The greater involvement of the nurse in the relationship leads to the bending of 'rules' if this is considered to be in the best interests of the patient. The patient comes to trust the nurse and as the relationship develops the nurse may come to assume the role of patient advocate in dealings with medical staff.

In all three types of relationship mentioned so far the nurse maintains a professional perspective. However, in the over-involved relationship the nurse and patient develop a close personal relationship. The nurse's commitment to the patient as a person takes precedence; it 'over-rides the nurse's commitment to the treatment regime, the physician, the institution and its need, and her nursing responsibilities toward other patients' (Morse, 1991, p. 459). Morse describes the various strategies nurses use to increase or decrease the level of personal involvement.

Good patient, bad patient

The principle of individualised care is an integral element in the philosophy of modern nursing. However, whilst nurses may strive to treat each patient as an individual, difficulties can be encountered when trying to realise this principle in practice. For example, in organisations where staff are engaged in providing a service for large numbers of people the pressure of daily work may lead to the emergence of informal working practices or routines based on a crude or simplistic categorisation of clients. This sorting of individuals into types or categories is seen by phenomenologists as a feature of everyday life (Schutz, 1967). A consequence of creating typifications of patients is that staff pay primary attention to the identifying characteristics of the type and overlook the individual characteristics of those patients who have been assigned to a particular category. In short, the typification process is a form of stereotyping. Reducing individuals to pre-existing stereotypes can result in the routinisation of care for specific groups of patients, allowing subtle individual differences to go unrecognised, thus ultimately working against the goal of individualised care.

Research reveals that two broad categories of 'good' patient and 'bad' patient are used by health workers in a variety of healthcare settings. Studies of nurse–patient interaction have identified a number of themes associated with positive or negative evaluations of patients. These themes include the nature of the illness or disease, aspects of patients' behaviour and the socio-biographical characteristics of patients (Kelly and May, 1982). Research suggests that staff can label a patient as a 'problem patient' and develop negative attitudes towards them purely on the basis of the nature of the illness. However, if the illness provides staff with an opportunity to practise their clinical or nursing skills then they are likely to view the patient in a more positive light (Simpson *et al.*, 1979). Patients can be categorised as bad if they fail to conform to the treatment regimen or constantly complain (Armitage, 1980). There is also evidence to suggest that nurses' attitudes towards patients can be influenced by non-clinical factors such as age, gender, social class and ethnicity (Kelly and May, 1982).

In one sense, the patients labelled 'good' are the ones who tend to conform to the image of the ideal patient held by the professional. For the general practitioner the 'good' patient is the one who knows when a medical consultation is appropriate and does not bother the doctor with trivial complaints (Robinson, 1971). As regards nurses, ideal patients are those who readily cooperate in their treatment, willingly conform to hospital rules, do not disrupt the ward routine and communicate well with staff. Stockwell (1972) observed that nurses were selective in their interaction with patients and would spend more time with, and undertake small favours for, those patients who behaved in accordance with the nurses' role expectations of the ideal patient. Those patients who failed to live up to the ideal were seen as unpopular. Stockwell observes that nurses used sanctions against patients who complained or grumbled or who expressed more suffering than nurses believed was warranted by their condition.

'Bad' patients are also 'problem' patients; patients who by their manner and behaviour make it difficult for nurses to carry out their work (Rosenthal et al., 1980). However, not all 'problem' patients are necessarily perceived as 'bad' patients. Lorber (1975) describes how nurses labelled some 'problem' patients as 'forgivable' and others as 'wilful'. Patients in the former category posed a problem in that they were very ill, complained about their condition and made heavy demands on staff time. However, because the nurses felt that these patients were not responsible for their illness and were openly appreciative of the nursing care they received they could forgive these aspects of their behaviour. In contrast, those patients who were not considered by the staff to have a serious illness but presented themselves as being gravely ill and demanded excessive attention did not warrant forgiveness and were labelled as 'bad' patients.

In a study of casualty staff working in three hospital accident and emergency departments in England, Jeffery observed that '. . . staff classify patients broadly into good and rubbish patients. The features of good patients which are attended to are medical in character, whereas rubbish is described in predominantly social terms' (Jeffery, 1979, p. 104). The good patients or interesting patients were described as such on the basis of their medical condition or cause of their injury. Patients labelled as good were those who provided medical staff with an opportunity to practise skills necessary for passing examinations, allowed staff to practise a chosen speciality or were considered to test their general competence. In essence, 'good patients . . . make demands which fall squarely within the boundaries of what the staff define as appropriate to their job' (Jeffery, 1979, p. 94).

In categorising casualty patients as 'bad' or 'normal rubbish' staff made reference to factors unrelated to the medical condition of the individual. The 'rubbish' patients were the ones they did not like dealing with. They fell into four broad categories: trivial cases, which did not constitute an emergency, drunks, overdoses and tramps. According to Jeffery these patients were seen as deviants.

In the eyes of the staff they were considered to have broken unwritten rules, similar to those contained in the classic definition of the sick role, and were therefore denied the status of 'good' patient. In contrast to 'good' patients, 'rubbish' patients were seen as being largely responsible for their condition, did not cooperate with staff in their treatment and did not display a desire to get better. Jeffery describes how staff 'punished' these patients by, for example, increasing the length of time they had to wait for treatment.

The notion that casualty staff distinguish broadly between 'good' and 'rubbish' patients has not gone unchallenged. According to one observer this categorisation constitutes:

> a serious oversimplification which overlooks the relatively disinterested and neutral attitude taken by staff to many of the large numbers of patients processed in the mundane working day.
>
> (Hughes, 1980, quoted in Dingwall and Murray, 1983, p. 131)

A further limitation of Jeffery's study is that it does not include children. As Dingwall and Murray (1983) contend, children break all the unwritten rules acknowledged by staff as being instrumental in constructing stereotypes of 'bad' patients. In the main, children bear some responsibility for the injuries they sustain and they can be uncooperative patients. However, although they break the rules they are not subjected to the type of punitive treatment experienced by some categories of adult patients (Jeffery, 1979). Furthermore, Dingwall and Murray suggest that initial categorisations of patients are not necessarily fixed; patients can be re-categorised during the course of treatment. Thus a patient originally assigned to a 'rubbish' category may later be diagnosed as having a clinical condition that is considered to be interesting and in this respect achieve the status of a 'good' patient.

From an interactionist or ethnomethodological perspective, health professionals and patients can be seen to be actively engaged in interactional work in the construction of social action. The categorisation of patients as 'good' or 'bad' is a normal and routine feature of health work. What is of particular interest to many sociologists is the nature of the criteria used for the purpose of moral evaluation and the process by which patient identities are formed. As previously described, some researchers see doctors' and nurses' evaluations of patients as taking place entirely within the context of the normative structure of the professional–patient relationship. Those who fail to conform to the role expectations of the ideal patient are considered to be 'troublesome' or 'problem' patients. However, there is also evidence that professionals' categorisations are influenced by factors not directly related to how well the individual performs in the patient role. Roth (1972) describes how care workers employ wider conceptions of moral worthiness when evaluating patients as troublesome. In a similar vein, Macintyre (1977) claims that medical staff draw upon cultural assumptions in the process of typifying patients. She suggests that when dealing with pregnant unmarried women, doctors invoke gender stereotypes and cultural notions of female sexuality to the extent that they categorise them as 'good girls' or 'bad girls' rather than 'good' or 'bad' patients.

The 'bad girls' are the ones who are considered to be 'easy-going' and promiscuous: whereas the 'good girls' are the ones who, according to the personal value judgements of the doctors, have been 'taken advantage of' and are treated as innocent victims. Macintyre points out that it is the 'good girls' who receive a more sympathetic response to a request for an abortion. Fisher and Groce (1985) also illustrate how value judgements enter into doctor–patient encounters in describing how cultural assumptions about women are negotiated within the context of the medical interview and have implications for the delivery of healthcare.

In summary, a brief review of the literature indicates that there is a general consensus of opinion among researchers that the categorisation of patients is a characteristic feature of medical encounters in a number of different clinical areas. However, when it comes to considering the origins of particular patient typifications, two broad themes can be identified. Firstly, there are those who claim that the criteria on which evaluations are made are heavily focused on factors such as patient cooperation and the perceived seriousness of the medical condition (Biener, 1983). According to this view, the evaluation of patients is necessitated by the need to manage the day's workload. In a study of cancer specialists, Murcott asserts that '. . . typifications are to be understood against a background of "getting through the day's work", not simply as matters of unreasonable prejudice . . .' (1981, p. 128). The problem patients are the ones who are perceived as making life difficult for the staff. Secondly, some researchers emphasise how evaluations of patients are partly influenced by the social attitudes, cultural beliefs and moral values which health workers bring to the job (Roth, 1972; Fisher and Groce, 1985).

Professional–patient interaction in pregnancy and childbirth

> In encounters including gynaecological examination, female physicians are perceived as more attentive and informative by their patients than their male colleagues.
> (Christen *et al.*, 2008, p. 1475)

Feminist sociologists have made a significant contribution to our understanding of the way in which pregnancy and childbirth have been subjected to increasing medical intervention. A major consequence of this development is that motherhood has become a 'medicalized domain' (Oakley, 1984). The management and control of labour and childbirth is now firmly in the hands of the medical profession. Historical studies reveal how doctors gradually came to dominate this area of medicine by restricting the activities of female midwives (Donnison, 1977). Childbirth is a highly technological affair, with the increasing use of equipment such as foetal heart monitors: 99 per cent of births now take place in hospital. As Stacey notes childbirth has moved 'from the private domain of the home under the control of experienced women to the public domain of the hospital under the control mainly of men' (1988, p. 236).

Studies of women's experiences of care received during the antenatal and early postnatal periods illustrate how many women feel they are not given an opportunity to exercise a choice as to the kind of maternity care they receive. Research dating back to the 1970s shows how women feel that they have very little control over what happens to them during the process of childbearing (Oakley, 1979, 1980). In order to be able to make choices it is essential that women are given the necessary information. Using data from interviews with mothers in London and York, Graham and Oakley (1986) report that frequently voiced concerns related to communication problems with doctors, such as not feeling able to ask questions and not being given sufficient information about their treatment.

The potential for conflict in doctor–patient relationships in this area is evident when it is realised that doctors and mothers have different perspectives on the nature of childbearing. As a result of the increasing medicalisation of reproduction, obstetricians are more inclined to view pregnancy as potentially pathological rather than see it as a normal physiological activity which can occasionally present problems. For the obstetrician the primary purpose of antenatal care is to look for any abnormalities (Arney, 1982). This medically oriented approach, which sees pregnancy as a problematic event, is contrasted with the mothers' view, which sees it as a natural biological process. However, according to Graham and Oakley this difference in the images of childbearing is not simply a difference of opinion over the routines and practices that feature in the medical management of pregnancy and childbirth. The difference is of a much more fundamental nature and is explained by using the concept of a 'frame of reference'.

> 'Frame of reference' embraces both the notion of an ideological perspective – a system of values and attitudes through which mothers and doctors view pregnancy – and of a reference group, consisting of a network of individuals who have significant influence upon these sets of attitudes and values.
>
> (Graham and Oakley, 1986, p. 99)

The two frames of reference are labelled medical and maternal. From a medical frame of reference pregnancy is treated as an isolated episode. As far as the obstetrician is concerned the patient career of the pregnant woman begins when she first attends antenatal clinic and ends when she is discharged from maternity care. Viewed from a woman's frame of reference having a baby is a major life event which leads to significant role changes. Becoming a mother has a major and lasting impact on a woman's lifestyle (Hart, 1977).

An understanding of the differences between the two frames of reference can help to explain why some women feel dissatisfied with the maternity care they receive. As Graham and Oakley (1986) state, women have a holistic view of childbearing; they see it as a personal experience, not simply a medical event. Consequently they may attach importance to physical and emotional changes in pregnancy which are considered insignificant from a medical perspective. Doctors may not be interested in listening to the minor physical discomforts encountered by their patients (Homans, 1985). Observations of doctor–patient consultations in antenatal clinics show how doctors attempt to focus the interview on matters concerning the medical management of the pregnancy and offer little opportunity for the discussion of social or emotional problems. Attempts by patients to introduce non-medical concerns produced irritated responses from the doctors (Oakley, 1980, pp. 30–1).

Patients want more information, particularly about the medical procedures they are subjected to. Kirke (1980) reports maternity patients complaining that staff did not always explain the reason for certain procedures, such as the use of ultrasound or the regular testing of urine samples. As in other areas of medicine patients are often reluctant to ask for information. One reason for this may be that consultations are sometimes conducted in a manner that discourages patients from asking questions. As Graham and Oakley (1986) comment, this is likely to be the case when medical encounters begin with the examining doctor entering a cubicle where the patient is already lying down on a couch ready to be examined. Even though patients are invited to ask questions they may still decline the offer, as observed by the following comment:

> The nurse says, 'Now, do you want to ask the doctor anything?' And more invariably than not you say 'no' because you just don't feel you can. The way they ask you, 'Right, do you want to ask the doctor anything?' you think, no. All you want to do is get up and get out.
>
> (Quoted in Graham and Oakley, 1986, pp. 109–10)

What is of particular note here is that presumably in the course of the examination the doctor addressed questions directly to the patient. However, it is the nurse who asks the patient if she would like to ask the doctor anything. This confirms the power imbalance in the doctor–patient relationship by highlighting the social distance between the two.

Controlling the amount and type of information they give to patients can help doctors to maintain their position of dominance. Graham and Oakley (1986) noted that doctors resorted to technical explanations in cases where patients were seen to be reluctant to agree to a course of action or form of treatment they were recommending. Also, the assumptions that doctors made as to why patients requested information determined the way the information was delivered. The widespread belief was that it was patient anxiety that led to a demand for information. Consequently they saw the aim of medical explanations as being to allay anxiety, rather than to provide patients with detailed information. Joking was often used as an anxiety-reducing device as the following interchange shows:

First doctor: You're looking serious.
Patient: Well I am rather worried about it all. It feels like a small baby – I feel much smaller with this one than I did with my first, and she weighed under six pounds. Ultrasound last week said the baby was very small as well.
First doctor: Weighed it, did they?
Second doctor (entering examination cubicle): They go round flower shows and weigh cakes, you know.
First doctor: Yes, it's a piece of cake really.

(Graham and Oakley, 1986, p. 114)

Within the medical frame of reference Oakley (1980) identifies two general typifications of women patients. The first portrays them in a mechanistic way, as 'reproductive machines' or vessels for producing children (Lewis, 1980). The female body is likened to a highly complex machine, which occasionally requires intervention to correct some malfunctioning. The purpose of obstetric practice is to search for and repair the fault. During this process the patient is expected to play a passive role and accept the fact that successful childbirth can only be achieved within a carefully controlled medical context. This has become known as the 'active management of labour'. Medical procedures or the administering of drugs are frequently used to accelerate labour in order to ensure that a 'normal' delivery takes place.

In the second typification of women, found in medical literature and practice, attention is drawn to what are perceived to be the biologically determined 'feminine' qualities of women. The truly feminine woman is the one who has a strong maternal instinct and who sees her main vocation in life as becoming a wife and mother. As Oakley contends, by being absorbed into the medical frame of reference these typifications will have an impact on how doctors evaluate their patients. What is more, there is an added gender dimension: given that over 80 per cent of obstetricians are men, the majority of obstetric encounters are male–female encounters. Thus in typifying women as a special category of patients, doctors make use of cultural images generated in a male-dominated society.

The medicalisation of pregnancy and childbirth has drawn criticism from a variety of sources. As described above, feminist theorists such as Ann Oakley have argued that medicine has become a controlling force in the lives of women. Concern has also been expressed by professional practitioners. The Association of Radical Midwives, formed in 1976, has made numerous recommendations for changes in the provision of maternity care. One of their demands was that women should have more say in how labour is handled (Flint, 1986). Wendy Savage (1986), a consultant obstetrician and advocate of holistic care, has also argued that women should be allowed to make informed choices throughout pregnancy and childbirth.

The doctor–nurse relationship

> Traditionally the doctors made all the decisions regarding the care of the patients, and imposed their authority over the work or decisions of other members of the team; work in which they had no particular training or skill. Modern practice has fortunately changed this relationship to one of complementary respect for roles.
>
> (Tweed *et al.*, 2008, p. 6)

Gender issues

Central to our understanding of how dominance and control feature in the doctor–nurse relationship is an appreciation of the role gender plays in the division of labour in healthcare. Basically, gender is significant in two main ways. Firstly, on a structural level, there is evidence of gender segregation both within and between the occupations of medicine and nursing. Secondly, as regards social interaction, gender can influence power relations and professional encounters between doctors and nurses in the day-to-day provision of healthcare.

Although gender inequalities in healthcare are apparent in the sexual division of labour, over recent decades there has been a significant growth in the proportion of women among new entrants to medical school. It is estimated that women now make up approximately 40 per cent of all doctors and that 42 per cent of general practitioners are women (Elston, 2009). In contrast, nursing is a predominantly female occupation with men forming less than 15 per cent of the workforce. However, as Porter notes, 'The successful entry of a male minority into nursing, rather than diluting gender as a major defining factor in occupational differentiation, has exacerbated it by adding male managers to the nurse's burden of male doctors' (1992, p. 512). Some observers maintain that nursing is increasingly becoming dominated by men as they begin to occupy a disproportionate number of the senior posts in nursing management (Hearn, 1987).

In medicine, there is an uneven distribution of women across the specialist areas. High concentrations of women are found in such fields as general practice, school health services, radiology and child psychiatry. Women are also underrepresented in senior posts. In 1990 only 15 per cent of all hospital consultant posts in England and Wales were held by women (Elston, 1993); however, by 2007 this figure had risen to 28 per cent in England (Elston, 2009). Women are not only channelled into certain areas of medicine but within those areas they can encounter male colleagues who expect them to deal with a specific category of patients or set of medical problems. In her study of the gendered experience of women doctors in general practice, Lawrence refers to this as 'ghettoism' (1987, p. 151). A number of the female family doctors she interviewed stated that because of their experience in male-dominated group practices they preferred to work as independent general practitioners. They had chosen general practice as opposed to hospital medicine because they did not want to specialise. Yet on entering group work they had found their male colleagues steering them towards dealing with 'women's problems'.

Gender is also important in understanding the nature of inter-occupational interaction and the construction of practitioner–patient relationships in healthcare settings. Gamarnikow (1978) describes the conceptualisation of the doctor–nurse–patient triad characteristic of the Nightingale era as strongly resembling the power relations between husband–wife–child in the patriarchal family of the Victorian period. The doctor was the one who exercised authority and control over both the nurse and the patient. In carrying out the orders of the doctor, the nurse was expected to be disciplined and deferential. Any authority the nurse had over the patient was delegated by the doctor. The nurse was there to assist the doctor and provide a comfortable environment for the patient. Thus, from a feminist perspective the patriarchal ideology and female subordination characteristic of family life were reproduced in the medical division of labour in the hospital setting: in terms of power relations the nurse–doctor role configuration was, in a structural sense, analogous to that of husband and wife. This view of the dominant doctor and the subservient nurse became the traditional model of the doctor–nurse relationship. As Dingwall and McIntosh assert, 'The Victorian ethos of male superiority reinforced the nurses' deferential attitudes to doctors far into the twentieth century . . .' (1978, p. 107).

The traditional dominant–subservient model of the doctor–patient relationship is based on an acceptance of the view that biological differences between the sexes provide a suitable foundation for the sexual division of labour that occurs in healthcare work. Supporters of the idea that gender role differentiation is biologically determined hold that women possess innate characteristics, such as a nurturative mentality, which makes them natural carers of sick people. In fact, 'The idea that nursing and mothering are natural activities of women is an ancient theme in western culture. The word "nurse" is derived from "nutririe", signifying to nourish and to suckle' (Turner, 1987, p. 150). This kind of thinking is central to our stereotypes of femininity and masculinity. Female sex-stereotypical roles are referred to as 'expressive', whereas male roles are defined as 'instrumental'. The assumption is that women in general are compassionate, caring, gentle and emotionally expressive. In contrast, men are more instrumentally oriented, on account of their natural aggression, decisiveness and rationality. The term 'patriarchal feminine' has been used to describe the female role as this captures the fact that the nurturing and caring aspects of the role are at the root of the problem of female subordination (Hearn, 1982).

The idea that the social roles performed by men and women are biologically determined is challenged by many feminist sociologists who maintain that there is nothing natural or inevitable about the sexual division of labour (Oakley, 1972; Gamarnikow, 1978). They argue that gender roles are social constructions and are not biologically given. What is considered appropriate gender behaviour can vary not only between societies at any one time but also within a single society over a period of time. It follows that if socially defined gender roles are not based on biological factors, but are acquired through the process of socialisation, then they are subject to change. As far as the division of labour in healthcare is concerned, we need to undertake a reassessment of the traditional dominant–subservient model of doctor–nurse interaction, in order to ascertain whether or not there has been any shift in the gender balance of power in the working relationship between doctors and nurses in the contemporary era.

The doctor–nurse game

In the 1960s, Stein (1978) conducted a small-scale study into communication and decision-making in doctor–nurse encounters, in which he argued that the working relationship has something of a 'game-like' quality about it. Hence, he refers to the 'doctor–nurse game'. He discovered that although nurses were subordinate to doctors within the professional hierarchy, they were able to exercise a degree of informal influence when it came to deciding what type of treatment patients should receive. What was important from Stein's observations was how nurses actually communicated their recommendations to doctors.

One rarely hears a nurse say, 'doctor, I would recommend that you order a retention enema for Mrs Brown'. A physician, upon hearing a recommendation of that nature, would gape in amazement at the effrontery of the nurse. The nurse, upon hearing the statement, would look over her shoulder to see who said it, hardly believing the words actually came from her own mouth. Nevertheless, if one observes closely, nurses make recommendations of more import every hour and physicians willingly and respectfully consider them. If the nurse is to make a suggestion without appearing insolent and the doctor is to seriously consider that suggestion, their interaction must not violate the rules of the game.

(Stein, 1978, p. 109)

The game takes the form of an elaborate ritual of verbal and non-verbal communication, where 'the cardinal rule . . . is that open disagreement between the players must be avoided at all costs' (Stein, 1978, p. 110). The nurse must convey her views to the doctor without appearing to be making a firm recommendation regarding treatment and the doctor must invite the nurse to offer an opinion without it seeming as though her advice is being sought. The game has rewards for both parties: the doctor benefits from the knowledge the nurse brings to the situation, while the nurse enjoys greater job satisfaction by being given the opportunity of extending her role. Although the idea of the doctor–nurse game challenges the traditional dominant–subservient model's basic assumption of 'unproblematic subordination', it 'still portrays nurses in the subservient position of having to co-operate in the construction of an elaborate façade, the function of which is to hide the degree of skills, knowledge and information they possess' (Porter, 1991, p. 729).

Recent research findings illustrate that nurses are not dependent upon subordinate modes of inter-occupational interaction to the extent suggested by the doctor–nurse game model. In a participant-observation study of doctor–nurse interaction in a hospital casualty department, Hughes (1988) concludes that it is important to consider the situated nature of medical dominance and nurse deference. Although he observed instances of nurses employing some of the subtle 'game-playing' tactics identified by Stein (1978), he found that, in general, nurses were more overtly involved in decision-making. One area in which this was evident was in the categorisation and processing of patients. In the department studied by Hughes, senior nurses played a central role in controlling the movement of patients from admission to treatment. Such was the volume of work that casualty officers would have been overwhelmed if decision-making had not been shared with other staff. In collecting information from patients and conducting preliminary physical examinations, nurses very often ended up making a provisional diagnosis. As Hughes observed:

Where nurses are reasonably sure that certain investigations such as ECGs will be required, they may themselves carry them out so that results are available by the time the doctor arrives. Similarly where nurses believe certain treatments such as stomach washouts or suturing to be required they may prepare the equipment and get the patient ready, even though the doctor has not yet become involved in the processing of the case.

(Hughes, 1988, p. 8)

What is represented here is a blurring of the point at which patient categorisation becomes diagnosis. Although nurses were engaging in diagnostic work they did not consider it as such because they were not the ones who actually informed the patient about the nature of his or her condition.

According to Hughes, experienced nurses acted as 'carriers and mediators of social knowledge' (1988, p. 18). They had a considerable fund of local knowledge about departmental procedures, administrative practices and contacts with other service providers. Newly qualified doctors or locums found such information useful and in some cases sought the advice of nursing staff. In one or two instances inexperienced casualty officers actually asked nurses for information regarding specific clinical procedures and techniques. Although nurses acknowledged the doctors' clinical authority, and on occasions used subtle non-verbal and cryptic verbal cues to convey their recommendations, they were not as fully committed to 'game-playing' as the doctor–nurse game model suggests. The nurses in Hughes' study did not appear to be immersed in what Dingwall and McIntosh refer to as 'the elaborate ritualized façade described by Stein' (1978, p. 108). They did not always try to disguise their advice-giving and were frequently observed offering advice in 'an open and straightforward way' (Hughes, 1988, p. 17).

Patterns of interaction

In order to explore patterns of interaction between medical and nursing staff, Porter (1991) undertook a participant observation study in an intensive care unit in a large metropolitan hospital in Ireland. Following a review of the literature on nurse–doctor interaction he identified four broad types of power relations, which formed the focus of his investigation into the nature and extent of the involvement of nurses in the decision-making processes surrounding patient care. The four major types of interaction are described in Box 9.4.

The first of the four types of interaction is labelled 'unproblematic subordination' and is a description of the traditional dominant–subservient model of nurse–doctor power relations in which the nurse simply obeys the orders of the doctor and has no influence in the decision-making process. Interestingly, Porter found that while on the surface nurse subordination appeared to be a feature in many nurse–doctor encounters, further analysis of the data revealed that the notion of unproblematic subordination overlooked some important aspects of this type of inter-occupational interaction. For example, he observed many instances where doctors did not simply issue orders but explained to nurses the reasoning behind their decisions. Thus he came to the view that the nurse–doctor relationship was more complex than the traditional model suggested and could not be understood in terms of the concept of unproblematic subordination. However, his analysis of encounters between nurses and senior medical staff did reveal evidence of subordinate modes of interaction. As he concludes, 'the only scenario where unproblematic subordination could be deemed to have occurred with any frequency was in the communications between consultants and nurses' (Porter, 1991, p. 732).

> ### Box 9.4   Definition
>
> #### Four types of nurse–doctor interaction
>
> - *Unproblematic subordination.* Nurses have no involvement in the decision-making process surrounding patient care, they obediently follow doctors' instructions and do not question decisions made by doctors.
> - *Informal covert decision making.* There is pretence of unproblematic subordination, nurses obey the rules of the 'doctor–nurse game' and do not openly disagree with doctors. Nurses make recommendations without appearing to do so.
> - *Informal overt decision making.* Nurses are assertive and freely express their views regarding patient care. The rules of the 'doctor–nurse game' do not apply.
> - *Formal overt decision making.* Nursing input into decision making is officially sanctioned in the form of the nursing process. Each patient has a nursing care plan based on detailed information about diagnosis and treatment. Care plans are revised daily. In theory the nursing process helps nurses to make decisions about care.
>
> *Source*: Porter, 1991

The other three types of nurse–doctor interaction distinguish between formal/informal and overt/covert characteristics of decision-making processes. Stein's doctor–nurse game model provides a good example of informal covert decision-making. However, Porter observed numerous episodes of nurse–doctor communication where the rules of the game did not seem to apply. Nurses did not display deference in all encounters and did not always refrain from making overt suggestions regarding patient care. The situation was different in the case of nurse–consultant interaction, where nurses tended to offer factual information only when requested to do so by a consultant. According to Porter, it was on the consultants' rounds, 'where exceptions to the rules of play are rare', that there was evidence of a deference game being played out (1991, p. 733).

Porter's data shows that nurses frequently indulged in informal overt decision-making and did not simply follow instructions without comment. This is illustrated in the following interaction between a male junior house officer (JHO) and a female staff nurse (SN).

JHO: Mrs Surname is a bit dehydrated. I want to erect some IV fluids.
SN: Well, we have been managing to get her to drink 100 ml an hour this morning. Why don't we try her for 24 hours?
JHO: That's fine, if we could try and get a litre and a half into her.

(Porter, 1991, p. 733)

This informal overt approach was identified as a commonly used nursing strategy. The nature and extent of its use varied according to the particular situational context and the status of the nurse involved.

Formal overt decision-making, in the form of the nursing process, apparently did little to increase nursing input into decision-making. As Porter concludes, 'formal decision making is of little significance compared with the informal strategies adopted by nurses' (1991, p. 734). Overall he claims that the use of these strategies goes some way towards reducing, but not eliminating, the power differential that exists between doctors and nurses. By and large, the four types of interaction are seen as stages in the increasing involvement of nurses in the decision-making process. 'From their initial subservience, nurses have progressed through an era where informal covert decision making appeared to be dominant to the present time when informal overt decision making is accepted as a valid nursing strategy' (Porter, 1991, p. 735). The fourth stage has yet to be attained.

As noted earlier in this section, gender plays an important part in understanding power relations between nursing and medical staff. Nursing, as an occupational activity, 'is almost wholly a woman's province' (Strauss, 1966, p. 61) and nursing work is often devalued on account of its being perceived as largely 'women's work' (Abbott and Wallace, 1990b). Porter (1992) describes how gender is an important factor in the everyday working lives of nurses. In his study of how gender affects inter-occupational interaction in the hospital, he found that although there was considerable variation in the behaviour of male doctors towards nurses in general, there was no indication that male nurses were treated any differently than their female counterparts. Porter argues that the failure of male nurses to gain an advantage over their female colleagues, given the gendered nature of workplace power relations, owes much to the social distance that exists between doctors and nurses and the fact that nursing is an occupation characterised by female subordination. However, while the gender of the nurse had little impact on the quality of doctor–nurse interaction, the gender of the doctor was found to be of some importance. According to Porter, 'it was generally true that most female doctors were considerably more egalitarian than most of their male counterparts' (1992, p. 517). Whether increasing the proportion of female doctors will bring about greater gender equality in the division of labour in healthcare and significantly reduce the role gender plays in the power relations between doctors and nurses remains to be seen.

Communicating with dying patients

As previously noted, good, effective communication between healthcare professionals and patients is essential in order to establish positive interpersonal relationships, facilitate the exchange of information and aid decision-making about treatment regimes and clinical interventions. Patient-centred communication is an integral component of high-quality medical and nursing care; it is vital to the success of patient-centred care. The principal features of the doctor–patient encounter create the basis for a complex interpersonal relationship:

> It involves interaction between individuals in non-equal positions, is often non-voluntary, concerns issues of vital importance, is therefore emotionally laden, and requires close cooperation.
>
> (Ong *et al.*, 1995, p. 903)

However, it should not be assumed that there is a single approach to patient-centred communication that applies in all cases. Health workers need to adopt a flexible style of interaction and adapt their behaviour to the specific needs of individual patients (Epstein *et al.*, 2005). It also needs to be remembered that some patients may feel uncomfortable with a patient-centred approach and in some settings and circumstances may favour a doctor-centred consultation style (Bradley *et al.*, 2000).

Some clinical settings are characterised by a heightened level of sensitivity and emotion, such as in 'bad news consultations', where a doctor is required to inform a patient that they have been diagnosed with a life-threatening illness. For many patients this consultation can determine how they perceive their illness and respond to future care and treatment. From the patients' perspective, the manner and demeanour of the medical practitioner who imparts the bad news is considered to be the most important factor in preparing them for their diagnosis (National Cancer Alliance, 1996). In a review of the literature on breaking bad news, Ptacek and Eberhardt (1996) provide a summary of the recommendations for conducting such consultations. They focus on two key dimensions: the physical and social setting of the doctor–patient consultation and the nature and content of the conversation. With regard to the former, emphasis is placed on the following: the choice of location (this should be quiet, private and peaceful); the timing and structure of the consultation (avoid interruptions and allocate sufficient time so that the patient is not rushed); the interpersonal behaviour of the doctor (sit close to the patient and maintain eye contact); the presence of significant others (ensure that the patient has someone with them if they so wish). Recommendations concerning the content of the message and how it is delivered are highlighted in Box 9.5.

As discussed in Chapter 7, there is now a more open dialogue when health professionals interact with terminally ill patients and their families. This is essential if dying patients are to experience a 'good death'. In the contemporary period, 'it seems the fear of death is being replaced by the fear of dying' (Clark, 2003, p. 174). Patients can suffer additional stress and anxiety when they feel that they do not have control over the circumstances of their dying. They can feel excluded from the decision-making process in relation to treatment and care near the end of life. Invasive therapies and aggressive treatments can seriously mar the quality of life of patients with a terminal illness. According to Hickman (2002), communication issues are at the very heart of many of the problems encountered by dying patients and their families. Health professionals are provided with guidelines for improving end-of-life communication, particularly in relation to the initial breaking of the bad news of a chronic illness or terminal prognosis. However, 'communication near the end of life is a *process*, not a one-time event' (Hickman, 2002, p. 256, emphasis added). In other words, communication at this phase of the life course embraces a wide range of issues including establishing treatment goals, deciding the circumstances in which life-prolonging treatment should be administered and discussing views and feelings regarding end-of-life decision-making.

Box 9.5   Research findings

Content of the 'bad news' message

What is said:

The doctor should:

- be fully prepared;
- 'give a warning shot';
- discover what the patient already knows;
- convey a measure of hope;
- acknowledge and explore the patient's reaction;
- allow the patient to express his or her emotions;
- summarise the discussion.

How it is said: with warmth, care, empathy and respect.

Language used: this should be simple, direct and free from medical jargon or technical diagnostic terminology. Words should be chosen carefully and euphemisms avoided.

Pace of delivery: the information should be delivered at a pace which the patient finds comfortable. The patient should be allowed to dictate what they are told.

Source: Ptacek and Eberhardt, 1996 (adapted from Macdonald, 2004, p. 65)

Whether or not a patient is aware of a terminal diagnosis, and how those who are aware respond, will have an impact on how health professionals interact with them. The disclosure of information is a key aspect of end-of-life care. There is research evidence to suggest that among hospital doctors and general practitioners disclosure has become a more commonly accepted practice over the last two decades (Seale and Cartwright, 1994; Field and Copp, 1999). However, despite this greater willingness for open communication, some studies have questioned how truthful doctors and nurses are when communicating with patients about death and dying and whether or not they indulge in a 'conspiracy of silence' in certain situations with particular types of patients (Costello, 2000; Davey, 2000). For example, Blackburn (1989) discovered poor communication between elderly patients and hospital doctors and nurses. Costello (2001) conducted a study of elderly hospital patients in three different ward settings: acute assessment, continuing care and rehabilitation. He identified among ward nurses a general lack of 'emotional engagement' with dying patients and an institutionalised non-disclosure of information. In explaining the perceived reluctance on the part of nurses to enter into an open dialogue with patients about dying, he explores the workings of the hospital ward culture. This culture contains a number of unspoken rules or tacit agreements that serve to foster and maintain a 'conspiracy of silence', which helps to preserve the 'sentimental mood' of the ward (Glaser and Strauss, 1965) and prevent disruption to its organisation and pattern of working. As he states:

> The truth is kept from the competent patient almost as if the prognosis were owned by professional staff who were reluctant to share it with the patient. In this way, as others have pointed out (Kelner and Bourgeault, 1993), doctors and nurses exert control over how a patient dies.
>
> (Costello, 2001, p. 65)

Costello also draws attention to the fact that many nurses work in a professional culture where the emphasis is on curative care and not palliative care. Consequently, their primary focus is on treatment and cure and not terminal care and death. Thus he concludes, '[i]t would appear that hospital culture and the mores, beliefs and ideologies that emanate from the biomedical model, significantly shape the experiences of older dying patients' (Costello, 2001, p. 59).

There are numerous reasons why health professionals tend to avoid engaging in conversations with patients about issues surrounding death and dying. Buckman (1992) and Morrison (1998) offer a number of possible explanations for this perceived reluctance; these include:

- not wanting to cause patients any distress;
- a lack of sufficient and appropriate training to handle end-of-life conversations in a clinical setting or caring context;
- anxiety over the possibility of being blamed by a patient for a poor prognosis;
- a wish to avoid uncomfortable encounters with patients and family members when discussing the availability and clinical efficacy of various treatment options;
- concerns that they might have difficulty coping with their own emotional responses.

Although the majority of deaths occur in institutional settings, most terminal care is delivered in the home. Thus, achieving a good death can depend fairly heavily on the quality of care provided by general practitioners and community nurses. Field (1998) reports positive responses from general practitioners when asked about their experiences of caring for the dying. Many of those interviewed described this aspect of their work as both rewarding and satisfying. Other studies highlight the need for more training in palliative and terminal care (MacLeod, 2001; MacLeod and Nash, 1991). In one national British study a third of general practitioners claimed to experience difficulty coping with their own emotional responses to patients' deaths (Seale and Cartwright, 1994).

Strategies to improve communication near the end of life need to be informed by the expressed needs of dying patients and their families. These needs are well documented in the research literature. Patients and families prefer bad news to be delivered in a quiet and private setting, with the doctor speaking in a straightforward manner but with sensitivity and compassion, and using non-technical language (Hanson *et al.*, 1997; Ptacek and Ptacek, 2001).

Summary

- The doctor–patient relationship can be examined from a functionalist or consensus perspective. Despite the fact that the existence of professional autonomy and medical dominance makes the relationship an unequal one, doctors and patients are identified as sharing a common value system and the roles they perform are seen as being complementary. The nature of the doctor–patient relationship may vary according to the type of illness and the situational context of the medical encounter.

- Some of the basic assumptions made by consensus theorists are rejected by those who adopt a conflict model of the doctor–patient relationship. Conflict theorists offer a radical critique of professional power. The existence of a gulf between formal medical models of illness and informal lay explanations of ill health can be one source of conflict. Whereas consensus theorists tend to view patients as passive and submissive, conflict theorists see them as active and critical.

- Medical consultations can be 'doctor-centred' or 'patient-centred'. The organisation and structure of the medical interview reflects the asymmetrical nature of the doctor–patient relationship. It is important to take social class, gender and ethnicity into account when evaluating practitioner–patient encounters.

- Morse (1991) identifies four basic types of mutual relationship in nurse–patient interactions: clinical; therapeutic; connected and overinvolved. The level of intensity and degree of involvement in the relationship varies from one type of relationship to the next.

- Research shows how nurses distinguish between 'good' and 'bad' patients. Their evaluations are based on a number of criteria including the nature of the illness, the response of the patient, the nurse's cultural beliefs and personal assessment of the patient's motives and moral worthiness.

- Feminist researchers have drawn attention to the medicalisation of reproduction whereby pregnancy and childbirth have become increasingly subject to medical control. Women's dissatisfaction with maternity care largely stems from the fact that 'medical' and 'maternal' models of childbirth differ.

- Gender inequalities are apparent in the division of labour in healthcare. Although the proportion of women in the medical profession has increased in recent years, there is an uneven distribution of women across the specialist areas of clinical practice. Given that nursing is a predominantly female occupation, women are underrepresented in senior managerial posts.

- Gender stereotypes feature largely in both the traditional dominant–subservient model and the doctor–nurse game model of the relationship between medical and nursing staff. Data from recent research into power relations between doctors and nurses indicates that when it comes to making decisions about the care of patients, nurses make a more overt contribution than is recognised by either of these models.

• Communication near the end of life can be problematic. Strategies to improve care at this stage of the life course need to identify barriers to good, effective communication and address the expressed needs of patients and their families.

Questions for discussion

1 Compare and contrast functionalist and conflict approaches to the study of the doctor–patient relationship.

2 What factors inhibit communication between health professionals and patients?

3 What can we learn about nurse–patient interaction from social science research?

4 Do doctors and mothers have different perspectives on childbirth?

5 How does gender affect the working relationship between doctors and nurses?

6 What are the barriers to good communication between health professionals and dying patients and their families?

Further reading

Bury, M. (1997) *Health and Illness in a Changing Society*, London: Routledge.

Davies, C. (1995) *Gender and the Professional Predicament in Nursing*, Buckingham: Open University Press.

Freidson, E. (1983) 'The theory of professions – state of the art', in R. Dingwall and P. Lewis (eds), *The Sociology of Professions*, London: Macmillan.

Freidson, E. (1986) *Professional Powers: A Study of the Institutionalisation of Formal Knowledge*, London: University of Chicago Press.

Macdonald, E. (ed.) (2004) *Difficult Conversations in Medicine*, Oxford: Oxford University Press.

Mackay, L. (1990) 'Nursing: just another job?', in P. Abbott and C. Wallace (eds) *The Sociology of the Caring Professions*, London: Falmer.

Riska, E. and Weger, K. (eds) (1993) *Gender, Work and Medicine: Women and the Medical Division of Labour*, London: Sage.

Roter, D. L. and Hall, J. A. (2006) *Doctors Talking with Patients/Patients Talking with Doctors: Improving Communication in Medical Visits*, 2nd revised edn, Westport, CT: Praeger Publishers.

Turner, B. (1987) *Medical Power and Social Knowledge*, London: Sage.

CHAPTER 10

Contemporary issues in healthcare

Professions in healthcare

The professions represent a special category in the study of occupations. There are certain unique characteristics associated with professions that distinguish them from ordinary occupations. Health professions represent a special case in that they involve a component of helping and caring not associated with other occupations. Professional occupations like healthcare often exert major control over other occupations.

(Thomas, 2003, p. 125)

What is a profession?

As described in the previous chapter, there is an imbalance of power within the doctor–patient relationship. The power and authority of doctors tend to pervade all aspects of the medical encounter. In order to appreciate fully the nature of the relationship between medical practitioners and their patients it is necessary to understand something about the professional organisation of medical practice. However, medical dominance is not just a feature of doctor–patient interaction; it is also a key element in the relationship between the medical profession and the other occupational groups in the healthcare field. Before we examine the concept of medical dominance we need to explore the basic attributes of a profession.

A profession can be described as 'a special kind of occupation' (Freidson, 1970a, p. xvii). There have been many attempts at identifying what special characteristics serve to distinguish a profession from an occupation. Millerson (1964) lists the six most important traits of a profession as follows: the possession of a specialised skill based on theoretical knowledge; provision of formal training and education; a system for testing the competence of members; a professional code of conduct; the existence of professional associations and a commitment to altruistic service. Barber (1963) identifies 'four essential attributes' of a profession: access to a body of systematic knowledge; a concern for the interests of the community rather than self-interest; control of behaviour by a code of ethics; the receipt of high rewards for their services. Goode (1960) differentiates between 'core' characteristics and 'derived' characteristics in defining professions. He identifies two core characteristics: 'prolonged specialised training in a body of abstract knowledge' and 'a collectivity or service orientation' (Goode, 1960, p. 903). The ten derived characteristics are outlined in Box 10.1. The first five of these refer to professional autonomy. It is 'legitimate organised autonomy' that

---

Box 10.1   Definition

Ten derived characteristics of a profession

1 A profession determines its own standards of education and training.

2 Professional practice is legally recognised by some form of licensure.

3 Licensing and admission boards are run by members of the profession.

4 Most legislation affecting a profession is shaped by that profession.

5 The professional practitioner is relatively free of lay evaluation and control.

6 The student professional goes through a more extensive socialisation experience than students in other occupations.

7 A profession gains in income, power and status and attracts high-quality students.

8 The norms of practice enforced by a profession are often more stringent than legal controls.

9 Members more strongly identify with and are more closely affiliated to their profession than are members of other occupations with theirs.

10 A profession is likely to be a lifetime occupation.

Source: Adapted from Goode, 1960, p. 903

gives professions their special character. As Freidson asserts, 'a profession is distinct from other occupations in that it has been given the right to control its own work' (1970a, p. 71). Elsewhere he describes the three characteristics of professional autonomy as the existence of a system of licensure and registration, the control of a specialised body of knowledge and the presence of a code of ethics (Freidson, 1970b).

At first glance it is clear to see why medicine has been referred to as 'the queen of the professions' (Hughes, 1963) as it possesses many of the characteristics outlined above. For example, doctors undergo a prolonged period of training during which they acquire a body of medical knowledge for use in the diagnosis and treatment of illness and disease. The education and training they receive is largely controlled by the General Medical Council in conjunction with other professional associations, namely the Royal Colleges, which represent various specialist interests within medicine. Since the introduction of the Medical Registration Act of 1858, doctors have required a licence to practise. The General Medical Council is authorised to issue licences on behalf of the state and is responsible for maintaining a register of qualified practitioners. It is not only in the area of training that professional autonomy is evident. The medical profession has a code of ethics, which is enforced through its professional associations. Any allegations of malpractice or misconduct are dealt with internally by disciplinary committees drawn from within the General Medical Council and the British Medical Association.

The fact that many of the characteristics of a profession are to be found in the occupation of medicine should come as no great surprise, especially given that medicine was one of the occupations theorists used when constructing trait or attribute models of professions in the first place (Morgan *et al.*, 1985). From a sociological perspective there is little to be gained from pursuing a universal definition in an attempt to construct a hierarchy of occupational status groups. Much more can be gained by exploring the social processes and historical conditions out of which the various professions have emerged. This is not to suggest that the characteristics of professions should be ignored in any sociological analysis but to recommend that they should be viewed within the context of a wider theoretical framework.

Barber's (1963) 'four essential attributes' are presented as part of a functionalist approach to the study of professions. According to this theoretical perspective, professions fulfil vital functions essential to the maintenance of the social system and thus make a significant contribution to the well-being of society. Doctors play a vital role in controlling illness and disease. Although the acquisition of specialist knowledge is a potential source of power, the medical profession has a code of ethics to ensure that expert knowledge is only used for the common good and not the personal benefit of the professional practitioner. Thus, it is assumed that the value placed on altruistic service acts as a safeguard against the abuse of power and the exploitation of patients. Consequently, the financial rewards, prestige and status accorded to members of the medical profession are viewed as a reflection of their contribution to society.

A number of criticisms can be levelled against the functionalist position in general and its application to medicine in particular. First, functionalism appears to ignore historical specificity by assuming that there is something timeless about the definition of a profession. Second, a functionalist account reads like a justification of the status quo. Third, there is an inherent assumption that occupations simply evolve into unified professions by means of some natural and inevitable process. This ignores the fact that an occupation can achieve professional status following a power struggle between competing interest groups. Finally, the functionalist tradition accepts without question the altruistic intentions and professional skills attributed to the doctor. On the whole, functionalism does not offer a critique of professional power and medical dominance.

Freidson (1970a, 1970b) provides an alternative explanation of the establishment of the professions. Unlike the functionalists, he emphasises how certain occupations use their distinctive characteristics, such as expert knowledge and professional autonomy, 'as ideological ammunition for attaining the powerful position of professional status, as well as for maintaining it' (Morgan *et al.*, 1985, p. 109). Occupational groups thus play an instrumental role in the process of professionalisation. Turner defines professionalisation as 'an occupational strategy to maintain certain monopolistic privileges and rewards' (1987, p. 154). Thus professional status can be viewed as something that is achieved following a period of political struggle and conflict. According to this view, members of a professional group may subscribe to an ethos of altruistic service but this does not prevent them from taking action to promote their own interests.

Professional dominance

The specialist knowledge to which professions lay claim is a key element in their ability to exercise power and control over their work. According to Abercrombie and Warde (1994, pp. 85–6), there are four key features to professional knowledge: (1) it must have scientific legitimacy; (2) it must be useful and capable of being applied to practical problems; (3) it must not be too narrow or easily converted into a set of practical rules or techniques that can be applied by untrained people; (4) it must allow practitioners to bring to bear their judgement when applying abstract knowledge in a particular client's case. These all apply in the case of medical knowledge.

In discussing the power of the medical profession, Elston (1991) observes that the concepts of dominance and autonomy are often used interchangeably, despite the fact that it is possible to distinguish between them on analytic grounds. She defines 'medical dominance' as 'medicine's authority over others' and professional autonomy as 'the legitimated control that an occupation exercises over the organisation and terms of its work' (Elston, 1991, p. 61). As regards medical dominance, Elston draws on Starr (1982) when she differentiates between two broad types of authority, namely social and cultural authority. The former takes the form of the ability of the medical profession to direct and control the actions of others by the issuing of commands, while the latter is said to occur when the specialist knowledge possessed by doctors is endorsed by others and accepted as valid. In the case of professional autonomy, this is a key concept that has a number of different dimensions. The right of doctors to set the level of professional fees is an example of economic autonomy. The power of the medical profession to control recruitment, determine the standards of performance, assess professional competence and discipline its own members is a reflection of its clinical or technical autonomy. Finally, there is political autonomy, as witnessed by the right of doctors, as experts on health issues, to make policy decisions (Elston, 1991, pp. 61–2).

Although the two dimensions of dominance and autonomy are conceptually distinct, they are closely related, as is evident in Turner's definition of medical dominance:

> We may define medical dominance as a set of strategies requiring control over the work situation, the institutional features of occupational autonomy within the wider medical division of labour, and finally occupational sovereignty over related occupational groups.
>
> (Turner, 1987, p. 141)

Medical dominance is a fundamental feature of the power the medical profession has over other occupations engaged in the delivery of healthcare. The collective strategies used by medical practitioners to establish and maintain power and control form an integral element in the process of professionalisation. A review of the social history of medicine reveals professionalism as an 'occupational strategy' designed to promote upward social mobility and improve the economic position of group members (Parry and Parry, 1976), thereby ensuring the dominance and superiority of the medical profession over other occupational groups allied to medicine.

Turner identifies three different modes of occupational domination within the division of labour in healthcare, which he labels subordination, limitation and exclusion. Subordination occurs where occupations allied to medicine undertake tasks that are delegated by doctors. Consequently, auxiliary occupations have limited scope for developing autonomy of practice. Nursing and midwifery are cited as examples. Occupational limitation refers to situations where medical dominance is used to restrict or limit the practice of other professional groups. As Turner states, 'These occupational limitations involve various forms of containment to a specific part of the body (as in dentistry) or to a specific therapeutic method (as in pharmacy)' (1987, p. 141). The medical profession is able to exert its influence through its representation on the registration boards of other professional bodies. Finally, medical dominance is also evident in the way the medical profession seeks to protect its monopoly by means of 'exclusionary closure' (Parkin, 1979). This refers to the use of licensing, registration and accreditation procedures to define what are regarded as legitimate forms of practice and control access to occupational positions.

The occupational domination of the medical profession has been increasingly challenged during the second half of the twentieth century. In the view of some observers, medicine has undergone a social transformation, on account of which medical practitioners have experienced a form of 'de-professionalisation' (Haug, 1973) or 'proletarianisation' (McKinlay and Arches, 1985). According to the de-professionalisation thesis medical knowledge has lost its exclusivity, which has brought about a decline in the cultural authority exercised by medicine. Lay people now have greater access to medical knowledge and patients have an increased awareness of the alternative therapies and treatments that are on offer. Furthermore, it is maintained that the increasing professionalisation of occupations allied to medicine has also weakened the medical profession's monopoly over health-related knowledge. Morgan *et al.* (1985) see the growing professionalisation of paramedical occupations as posing the most serious threat to medical autonomy.

In contrast to the de-professionalisation argument, the proletarianisation thesis concentrates on the changing working conditions of doctors and the increasing bureaucratisation of the healthcare system as the main factors responsible for the erosion of the power and authority of the medical profession. Supporters of this thesis claim that technological innovations and the routinisation of much medical work have culminated in the de-skilling of medical labour. At the organisational level, the introduction of new managerial structures and bureaucratic practices is thought to have impinged on medical autonomy and diminished the power of the profession.

In addressing the question of the relevance of these two approaches to understanding the state of the medical profession in Britain, Elston concludes that 'neither of these two alternative accounts of diminishing medical power can be regarded as satisfactorily developed theories amenable to rigorous testing' (1991, p. 65). She sees their role as a much more modest one, that is helping to frame research questions and encourage debate about the impact of changes in the organisation of medicine on the future of the medical profession.

Is nursing a profession?

Nursing appears to possess many of the characteristics that serve to distinguish a profession from an occupation. For example, nurses undergo a programme of specialised training and their competence is assessed by formal examinations. Nursing has its own professional associations and a professional code of conduct (United Kingdom Central Council for Nursing, Midwifery and Health Visiting, 1984). Commitment to the principle of service to others is also a core feature of nursing. However, despite these attributes some theorists feel that nursing falls short of full professional status on two main counts. First, it does not have a separate and distinct scientific body of knowledge and, second, there is limited scope for exercising professional autonomy. Consequently, nursing has been described as a 'semi-profession' (Etzioni, 1969).

Nursing is seen as being heavily dependent on medicine in a number of respects. For example, Goode maintains that nurses receive 'a lower-level medical education' and rely on medicine for their knowledge base (1960, p. 903). However, this is disputed by more recent commentators who assert that nurse education and training has been transformed of late. Nurse educators and researchers claim that nursing now has its own body of specialised knowledge, which is continually being updated by means of scientific research into nursing practice and the development of theoretical models of nursing activity (Ellis and Hartley, 1992; Hamilton, 1992). As regards professional autonomy, Freidson believes that in nursing 'autonomy is only partial, being second-hand and limited by a dominant profession' (1970a, p. 76). By and large, doctors are in overall control of diagnosis and treatment and can direct the kind of nursing care a patient receives.

Within the hierarchical division of labour in healthcare, overcoming the occupational subordination of nursing to medicine is a fundamental objective in the campaign for full professional status. As Carpenter suggests, 'nurse subordination is not an established fact, but something that has to be constantly recreated', and therefore it is open to challenge (1993, p. 115). Indeed, as the social history of the development of nursing reveals, professional autonomy and self-government have been key issues in the nurses' professional project for many years. A professional project is defined as a labour market strategy adopted by an occupational group with the aim of acquiring a monopoly over the provision of a particular service (Witz, 1990). In this context, Carpenter identifies three distinct but overlapping stages in the development of professionalism in British nursing. First, there was the Nightingale era, covering the period from the mid-nineteenth century to the second decade of the twentieth century. This witnessed the social creation of the deferential nurse. Nursing was presented as a vocation and although an attempt was made to identify an autonomous occupational role for the nurse, it was made explicitly clear that the nurse was subservient to the doctor. As Davies notes, a 'good nurse', in Florence Nightingale's view, 'should be restrained, disciplined and obedient. She should carry out the orders of doctors in a suitably humble and deferential way' (Davies, 1977, p. 481).

The second stage in the reform of nursing began in the closing decades of the nineteenth century and lasted until the 1960s. This was a period of professionalisation, which started in the late 1880s with a campaign by nurses for the introduction of a state-supported registration scheme, led by Ethel Bedford-Fenwick who founded the British Nursing Association in 1887. As Witz remarks, the 'demand for "self-government" was the nub of their strategy of professionalisation, and it was posed as an alternative to the "subjugation" of nurses' (1990, p. 686). Campaigners saw achieving occupational control through exclusionary closure as the best way of securing professional autonomy and improving the status of nursing.

The early 1970s saw the rise of the third phase of professionalisation, which Carpenter describes as 'the new professionalism'. This marked a renewed effort to achieve full professional status. However, this differs from previous attempts at professionalisation in a number of important ways. First, whereas the earlier professional project embraced all nurses, the emphasis was now on making clinical nursing an exclusive activity by drawing a distinction between basic care and clinical care. According to Carpenter, 'a significant amount of basic nursing care is now being defined as the work of "others", and nursing itself is increasingly being redefined to mean primarily clinical nursing' (1993, p. 122). For example, healthcare assistants are now performing what used to be basic nursing tasks, under the supervision of trained nurses. A second distinguishing feature of the new professionalism is the attempt to re-negotiate the role of the clinical nurse within the professional division of labour in the healthcare setting, an aspect of which has been the attempt to formulate an expert knowledge base unique to clinical nursing. Thirdly, the development of 'new nursing' in the 1980s and 1990s, in the form of the introduction of 'primary nursing', 'nurse consultants' and 'nurse practitioners', created an opportunity for clinical nurses to challenge their subordinate role by taking on new responsibilities in the areas of diagnosis and treatment. For example, the Medicinal Products Act 1992 extended to nurses the right to prescribe a limited range of drugs.

Many of the supporters of the professional project in nursing seem to regard the major attributes of the established professions with unqualified approval and focus their attention on addressing the problems and difficulties encountered by nursing in its quest for professional status (Keogh, 1997). Advocates of professionalisation give little, if any, consideration to the potential disadvantages associated with the traditional model of professionalism. As Davies comments in relation to nursing:

> The standard textbooks, by and large . . . do not debate the pros and cons of professionalism *per se* or question the justifiability of the power which professionalism brings. Energies are more often expended in arguing either that nursing is already a profession, or that it is vital that it should become one, in order to control its own work and to realize the unique function of the nurse in the process of health and healing . . .
>
> (Davies, 1995, p. 134)

It is important that nurses take a more critical look at what professionalisation actually entails. As Salvage (1985) argues, it is not so much a case of deciding whether or not nursing is a profession but more one of asking whether it should be a profession and if so what form it should take. Schrock (1982) makes a similar point in relation to health visiting, when she states that, while it is becoming a profession in the traditional sense, the question health visitors should be asking is what kind of a profession do they want to create?

For an insight into some of the potential disadvantages associated with professionalisation one has only to consider the experience of medicine. Critics such as Illich (1977) have warned against the dangers of the 'over-professionalisation' of medicine. As noted earlier in this chapter, professionalisation can have an adverse impact on the nature and quality of the doctor–patient relationship. The fact that doctors have access to a specialist body of knowledge creates a 'competence gap' between them and their patients. This social monopoly of knowledge forms the basis of the medical profession's claim to authority and helps both to create and to exacerbate the social distance between the doctor and the patient. This form of professionalism could prove to be socially divisive within nursing. If the nurses' professional project is inspired by an orthodox view of professionalism, an exclusionary strategy may be employed, whereby education and training are used to create an elite group of professional nurses. This may have negative consequences, such as distancing nurses from untrained auxiliary healthcare workers, patients and their relatives (Salvage, 1985). The solution may be for nursing to embrace a new type of professionalism, which has been termed 'new professionalism' or 'democratic professionalism' (Hugman, 1991). This advocates the creating of equal partnerships both between the different groups engaged in the delivery of healthcare and between practitioners and their patients.

Health promotion

What is distinctive about health promotion is the attention that it gives to the *facilitation* of healthy lives: the idea that it is no good just telling people that they should change their lifestyles without also altering their social, economic and ecological environments. People must be *able* to live healthy lives. Health promotion aims to work not only at the level of individuals but also at the level of socio-economic structures and to encourage the creation and implementation of 'healthy public policies' such as those concerned with transport, environment, agriculture and so on.

(Burrows *et al.*, 1995, p. 2, emphasis in original)

The emergence of health promotion

It is only during the last two decades that health promotion has emerged as a key theme in healthcare policy, as illustrated by the switch in emphasis from cure to prevention in major policy statements made since the mid-1970s. One of the first official publications to draw attention to the importance of preventive measures in reducing illness and disease was *Prevention and Health: Everybody's Business* (DHSS, 1976). The policy objective of promoting good health was a feature of a number of policy documents throughout the 1980s and 1990s. For example, *Promoting Better Health* (DHSS, 1987) outlined the role of the primary healthcare team in health promotion. The White Paper entitled *The Health of the Nation* (Department of Health, 1992) also emphasised prevention of illness as a central policy issue and identified five key areas in which improvements in health could be achieved. One of these areas included lifestyle factors such as smoking, diet and alcohol consumption.

This change in the focus of healthcare policy increased the volume of health promotion work by extending existing services and introducing new initiatives. For example, following the introduction of the new General Practitioner Contract in 1990 funds were made available for the provision of health promotion clinics. This initiative, along with other illness-prevention activities, increased the amount of health promotion work undertaken in general practice (Hannay *et al.*, 1992). Promoting good health has become an integral part of the role of the practice nurse (Bradford and Winn, 1993). In the case of nursing in general, there is evidence of a growing emphasis on health as opposed to illness. According to

Macleod Clark (1993), nursing practice is witnessing the beginnings of an evolution from 'sick nursing' to 'health nursing'. The former is characteristic of the traditional model of nursing, in which health professionals use their expert knowledge to diagnose a disease or illness and decide on an appropriate course of treatment. The patient does not participate in the decision-making process and is expected to willingly comply with whatever treatment is imposed. In contrast, health nursing represents an attempt to empower patients by providing them with the knowledge and information they need in order to take responsibility for their own health. The conceptual distinction between the two approaches to nursing is captured in the following:

> Health nursing is thus the process of promoting health through nursing care. It is vital to emphasise here that it is not what a nurse does that defines sick nursing or health nursing – it is how she does it. The move from sick nursing to health nursing is a philosophical move, not merely a tacking on or a change in the activities of nursing. This is an important point for, by and large, traditional nursing work retains its validity. There remains and will always remain a need to care for the acutely and chronically sick and the dying, and there will always be a requirement to help patients to meet needs they cannot meet themselves. The problem is that the sick nursing approach to providing such care is no longer tenable or appropriate. Sick nursing must evolve into health nursing in order to respond to future health care needs.
>
> (Macleod Clark, 1993, p. 258)

These two approaches to nursing practice have clear implications for nurse–patient interaction. From a sick nursing perspective the nurse–patient relationship is seen as being characterised by professional dominance and patient passivity, whereas the philosophy of health nursing is founded on the belief that it is essential that nurses work in partnership with patients and enable patients to participate in their own healthcare.

Health promotion work is undertaken by all types of healthcare workers. What they actually do and how they do it is largely determined by a host of factors including the type of healthcare context in which they work, the primary healthcare needs of their patients/clients, their knowledge of health promotion techniques, the level of support they receive from allied services and their own attitudes towards health promotion. Despite variations such as these it is possible to identify some fundamental principles underlying the concept of health promotion, although, as the next section illustrates, the very notion of health promotion is 'the subject of fierce and incessant disputes among professional practitioners and policy makers' (Beattie, 1991, p. 162).

The concept of health promotion

There is no one agreed definition of health promotion. As Cribb observes, the concept has an elastic quality: 'health promotion denotes a conceptual space rather than a clear professional policy or institutional domain . . . it is a space of debate, uncertainty and ambiguity' (1993, p. 29). Since its introduction in the late 1970s there have been many attempts at providing a definition. One of the

Box 10.2   Definition

Health promotion

Health promotion is the process of enabling people to increase control over, and to improve, their health. To reach a state of complete physical, mental and social well-being, an individual or group must be able to identify and to realize aspirations, to satisfy needs, and to change or cope with the environment. Health is therefore seen as a resource for everyday life, not the objective of living. Health is a positive concept emphasizing social and personal resources, as well as physical capabilities. Therefore, health promotion is not just the responsibility of the health sector, but goes beyond healthy lifestyles to well-being.

Source: Ottawa Charter for Health Promotion (World Health Organisation, 1986) quoted in Breslow, 1995, p. 377

most broad-ranging and widely quoted definitions of health promotion originates from the *Ottawa Charter for Health Promotion* (World Health Organisation, 1986) and is reproduced in Box 10.2.

A number of features of this definition warrant special mention. Firstly, as the purpose of health promotion is to promote health, how health is defined will undoubtedly determine the nature and scope of health promotion work. The definition of health embraced by the World Health Organisation (WHO) is a positive, holistic one. As stated in the Ottawa Charter, health is more than the absence of disease, it is 'a resource for everyday life' and is identified as 'a state of complete physical, mental and social well-being'. According to this approach, health promotion is about the maintenance of health in its broadest sense and is not restricted to the prevention of specific diseases. The distinction between health promotion and disease prevention is neatly summarised in the following:

> The relationship between health promotion and disease prevention may best be portrayed as a continuum ranging from extreme infirmity to bounding health. Every person's degree of health may be found somewhere on the continuum. Promotion of health means facilitating at least the maintenance of a person's current position on the continuum relative to age and, ideally, advancing toward its positive end. Disease prevention, on the other hand, means avoiding specific diseases that carry one toward the negative end.
> (Breslow, 1995, p. 379)

Preventing disease is thus one aspect of health promotion. Primary prevention strategies such as childhood immunisation programmes reduce the risk of disease and therefore are part of the practice of health promotion.

A second feature of the Ottawa Charter's definition of health promotion is that it emphasises the importance of helping people, either as individuals or in groups, to gain control over their health and adapt to the environments in which they find themselves. The underlying philosophy is one of enabling, and not coercing, individuals or communities. Empowerment constitutes a key element in the ideology of health promotion. Thirdly, it is not only recognised that people's health is not purely an individual responsibility but also acknowledged that health promotion is not the province of the healthcare sector alone. Social and environmental factors, largely beyond the control of individuals, can have a detrimental effect on health. Therefore, health promotion needs to be viewed within the wider context of public policy in general. A 'healthy public policy' is at the centre of health promotion and is one that uses legislation and policy statements to help to create a health-promoting environment (Tones, 1993). For example, environmental legislation to reduce the levels of pollution and policies to address the substantial social and economic inequalities that exist between social groups can go some way towards creating the conditions necessary to support healthy lifestyles.

Within the literature a distinction is drawn between health promotion and health education. As is the case with health promotion, there have been numerous attempts at defining health education. In general, health education is seen as having three fundamental features: the dissemination of information, empowerment and the promotion of collective action in the interests of community development (French and Adams, 1986). Some theorists have attempted to construct typologies of health education. For example, Draper (1983) describes five broad types on the basis that they provide education about:

1 the body and how to look after it;
2 available health services and how to use them;
3 the environment and how it affects health;
4 the politics of health, including issues of power and accountability;
5 the ethics and effectiveness of health education.

Early health education initiatives were founded on the idea that information leads to knowledge and the acquisition of knowledge enables people to make rational choices to safeguard their future well-being. In other words, the central assumption is that once people are made aware of the health risks and health benefits associated with certain actions or lifestyles they will change their behaviour accordingly. However, such behaviourist and individualistic approaches tend to create a victim-blaming ideology by ignoring how economic conditions and social circumstances can effectively restrict the lifestyle options available to specific groups in the population (Crawford, 1977). It is from critiques of conventional approaches to health education that the concept of health promotion eventually emerged (Nettleton, 1995). Health education is very much a part of the much broader field of health promotion. As Tones asserts, '*Health Promotion = Health Education × Healthy Public Policy*' (1993, p. 3, italics in original).

Beattie's fourfold structural map (Figure 10.1) illustrating the repertoire of health promotion strategies is a useful device for exploring the concept of health promotion and developing an understanding of some of the broad policy issues involved in the promotion of health. The framework provided by Beattie locates the different strategies on two bipolar dimensions; one labelled the 'mode of intervention' and the other the 'focus of intervention'. The former is the authoritative/negotiated dimension. While authoritative strategies are 'top down'

Mode of intervention

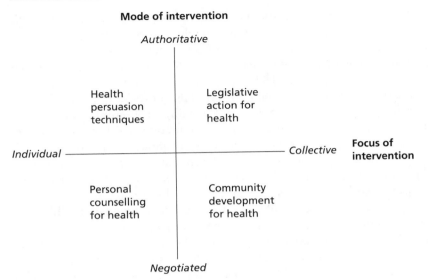

Figure 10.1 Strategies of health promotion

Source: Beattie, A. (1991) 'Knowledge and control in health promotion: a test case for social policy and social theory', in J. Gabe, M. Calnan and M. Bury (eds.) *The Sociology of the Health Service*, Routledge (p. 167)

and prescriptive, negotiated strategies are 'bottom up' and involve more parti-cipatory forms of intervention. In terms of the focus of intervention, health promotion strategies can focus on the individual or the group or community.

'Health persuasion techniques' are located in the top left-hand corner of the structural map. Beattie uses this term to describe the 'cluster of interventions which employ the authority of public-health expertise to re-direct the behaviour of individuals in top-down prescriptive ways' (1991, p. 168). Health promo-tion campaigns on alcohol consumption, smoking, healthy eating and human immunodeficiency virus/acquired immunodeficiency syndrome fall into this category. Despite the fact that research evidence suggests that such campaigns are not particularly successful at bringing about changes in individual lifestyles, many politicians and health promoters nevertheless enthusiastically support them.

'Legislative action for health' is another type of intervention strategy that has an authoritative or top-down approach. However, in this case health promotion activity is collectively focused. This applies where health promotion profession-als and public health experts use their knowledge and authority to campaign for the introduction of legislative measures designed to have a positive impact on the health of large groups of people. Examples include campaigns to introduce legislation to control the advertising of cigarettes.

'Personal counselling for health' is an individually focused health promotion strategy located at the 'negotiated' end of the mode of intervention continuum. As a strategy this approach emphasises the use of personal or group counselling techniques to help people to recognise the health risks associated with their current lifestyle and encourage them to make healthy lifestyle choices in the interests of future well-being. Beattie notes that although compared with health persuasion tactics this strategy casts the individual in an active role: '. . . its emphasis is clearly and almost exclusively on helping individuals to learn to cope (rather than to change their circumstances), and it therefore does not escape the charge of "victim-blaming" . . .' (1991, p. 175).

Finally, the strategy labelled 'community development for health' is a relatively new approach, which, as its name implies, is essentially a collectively focused form of health promotion. As a strategic option, community development projects have for many years featured widely in countries throughout the developing world. In recent times relatively small-scale local community health projects, with a community development approach, have been introduced in many developed countries, particularly in deprived urban areas. In Britain there are examples of such projects designed specifically for minority ethnic populations (Blenner-hassett *et al.*, 1989). The idea behind community-based health projects is that the community, or representative groups within the community, have an active and instrumental role to play in identifying local health problems and determining how they might be best addressed. This constitutes a form of participatory health promotion, whereby professional health workers do not simply provide expert information and knowledge but use their skills to empower local groups and develop health promotion partnerships in which members of the local community are encouraged to participate. It is not only minority ethnic groups that can benefit from a community development approach. Community development health projects have proved to be an important strategy in meeting women's health needs (Rodmell and Watt, 1986).

Beattie's conceptual framework is useful for analysing health promotion; however, it needs to be noted that his structural map constitutes an analytic device and the four models of health promotion it identifies are ideal types, which are unlikely to be encountered in their pure form in actual practice. It is highly likely that a successful health promotion programme would incorporate a mixture of health promotion strategies.

Sociology of health promotion

There is an important distinction to be made between a sociology *for* and a sociology *of* health promotion (Thorogood, 1992). In the case of the former, sociology can be seen as providing knowledge and information to enable health professionals to improve and develop their health promotion techniques and practices. For example, from a general point of view, sociological studies have done much to help us to appreciate how social divisions, cultural diversity and economic inequality can have a profound effect on the way in which people live their lives. If health promoters wish to change people's behaviour then they must understand what influences their behaviour in the first place.

There is more to changing behaviour than simply providing factual information about the health risks associated with certain behaviours and then expecting those informed to voluntarily choose the 'healthy' course of action. As Graham (1984) has shown in her study of health in families, lifestyle choices are seldom that simple. Choices need to be viewed within the wider context of the social structure in which individuals and families are located. As such, lifestyle decisions are influenced by the material resources available. According to Graham, 'The barriers to change are represented by the limits of time, energy and income available to parents. In such circumstances, health choices are more accurately seen as health compromises, which, repeated day after day, become the routines which keep the family going' (1987, p. 187). By providing an insight into how health choices are made in specific contexts, sociological research can provide important pointers for those engaged in the planning and delivery of health promotion programmes.

Structural factors are also important within the context of minority ethnic groups. Socio-economic disadvantage and racial discrimination can both have a detrimental impact on physical and mental health. Research evidence suggests that there is a mismatch between health professionals' perceptions of the health concerns of minority ethnic groups and the evidence available from epidemiological surveys (Bhopal and White, 1993, p. 142). Consequently, health promotion campaigns have been poorly focused, concentrating on aspects of the culture of origin of particular minority ethnic populations rather than the problems that they encounter living in contemporary Britain. According to Nettleton, 'Some campaigns have emphasised cultural difference to the neglect of structural constraints, with the consequence that institutional racism goes unacknowledged' (1995, p. 236). Sociological studies of the relationship between the socio-economic environment, ethnicity and health can provide health professionals with information on how to undertake effective health promotion work in cross-cultural settings. This involves more than developing sensitivity to cultural differences. In practice, health professionals need to work in partnership with minority ethnic communities, sharing knowledge and expertise, and actively involving community members in health promotion initiatives.

Studies of the structure and content of lay health beliefs and the workings of the lay referral system, as described in Chapter 2, are a good example of how sociology can be seen to contribute to health promotion. Research findings provide health professionals with much useful information about the lay logic behind ideas about health maintenance and disease prevention. It is important that the beliefs, experiences and perspectives of clients are considered when designing health promotion initiatives. This knowledge can help to create a form of 'reflective practice' (Schon, 1991), which enables health workers to elicit and promote client or patient participation more successfully. Individuals do not passively accept either the advice provided by health promoters or the authoritative statements produced by health promotion campaigns, without first attempting to make sense of such advice within the context of the values and beliefs they already hold about health and illness. As observed by Nettleton and Bunton, 'The literature on lay health beliefs, for example, has illustrated the need for health promoters to take account of, and be sensitive to, the language and concepts of those audiences whom they wish to reach' (1995, p. 42). In other words, in order to be effective, health promotion interventions must acknowledge the existence and complexity of lay health beliefs.

In contrast to a sociology *for* health promotion, a sociological analysis *of* health promotion takes a critical stance towards the very activity of health promotion itself. Nettleton and Bunton identify three broad sociological critiques, which they refer to as socio-structural, surveillance and consumption. In essence the structural critique maintains that many programmes to promote health ignore the nature and extent of material deprivation and underestimate the impact socio-economic factors can have on health status. Promoting good health and combating illness and disease are not only about encouraging people to change their behaviour but involve addressing wider social, economic and political issues surrounding structural inequalities, unemployment, poverty and pollution. A structural perspective serves to challenge those approaches to health promotion that neglect such wider issues and appear to blame the victim by focusing on promoting health through changing lifestyles. Such a critique illustrates how values and ideology feature in health promotion programmes. By and large, 'It draws attention to the fact that ideas about healthy living are promulgated by those who are white, middle-class and often work within sexist, racist and homophobic value systems' (Nettleton and Bunton, 1995, p. 45). Consequently, some groups can become negatively stereotyped and socially marginalised as a result of being singled out by campaigns to improve health and prevent disease.

Nettleton and Bunton use the term 'surveillance critiques' when referring to those perspectives that view health promotion as a technology of control. With the strategic focus on prevention, the monitoring of health-related behaviour has become something of a priority. Health promotion pervades all parts of the health service and is also encountered in the school and workplace. For Cribb, '"surveillance" acts as a technology of control irrespective of the intentions of professionals because it embodies standards of good and bad, and it brings them into the public domain and into the self-consciousness of the governed' (1993, p. 33). New forms of self-regulation and self-monitoring have emerged as part of the growing technology of health promotion in recent years. A good example is the use of health and lifestyle diaries in which individuals are encouraged to keep a daily record of their diet and physical activities. In this way individuals themselves become part of the surveillance process. Not only are they required to monitor those aspects of their behaviour which have implications for their health and general well-being but they are held to account for their actions. This represents 'a shift in the form of social regulation in relation to health from an external to an internal approach' (Nettleton, 1995, p. 240). It is not simply a case of health professionals telling people how they should behave (i.e. external regulation) but more a case of regulation coming from within the individual by means of personal control and self-discipline.

Health promoters use self-monitoring techniques, along with practitioner-based techniques such as observation and in-depth qualitative interviewing, to monitor different aspects of people's lives. All in all, this surveillance activity is underscored by a health-promoting ideology that stresses the importance of individuals accepting responsibility for preserving and maintaining their own health, an approach which has led to the creation of a new identity, that of the 'health promoting self' (Nettleton and Bunton, 1995, pp. 47–8).

The third sociological critique of health promotion draws on the sociology of consumption. Consumer culture is about the construction of social identities by means of lifestyle choices. The goods which people buy are marketed as reflecting something about the lifestyle of the buyer. Advertising promotes the idea that certain branded products are indicative of successful and desired lifestyles. Their ownership is deemed to be a symbol of social status: something that serves to distinguish one social group from another. According to this critique, in recent times health has come to be seen as an aspect of lifestyles, with the result that health promotion can now be viewed as part of a wider cultural process. As Nettleton and Bunton observe, two features are worthy of note in this respect. Firstly, there has been a general blurring of the boundaries between the health promotion literature produced by health professionals and the commercial literature on health maintenance and lifestyles. There are many commercial sector organisations involved in what may be loosely termed the health and lifestyle industry, producing a diverse range of goods including herbal cures, body care products and exercise equipment.

Secondly, what Nettleton and Bunton describe as a 'decentring of health' has occurred (1995, p. 49). In other words, advice about health maintenance is no longer solely provided by healthcare professionals working primarily within medical settings such as health centres or clinics. Individuals acquire knowledge and information from a variety of sources and in a number of different locations. Community centres, health and fitness clubs, slimming groups, leisure centres, specialist television programmes, newspaper articles and magazine features are some of the main sources of health promotion information available outside the health service sector. The increasing involvement of commercial organisations in health promotion work has led to the 'commodification of health products' (Featherstone, 1991) and the emergence of the image of the individual as a 'consumer of health' (Grace, 1991).

Health service: reforms and research

> . . . Britain's National Health Service, which established health care as a right, has been progressively dismantled and privatised by successive governments over the past quarter-century.
>
> (Pollock *et al.*, 2004, p. vii)

Health service reforms since the early 1990s

Public sector health and social welfare provision experienced the beginnings of a major ideological transformation during the 1980s. In political terms this decade belonged to the New Right. It was a period in which the centrist consensus politics characteristic of Britain in the post-war era lost out to the new radical neo-conservative political philosophy championed by Margaret Thatcher (Midgley, 1991). The 'conviction politics' of Thatcherism provided the basis for a new and radical political programme (Deakin, 1994, p. 110). A fundamental feature of this approach was a belief that the welfare state was a stultifying institution, which undermined individual responsibility and created a culture of dependence. The attack on state-provided welfare services was not merely a pragmatic cost-cutting exercise at a time of worsening economic conditions but was motivated in part by a wider ideological critique of the role of the state, coupled with a belief that healthcare and social welfare provision would benefit from being opened up to free market forces. Thus the liberal consensus with its support for an interventionist state was abandoned; the radical right advocated a minimalist state. The reforms drawn up in the 1980s and implemented in the early 1990s represented a 'rolling back of the frontiers of the state'.

At the forefront of the shift towards a market economy model of welfare was the adoption of a case management system in social care. The nomination of case managers was recommended in the White Paper, entitled *Caring for People* (Department of Health, 1989). Their role was envisaged as one of ensuring that the needs of individual clients are regularly reviewed, services are planned to meet specific needs and resources effectively managed. Among the many proposals contained in the NHS and Community Care Act 1990 was the introduction of a case management and assessment system, through which all those in need of community care must pass if they are to be deemed eligible for services funded by public money. Thus, case or care managers were given a gatekeeping function, as well as being responsible for negotiating and organising packages of care and monitoring both service expenditure and delivery.

The 1990 Act widened the role of managers within the NHS. A principal objective of the health reforms was to reorganise the financing of healthcare in order to ensure a more cost-effective use of resources. The idea was that this would be achieved by introducing an element of competition and tighter managerial control by means of the establishment of a quasi-market in healthcare. A key feature of the new arrangement was the creation of internal markets, which involved separating the functions of *purchasing* and *providing* healthcare services. Health authorities became one of the primary purchasers, responsible for buying health services to meet the needs of the local population. Funded by central government they negotiated contracts with both public and private sector agencies. The competition for scarce resources by the different provider units was seen as a way of ensuring that healthcare was provided on a cost-effective basis. Self-governing NHS trusts were set up and were free to tender for contracts in different health authorities. The purchaser–provider split was not so marked in the case of general practice. While all general practitioners provide primary healthcare, some of those in the larger general practices also became fundholders, which meant that they were able to purchase certain hospital services for their patients.

Supporters of the reforms argued that adopting the practice and principles of private enterprise would ensure that health and welfare services were not only provided more efficiently but would also be more responsive to the needs of individual clients. Individuals became 'consumers of care' and under free market conditions were expected to experience greater choice and control over the services they received. If service providers failed to offer consumers what they wanted, at a price that they could afford or were willing to pay, then they would go out of business. The underlying assumption was that healthcare and social welfare provision can be treated like any other consumer item bought from a retail outlet. In this context, increasing privatisation is seen as ensuring diversity and choice in community care provision. Indeed the notion of consumer choice is given considerable emphasis in the policy literature. In *Caring for People*, 'choice' is defined as 'giving people a greater individual say in how they live their lives and the services they need to help them' (Department of Health, 1989, p. 4). There is a distinction to be made between choice of service and choice of provider. Ideally individuals should be able to choose between different types of services according to their needs and personal preferences. An example of this would be an elderly person choosing between either going into residential accommodation or receiving a package of community support services which would enable them to live at home. In this context consumer choice can foster independence. When there is more than one provider, consumers benefit from the range and diversity of provision on offer. The creation of a mixed economy of welfare is presented as a way of breaking the monopoly power of the state and freeing individuals to make their own decisions as to how they will be cared for.

While supporters of privatisation extol the virtues of consumer choice and user control, there are those who have expressed doubt concerning the appropriateness of the application of a consumerist ideology to the fields of healthcare and personal social services.

> Visitors to NHS hospitals today are struck by the way more and more of their forecourts look like cramped shopping malls, cluttered with outlets of W. H. Smith and café chains. NHS hospitals have become yet another outlet for the fast food industry, adding to the very problems of obesity and heart disease that the NHS exists to combat. This transformation began after the introduction of the internal market, when hospitals were expected to supplement their income from commercial retail rentals and private patients.
>
> (Pollock *et al.*, 2004, p. 18)

Critics maintain that the concept of consumer sovereignty, which features so prominently in policy rhetoric, has not been satisfactorily transformed into action. Walker (1993), quoting a study of private residential care for the elderly by Bradshaw (1988), maintains that genuine choice is often never exercised. Many elderly people who enter residential care do so because of a sudden breakdown in the informal support network and therefore do not have the time to consider the various options available. There is also evidence to suggest that once they have been admitted, residents have very little say in changes made in private homes. They can find changes being imposed on them without consultation, such as having to share a bedroom with other residents.

The concept of consumerism may be misleading when applied to health and social care:

> The Griffiths Report, White Paper and National Health Service and Community Care Act all derive from the limited form of supermarket-style consumerism which assumes that, if there is a choice between 'products', service users will automatically have the power of exit from a particular product or market. Of course, even if this is true in markets for consumer goods, in the field of social care many people are mentally disabled, frail and vulnerable; they are not in a position to 'shop around' and have no realistic prospect of exit.
>
> (Walker, 1993, p. 221)

Although the policy literature refers to user involvement with such phrases as 'user control' and 'money following the patient', the consumer-oriented model gives little guidance as to how service users can become truly empowered. Heginbotham (1993) suggests a distinction between 'material consumerism' and 'welfare consumerism'. The former is supermarket-style consumerism; individuals with adequate financial resources make free choices from a wide range of available products, whereas the latter means 'that the consumer must be involved to some degree in the creation of the product or service' (Heginbotham, 1993, p. 179). The suggestion is that welfare consumers should not merely be consulted but should be given the opportunity to play a more active part in the planning and organisation of services.

The NHS has undergone considerable change over the last two decades. The beginning of this century saw major structural changes with the introduction of the Private Finance Initiative and Primary Care Groups. The NHS Plan published in 2000 (Department of Health, 2000) introduced a wide range of reforms designed to modernise the NHS. New Labour set out a number of detailed and ambitious targets in terms of service provision and the allocation of resources. The relentless pursuit of a mixed economy approach to healthcare saw privatisation extended to the provision of clinical services. Overall, the policy changes have massively transformed the NHS. In some senses the NHS is now much less of a direct provider of health services and has increasingly come to adopt a 'franchising' role as a government-funded payer for services provided by a variety of public and private sector organisations (Talbot-Smith and Pollock, 2006).

The Department of Health is responsible for setting the national strategy for the NHS and making key decisions regarding the distribution of resources. The current aims and objects of the Department of Health and the core priorities of the NHS are outlined in Boxes 10.3 and 10.4 respectively. The Department of Health has a wide remit covering both health and social care. While it does not have a direct role in the day-to-day running of the NHS, it is responsible for setting national standards and reporting to Parliament on the general performance of the NHS.

The document published in 2000 outlining the plan for the modernisation and reform of the heathcare system noted that '[t]he NHS is a 1940s system operating in a 21st century world' (Department of Health, 2000, p. 10). Particular

Box 10.3   Definition

Aims and objectives of the Department of Health

Aims

The Department of Health's overall aim is to improve the health and well being of the people of England by:

- supporting activity at national level to protect, promote and improve the nation's health;
- securing the provision of comprehensive, high quality care for all those who need it, regardless of their ability to pay or where they live or their age;
- securing responsive social care and child protection for those who lack the support they need.

Objectives

The key objectives in pursuing these aims are to:

- reduce the incidence of avoidable illness, disease and injury in the population;
- treat people with illness, disease or injury quickly, effectively and on the basis of need alone;
- enable people, who are unable to perform essential activities of daily living, including those with chronic illness, disability or terminal illness, to live as full and normal lives as possible;
- maximise the social development of children within stable family settings;
- assure performance and support to Ministers in accounting to Parliament and the public for the overall performance of the NHS, Personal Social Services (PSS) and the Department of Health.
- manage the staff and resources of the Department of Health so as to improve performance.

Source: Adapted from Department of Health, 2004b, p. 12

attention was drawn to the overcentralised structure of the NHS, the absence of national standards and the lack of clear incentives for improving performance. The goals and recommendations are both detailed and extensive. A set of core principles are described as underpinning the plan for change; some of these are seen to 'restate the founding values of the NHS' (Department of Health, 2000, p. 3). However, some of the reforms and policy changes of recent years may be viewed as ideologically driven and constituting a threat to some of the founding principles of the NHS. In commenting on the current state of what they refer to as 'NHS plc', Pollock *et al.* (2004) maintain that the original principles of comprehensiveness, universality and equity have been abandoned or eroded. With regards to comprehensiveness, the 1980s witnessed the closure of many long-term care beds and the discontinuation of routine eye examinations. Changes to the funding of dental services resulted in fewer people having access to NHS dental care. By the beginning of this century more than half of all dental care was paid

> ### Box 10.4   Definition
>
> #### NHS core principles
>
> 1 The NHS will provide a universal service for all based on clinical need, not ability to pay.
>
> 2 The NHS will provide a comprehensive range of services.
>
> 3 The NHS will shape its services around the needs and preferences of individual patients, their families and their carers.
>
> 4 The NHS will respond to different needs of different populations.
>
> 5 The NHS will work continuously to improve quality services and to minimise errors.
>
> 6 The NHS will support and value its staff.
>
> 7 Public funds for healthcare will be devoted solely to NHS patients.
>
> 8 The NHS will work together with others to ensure a seamless service for patients.
>
> 9 The NHS will help keep people healthy and work to reduce health inequalities.
>
> 10 The NHS will respect the confidentiality of individual patients and provide open access to information about services, treatment and performance.
>
> *Source*: Department of Health, 2000, pp. 3–5

for directly by patients. As for universality, this too has come under threat as both primary and secondary care services can vary from place to place. While the amount of money spent on treating certain health conditions may vary across primary care trusts, this is only partly explained by factors such as differences in the age profiles and needs of local populations. Access to certain drugs, treatments and surgical procedures has been described as a 'postcode lottery' (Bungay, 2005). In terms of equity, the original principle was that access to care should be according to need and not based on the ability to pay. According to Pollock *et al.*, 'this has been steadily eroded both through the abandonment of comprehensiveness – so that many quite poor people now have to pay as much as the affluent for long term care, optical care, domiciliary services etc. – and through charges . . . for prescriptions, dentistry, and non-clinical hospital services . . .' (2004, p. 79).

There is no doubt that the various health reforms have influenced the research agenda in healthcare over recent years. The emphasis placed on the need to control expenditure and obtain value for money produced a call for more evaluation of medical interventions and clinical procedures. Essentially the assumption was the more we know about the relative effectiveness of different types of treatment, the easier it is to extract the maximum benefit from limited resources, the underlying belief being that 'Evidence-based medicine was seen to provide purchasers with a mechanism to establish what healthcare is the "best buy"' (Allsop, 1998, p. 289). In addition to a concern over the cost-effectiveness of health services, the new reforms also addressed the issue of the quality of the services provided for patients. As Ellis and Whittington assert, 'Quality assurance in the National Health Service has thus become not just a matter of professional concern or enthusiasm but a mandatory part of service provision' (1993, p. 18). A wide range of social research methods including self-completion questionnaires, in-depth interviews and qualitative observation has been used by health researchers to monitor the quality of care and measure levels of patient satisfaction. The nature, scope and limitations of evaluative health research are covered in the following sections.

The role of research in healthcare

Politicians, policy-makers, managers and healthcare practitioners are all involved, albeit in different ways and at different levels, in making decisions about the nature, organisation and delivery of healthcare services. In broad terms, decision-making in the health services is influenced by three sets of factors: the values held by those making the decisions, the resources they have at their disposal and the evidence provided by research studies (Gray, 1997). Much of the research undertaken to aid policy-making and inform individual professional practice involves some form of evaluation.

Three broad dimensions of healthcare provision provide a focus for evaluation. Donabedian (1980) refers to these as structure, outcome and process. Structure, in this context, refers to the physical surroundings and organisational settings in which healthcare is provided. This takes into account the amount of resources, equipment and personnel available. Outcome evaluation is concerned with measuring the impact of a treatment or service on the health status of patients and communities. The idea is to provide information about the effectiveness of a particular diagnostic procedure, medical treatment or caring service. Process evaluation is not concerned with issues of effectiveness but with how services are organised and delivered. This involves everything from measuring patient throughput to studying the behaviour of healthcare professionals towards individual patients in clinical settings.

Coulter (1991) identifies four levels of evaluation in health services research (Box 10.5), all of which have been engaged in by social researchers. The purpose of healthcare evaluation research is not merely to ascertain what medical therapies, clinical interventions, care programmes or types of service delivery are the most effective. Given that health service resources are finite and never likely to keep pace with the demand for healthcare, it is important to know not only whether a treatment or service has the desired impact but also whether it is cost-effective. Weighing the costs and benefits associated with a particular service is not solely about making an economic evaluation but also means taking into account social and clinical criteria. Consequently, healthcare evaluation is a multi-disciplinary research activity involving researchers from a variety of disciplines including medicine, epidemiology, economics, psychology and sociology.

> ### Box 10.5   Definition
>
> **Four levels of healthcare evaluation**
>
> 1 Evaluation of *specific treatments*, e.g. drug therapies or surgical procedures.
>
> 2 Evaluation of *patterns of care for particular patient groups*, e.g. the organisation of antenatal care or the care of patients with chronic conditions such as diabetes.
>
> 3 Evaluation of *organisations*, e.g. a hospital or a day centre.
>
> 4 Evaluation of *health systems*, e.g. the effects of different methods of payment for healthcare.
>
> *Source:* Coulter, 1991, p. 116

Evaluation research draws heavily on social science research methods and methodologies. It has been described as an activity that consists of 'the systematic application of social research procedures' (Rossi and Freeman, 1993, p. 5), while also making use of some of the theoretical insights and empirical generalisations found within the social sciences (Berk and Rossi, 1990). In this sense, sociologists contribute to evaluations of healthcare services through their understanding of data collection methodology, research design, data analysis and knowledge of the substantive findings of sociological research into health, illness and patterns of interaction between healthcare workers and patients. However, while sociologists can make a positive contribution to both outcome and process forms of evaluation, sociological analysis also provides the basis for a critical appraisal of the logic and practice of evaluation and the interpretation of research findings. Aspects of this dual contribution are evident in the following sections, which raise general issues about the evaluation of healthcare interventions.

Evaluating effectiveness

The first choice research design for the evaluation of clinical procedures is the randomised controlled trial (RCT), which is the medical equivalent of the classic scientific experiment (Cochrane, 1972). It has been described as the 'gold standard' in medical evaluation (Shepperd *et al.*, 1997, p. 26). Clinical trials are widely used to determine the efficacy of medical therapies. As St Leger *et al.* (1992) assert, in clinical terms, a therapeutic technique or procedure can be considered to be efficacious if on average it can be shown to have a beneficial impact on prognosis or suffering. In its simplest form, this research procedure involves the random allocation of individuals to one of two groups: a treatment, study or experimental group and a non-treatment or control group. It is possible that individuals in the control group or comparison group are not left untreated but continue to receive the standard form of treatment normally prescribed for their condition. By comparing the two groups on the basis of a number of pre-determined outcome measures the researcher is able to conclude whether the new treatment is more effective than the old one. The idea behind the random allocation of subjects is that it can be assumed that any patient characteristics likely to influence the response to the new treatment are evenly distributed between the treatment and comparison groups, thus making it more likely that any observed differences between the groups are a result of the treatment they received.

The RCT method is not restricted to the evaluation of drug trials, medical therapies and surgical interventions but can, in principle, be extended to areas such as nursing care, health promotion campaigns and most forms of service provision. Whatever the context, the logic and basic procedures behind RCTs are the same. With this method it is particularly important that steps are taken to reduce the possibility of any bias in the observation and interpretation of outcomes. Bias can originate from both the subject and the observer or experimenter. In the case of the former, patients may be affected by the knowledge that they are participants in a treatment group. This is especially a problem when subjective outcome measures are used, such as self-reported health status or general psychological well-being, as patients may be more inclined to report positive responses if they feel that they are receiving a 'state of the art' treatment. In drug trials, to guard against this eventuality, control group subjects are given a placebo, which is a chemically inert substance in the shape of the drug that is actually being evaluated. As for observer or experimenter bias, this can occur when the researcher or health professional responsible for collecting outcome data is able to distinguish the 'study' patients from the 'control' patients. For example, belief in a new healthcare technology can pose a threat to objectivity when it comes to making judgements about its impact on patients.

One of the most effective ways of minimising bias is through the construction of what are known as 'blind' trials. In the evaluation of a medical intervention or treatment programme there are three main groups: the patients, the health professionals who provide the care and the researchers who conduct the evaluation. Any of these three can be blinded to some aspects of an evaluation. If this applies in the case of only one group then the term 'single-blind' trial is used. Frost *et al.* (1995) used a single-blind RCT in their study of the effectiveness of an outpatient fitness programme for patients with chronic low back pain. The research procedure was conducted as follows. Those patients who were referred to the physiotherapy department by orthopaedic consultants because they were experiencing moderate disability as a result of their condition were asked whether they were willing to take part in the study. The patients who gave their consent were randomly assigned to one of two groups, a treatment group (i.e. outpatient fitness programme) or a control group. Both groups were given advice and information about back problems and also attended practical workshops to learn relaxation techniques. Only those patients assigned to the treatment group attended the special fitness classes. Patients were assessed before and after treatment by a single 'blind' observer who was unaware as to which of the two groups the subjects had been assigned.

Probably the most common form of blind trial is the 'double-blind' version. A double-blind RCT was used by Mynors-Wallis *et al.* (1995) in their study of the treatment of major depressive disorders in the primary care setting. The aim of the study was to evaluate the effectiveness of a psychologically focused problem-solving approach to treatment. Patients were randomly allocated to one of three groups. One group was treated with an anti-depressant drug and another received a placebo. Both patients and therapists were unable to distinguish the active drug from the placebo. Subjects assigned to the experimental group did not receive any medication but had sessions with a trained therapist, over a three-month period, in which the emphasis was on solving the patient's problems. The progress made by patients in all three groups was compared at the end of the experimental period.

The experimental model of controlled evaluation of medical interventions and therapeutic strategies is considered by many to be the single most scientifically valid way of evaluating healthcare. However, one should not overlook the problems encountered when trying to replicate the 'true' experimental research design, especially in healthcare settings. As Coulter maintains, 'Sociologists have tended to reject the experimental approach to evaluation, arguing that goals and outcomes are often hard to define and measure and that the approach assumes a greater degree of control over extraneous variables than is usually possible or desirable in social research' (1991, p. 122). Indeed, there are aspects of the social world of healthcare provision that militate against the use of RCTs. For example, the requirement that patients are randomly allocated to treatment and control groups can pose ethical dilemmas for those responsible for delivering care. Health professionals may feel that patients who are assigned to control groups are effectively being denied access to the treatment they deserve. In this respect, Oakley (1990) describes the concerns expressed by a number of midwives who took part in a controlled intervention study to determine whether women benefited from additional social support during pregnancy. What was an important issue for the midwives was the apparent conflict between the consequences of randomisation and the professional principles of midwifery. The random allocation of their clients to treatment or control conditions meant that in some instances midwives saw women assigned to the control group, when in their professional opinion they needed the additional support offered in the study group. Oakley found that the midwives tried various ways of influencing the randomisation process in order to ensure that their clients received the care they needed. For example, they tried to identify a pattern in the allocation of women so as to ensure that those whom they considered needed additional care were assigned to the treatment group.

Health economics

Evaluations of healthcare are not only concerned with determining service effectiveness and ascertaining the impact of clinical interventions but they also raise questions about the efficiency and economy of different services and treatment regimes. During the last twenty years or so economists have come to play an increasingly important part in the evaluation of health service care. This is partly due to the emphasis placed on controlling public expenditure and obtaining 'value for money' from public services by central government since the early 1980s. It is also a consequence of the need for information to help to provide a more equitable way of allocating resources and rationing healthcare. Although in the context of health the word 'rationing' attracts an emotive response, it is widely acknowledged that rationing is inevitable (New, 1997) and 'has in fact been practised within the NHS since its infancy' (Harrison and Hunter, 1994, p. 1). As economics deals with the problem of the allocation of scarce resources it is not surprising that economists have turned their attention to healthcare provision.

Health economics is about the costs and benefits of alternative allocations of scarce healthcare resources. There are three chief techniques of economic evaluation: cost–effectiveness analysis, cost–benefit analysis and cost–utility analysis. The first of these has been described as the 'most powerfully persuasive tool' in healthcare evaluation at the present time (Daly and McDonald, 1992, p. 5). Cost–effectiveness analysis is only one of a number of techniques used by health economists to measure efficiency. Basically it involves calculating the financial cost to the health service of providing a clinical procedure or treatment and then relating this to the health outcomes achieved. This method is particularly useful for comparing the relative efficiency of different types of treatment that have a common goal. However, before such an analysis can be attempted it is necessary to find a suitable way of measuring outcomes. Standard indicators of clinical outcome are used in cost–effectiveness analysis. For example, some interventions are evaluated by calculating the impact on life expectancy, i.e. the number of life years saved as a result of the treatment. In order to compare alternative forms of treatment the financial costs per unit of outcome (i.e. life year saved) are ascertained. A cost-effective treatment is one that either produces an agreed level of health benefits at the lowest financial cost or provides the maximum health gains for a fixed amount of resources.

Cost–benefit analysis differs from cost–effectiveness analysis in that a monetary value is attributed to both the costs and the benefits of different treatments in order to calculate the net benefit (i.e. benefit minus cost) or the ratio of cost to benefit. Quantifying benefits in this way does not restrict comparative analysis to alternative treatments for the same complaint but enables comparisons to be made between different treatments producing different benefits. However, this form of analysis can be expensive to undertake and not all costs and benefits can be readily assigned a monetary value.

Instead of measuring the value of an intervention on a monetary scale, cost–utility analysis measures benefits in terms of utility. The 'quality-adjusted life year' (QALY) technique is a good example of a utility measure (Rosser and Kind, 1978). In this type of analysis account is taken of qualitative as well as quantitative health outcomes when calculating the costs and benefits of a specified treatment. Thus it not only takes into consideration the life expectancy of a patient following treatment but also attempts to measure the quality of life they are likely to experience. The quality of life is measured on a scale from 0 to 1. Perfect health (i.e. the absence of any disability or distress) is assigned a value of 1, death is valued at

0 and a figure of less than 1 indicates a year of life of less than optimal health. Therefore, QALYs = expected life years × an index of 'utility'. In other words, the change in the duration of life (i.e. 'life year') is weighted by a factor deemed to represent the change in disability and distress (i.e. 'quality adjusted'). For example, if a given condition has a health-related quality of life score of 0.7, then a patient who can be expected to survive for six years following treatment will have the equivalent of 4.2 QALYs (0.7 × 6). In theory QALYs can be used to compare the benefits of different treatments. Furthermore, by calculating the costs per QALY it is possible to determine which are the most cost-effective interventions. QALY data may also be useful in helping healthcare managers make resource allocation decisions when there are a number of projects or initiatives competing for funding.

As illustrated in Box 10.6, quality of life is represented in two dimensions: disability and distress. In order to create an index of utility, researchers asked a group of 70 respondents, including doctors, nurses, patients and 'healthy volunteers', to provide scores for the various levels of disability and distress (Kind *et al.*, 1982, 1994). These scores were transformed to produce a valuation matrix (Box 10.7).

Health economics is not a perfect science. Good, accurate cost–benefit data are not always readily available and there are many unresolved issues surrounding the assessment of healthcare provision in general and the choice of outcome

Box 10.6 Definition

Classification of states of sickness

Disability

1 No disability.

2 Slight social disability.

3 Severe social disability and/or slight impairment of performance at work. Able to do all housework except very heavy tasks.

4 Choice of work or performance at work very severely limited. Housewives and old people able to do light housework only, but able to go out shopping.

5 Unable to undertake any paid employment. Unable to continue any education. Old people confined to home except for escorted outings and short walks and unable to do shopping. Housewives only able to perform a few simple tasks.

6 Confined to chair or to wheelchair or able to move around in the home only with support from an assistant.

7 Confined to bed.

8 Unconscious.

Distress

A None   **B** Mild   **C** Moderate   **D** Severe

Source: Rosser and Kind, 1978

Box 10.7   Research findings

Quality of life values

| Disability | Distress | | | |
	A	B	C	D
1	1.000	0.995	0.990	0.967
2	0.990	0.986	0.973	0.932
3	0.980	0.972	0.956	0.912
4	0.964	0.956	0.942	0.870
5	0.946	0.935	0.900	0.700
6	0.875	0.845	0.680	0.000
7	0.677	0.564	0.000	−1.486

Notes: dead = 0   perfect health = 1

Source: Kind et al., 1982

measures in particular. Since its introduction the QALY method has been the subject of much critical comment and debate (Baldwin et al., 1994). Some fundamental criticisms have been levelled by sociologists at the nature of the measurement procedures used in constructing the quality of life valuation matrix. According to Mulkay et al. (1987), the procedures are based on a number of contentious assumptions. For example, they question the implicit assumption made by health economists that the categories used in scaling levels of distress and disability actually capture the valuations people make in normal everyday circumstances. As they assert, 'ordinary people are only able to express their preferences through a measurement procedure which is constructed in terms of social scientist's preconceptions' (Mulkay et al., 1987, p. 557). Furthermore, Mulkay et al. challenge the notion that the valuations individuals make remain stable over time. They maintain that when 'we come to recognise the social character of the research process and the socially generated nature of subjects' responses, the assumption that the social researcher is eliciting relatively stable and context-free evaluations becomes much less plausible' (Mulkay et al., 1987, p. 556). In essence, the measurement procedure producing the smooth distribution of scores in the valuation matrix is seen as being artificial in nature. Quality of life scores are viewed as an artefact of a measurement process in which the numerical assessments made by respondents do not reflect the pre-existing values of ordinary people but are 'a result of respondent's recognition of a quantification already implicit in the analyst's (health economist's) pre-arranged categories' (Mulkay et al., 1987, p. 556).

Fundamental questions about the methodological thinking behind the construction of quality of life indicators have been raised by critics from a number of different disciplinary backgrounds. The view has been expressed that the phenomenon of the quality of life is much too complex to be captured by a single scale (Carr-Hill, 1991). Goodinson and Singleton (1989) question whether the original sample of 70 respondents used by Rosser and Kind (1978) was sufficiently representative of the general population to produce a valuation matrix for universal use. Some studies report marked differences between the assessments of the quality of life made by patients and doctors (Spitzer et al., 1981; Slevin et al., 1988).

Ethical objections have also been raised against using QALYs to help to make decisions about the allocation of healthcare resources. Using the cost-per-QALY approach is seen as being potentially iniquitous on account of the fact that it seems to reject the principle of equal access to resources according to need, in favour of a policy of distributing resources on the basis of the benefits obtained per unit of cost. Consequently, certain categories of patients may be discriminated against, such as those who are terminally ill or suffer from rare medical conditions that are relatively expensive to treat. The situation is exacerbated if resource allocation policy emphasises the economic goal of maximising the number of QALYs to be gained from an intervention or treatment. In the case of life-saving interventions, a QALY maximisation approach would give young patients priority over older patients, as the survival rate and life expectancy of the former are likely to be greater. However, if the objective is the wider goal of maximising total utility (i.e. distributing resources in such a way as to achieve the greatest benefits) greater weight may be given to the QALYs of some individuals or groups depending on their circumstances. For example, if there are two individuals suffering from the same medical condition and both are expected to gain the same number of QALYs following treatment, but one is a parent with young children and the other a single person with no dependants, then, all things being equal, total utility will be maximised if preference is given to the person with dependants (McKie et al., 1998, p. 52).

Concepts from health economics have been introduced into healthcare evaluation with increasing regularity over recent years as questions of cost-effectiveness, efficiency and equity have been addressed. The growing debate over the rationing of healthcare resources has also led to attempts to refine, modify and develop measures like QALYs. Much work remains to be done in this area. No matter what new techniques of measurement are devised in the interests of objectivity and rationality, ethical and political judgements will still be part of the decision-making process.

Summary

Professions

- The process by which an occupation develops the characteristics of a profession is referred to as 'professionalisation'. According to the trait theory approach professions have the following attributes: a specialised body of knowledge; autonomy of action; a code of ethics; a commitment to altruistic service. There is some debate as to whether or not nursing qualifies as a 'full' profession; it has been labelled a 'semi-profession' or 'para-profession'.

- Professions adopt collective strategies of occupational domination such as subordination, limitation and exclusion in order to maintain their power and influence. The de-professionalisation thesis and the proletarianisation thesis have been advanced by some theorists to account for the changing nature of the power relations between medical practitioners and other health professionals.

- Three broad overlapping stages in the development of professionalism in nursing have been identified. First there was the deferential nurse characteristic of the Nightingale era. Second, the early days of the professional project in nursing saw an attempt to create professional autonomy by means of exclusionary closure. Finally, there came the rise of the new professionalism, which emphasised the clinical nurse role and witnessed the creation of such specialist roles as 'nurse practitioner', thus effectively challenging the subservient role traditionally assigned to nursing.

Health promotion

- Health promotion relates to all aspects of life and lifestyle. It is about changing the behaviour of individuals and improving the social and environmental conditions in which they live. In broad conceptual terms health promotion activities can be identified as being primarily individually or collectively focused and as featuring a mode of intervention that is authoritative or negotiated. According to one classification there are four main strategies of health promotion: health persuasion techniques, personal counselling for health, legislative action and community development.

- It is possible to distinguish between sociological analyses *for* and sociological analyses *of* health promotion. In the case of the former, information and knowledge from sociological research can be used to inform policy and practice in health promotion. For example, studies by sociologists reveal how social norms and cultural values can influence the way people live their lives. Research in the sociology of health has also provided a rich vein of information on the nature of lay health beliefs and the workings of the lay referral system. As for the sociology *of* health promotion, this offers a critical analysis of the techniques and values underlying policy and practice. An ideology of individualism, coupled with a failure to appreciate that health is influenced by economic, social and environmental factors outside the direct control of the individual, can lead to victim blaming.

Health reforms and research

- The reforms contained in the NHS and Community Care Act 1990 were primarily aimed at improving efficiency through the introduction of a new style of public management. These reforms strengthened the role of managers, provided incentives to encourage collaboration with private sector organisations and paved the way for the creation of a competitive internal market. Supporters argue that the reduction of state intervention and the introduction of market principles return to individuals the power to take responsibility for their own lives and make choices in the marketplace for healthcare services. Critics maintain that the notion of consumer sovereignty is a feature of policy rhetoric but has yet to be realised in practice. The effects of these health reforms in terms of equity, efficiency and consumer choice will need to be closely monitored over the coming years.

- Following the health reforms of the early 1990s there has been a growing demand for information on the effectiveness, cost and quality of treatments and services. The RCT is a well-established research method in healthcare evaluation; however, difficulties can be encountered when trying to conduct such trials in certain treatment or health service contexts. Making decisions about the allocation of scarce resources requires good-quality objective information. The emphasis on cost-effectiveness means that economic concepts have been applied to healthcare issues with increasing enthusiasm over the last two decades. While health economists have developed some innovative measures, such as QALYs, these should not be taken at face value but consideration needs to be given to the methodological assumptions and value judgements on which they are founded.

Questions for discussion

1 What are the main characteristics of a profession? Which of the occupational groups in the healthcare sector are established professions and which, if any, are semi-professions? What are the disadvantages of professionalisation?

2 How is medical dominance defined and what are its essential features?

3 Do the policies and practices of health promotion constitute a technology of control or a form of individual/community empowerment?

4 How healthy is the *National* Health Service?

5 How might sociology make a contribution to the evaluation of healthcare services?

6 What role is there for the QALY method in the rationing of healthcare resources?

Further reading

Baldwin, S., Godfrey, C. and Propper, C. (eds) (1994) *Quality of Life: Perspectives and Policies*, London: Routledge.

Bunton, R., Nettleton, S. and Burrows, R. (1995) *The Sociology of Health Promotion*, London: Routledge.

Clarke, A. (1999) 'Evaluating healthcare', in *Evaluation Research: an Introduction to Principles, Methods and Practice*, London: Sage, Chapter 5, pp. 124–55.

Davies, C. (1995) *Gender and the Professional Predicament in Nursing*, Buckingham: Open University Press.

Freidson, E. (1983) 'The theory of professions – state of the art', in R. Dingwall and P. Lewis (eds), *The Sociology of Professions*, London: Macmillan.

Freidson, E. (1986) *Professional Powers: a Study of the Institutionalisation of Formal Knowledge*, London: University of Chicago Press.

Jenkinson, C. (1997) *Assessment and Evaluation of Health and Medical Care: a Methods Text*, Buckingham: Open University Press.

Mackay, L. (1990) 'Nursing: just another job?', in P. Abbott and C. Wallace (eds), *The Sociology of the Caring Professions*, London: Falmer Press.

Phillips, C., Palfrey, C. and Thomas, P. (1994) *Evaluating Health and Social Care*, London: Macmillan.

Riska, E. and Weger, K. (eds) (1993) *Gender, Work and Medicine: Women and the Medical Division of Labour*, London: Sage.

Talbot-Smith, A. and Pollock, A. M. (2006) *The New NHS: A Guide*, Abingdon: Routledge.

Glossary

Aetiology: The study of the cause of diseases.

Ageism: Refers to the stereotyping of individuals or groups of people on account of their age and unfairly discriminating against them as a result.

Amenable mortality: Deaths occurring before 75 years of age from causes that are considered amenable to medical intervention (e.g. breast cancer, leukaemia and hypertensive disorders).

Birth rate: The number of live births per 1,000 of the population over a period of time, usually a year.

Crude death rate: The simplest form of mortality rate, derived by dividing the number of deaths for an area by the population of that area. The area in question may be a country, city, town or local electoral ward or administrative district.

Culture: Socially transmitted values, attitudes, beliefs and patterns of behaviour shared by a population or society.

Disability-free life expectancy: Expected years of life free from limiting long-standing illness or disability.

Dizygotic twins: Commonly known as fraternal twins, begin life as two eggs fertilised by two separate sperm.

Doctrine of specific aetiology: The belief that a specific disease always has a specific cause.

Enacted stigma: The actual discrimination faced by individuals and groups in society on account of the perceived social unacceptability of their condition.

Epidemiology: The study of the distribution, causes and control of diseases in populations.

Ethnicity: Indicates identification with a particular group of people through a common heritage. Members of an ethnic group share common characteristics (e.g. language, religious faith and cultural traditions).

Ethnocentric: Believing that the people, traditions, customs and cultural practices of your own nationality, race or ethnic group are superior to those of other groups.

Felt stigma: Refers to both the shame associated with being labelled as socially unacceptable and the fear of enacted stigma.

Fertility rate: The number of births per 1,000 women aged 15–49 years in a given year.

Gerontology: The branch of medical science that deals with diseases and problems specific to old people. In its broadest sense the term is used to refer to the scientific study of the biological, psychological and socio-cultural aspects of the ageing process.

Healthy life expectancy: The measure of the balance between length of life and quality of life. It focuses on the 'quality-of-life' experienced by the individual, rather than concentrating on the mere presence or absence of disease.

Ideology: An organised body of beliefs, ideas and values that form the basis of a political or economic system: also used to refer to a body of ideas that reflect the social needs and aspirations of a group or class of people.

Infant mortality rate: Number of deaths during the first year of life per 1,000 live births.

Lay referral system: Refers to the social network of personal contacts that may influence an individual when he or she is deciding what action to take regarding a particular symptom episode.

Life course: An individual's passage through life, viewed as a sequence of significant life events, including birth, marriage, parenthood, divorce and retirement.

Life cycle: An individual's passage through age-based stages of development.

Life expectancy: The average number of years of life remaining at a given age.

Lifestyle: Refers to the general manner in which people live their lives; it encompasses their interests, attitudes, activities and actual behaviour. It is a feature that is focused upon when assessing the quality of life and promoting healthy behaviour.

Limiting long-standing illness: Chronic illness that the individual feels restricts his or her activities in some way.

Longitudinal study: A study which is based on collecting the same data at different points in time to enable the monitoring of change over time.

Monozygotic twins: Commonly known as identical twins, they begin life as one egg, which becomes fertilised by one sperm and divides into two eggs early in the gestational period.

Morbidity: The relative incidence of a particular disease.

Neonatal mortality: Deaths during the first four weeks of life.

Old-age dependency ratio: The number of people aged 65 years and over in comparison with the number of people of working age (i.e. 16 to 64 years of age).

Parasuicide: Non-fatal deliberate self-harm (i.e. attempted suicide).

Perinatal mortality: Stillbirths and deaths occurring during the first week of life.

Postneonatal mortality: Deaths after the first 28 days but before the end of the first year of life.

Preventable mortality: Deaths occurring before 75 years of age from causes that are considered to be preventable either through individual behaviour (e.g. lifestyle choices) and/or public health measures (e.g. immunisation programmes).

Primary deviance: Refers to those initial deviant acts or occasional transgressions, which arise from a variety of psychological and socio-cultural sources, and are explained away as a temporary aberration and do not lead to the development of a deviant identity or self-image.

Process of infantilisation: When the language and ideology of childhood is simply applied to other dependent groups.

Race: A group of people who are believed to be distinct from others on account of their physical characteristics. Racial classifications are based on biological criteria and morphological features. This contrasts with ethnicity where the emphasis is on social traits and not physical characteristics.

Racism: A distinction can be made between direct, indirect and institutional racism. *Direct racism* refers to situations in which people are treated less favourably (i.e. discriminated against) because of their race or ethnic background. *Indirect racism* occurs when services that are supposedly provided equally to all people are actually provided in a way that favours some ethnic groups at the expense of others. Institutional racism describes endemic indirect racism in an organisational setting where ignorance, prejudice or negative stereotyping becomes a feature of institutional processes and procedures.

Sample survey: A methodology employing questionnaires to collect data from a statistically representative sample selected from a larger population.

Secondary deviance: Arises as a result of the way in which the labelled individual or group responds to the reactions of others to their initial rule-breaking behaviour.

Secularisation: Has a number of meanings but generally refers to a situation where, at a societal level, religious values lose their social significance, there is a decline in religiosity and religious institutions come to have less authority.

Sick role: A socially prescribed role for the sick person.

Socialisation: The process by which individuals learn the normative patterns of behaviour, social values and beliefs characteristic of the group/society/culture in which they live.

Social capital: Refers to a feature of social structure and is considered to be a property or characteristic of a group or social network. Being part of a wider social network of contacts has social and economic benefits in that it provides a person with a sense of identity, security, safety and friendship. Social relationships and family connections can open up opportunities and life chances for the individual.

Social mobility: Movement one social class or social status group to another. This movement may be upwards (to a higher social group) or downwards (to a lower social group).

Social stigma: The result of severe societal reaction and social disapproval directed towards individuals or groups whose characteristics and beliefs are perceived to go against normative patterns of behaviour and culturally accepted practices.

Somatisation thesis: The idea that bodily symptoms can mask a real mental illness.

Standardised mortality ratio (SMR): The ratio of the *observed* number of deaths in an area to the number of deaths *expected* if the age-specific death rates for the standard population (e.g. the whole country) were applied to the population of the region.

Subculture: A social group within a society or national culture that has a distinctive lifestyle, patterns of behaviour and beliefs.

Sudden Infant Death Syndrome (SIDS): A sudden, unexpected death of an apparently healthy infant, usually during sleep; also referred to as 'cot death'.

Unavoidable mortality: Deaths occurring before 75 years of age from causes that are considered both not amenable to medical intervention and not preventable through changes in individual lifestyle or public health measures (e.g. cancers of the pancreas, ovary, and prostate).

References

Abbott, P. A. and Sapsford, R. J. (1987) *Women and Social Class*, London: Tavistock.

Abbott, P. and Sapsford, R. (2005) 'Living on the margins', *Policy Studies*, 26, 1: 29–46.

Abbott, P. and Wallace, C. (1990a) *An Introduction to Sociology: Feminist Perspectives*, London: Routledge.

Abbott, P. and Wallace, C. (eds) (1990b) *The Sociology of the Caring Professions*, London: Falmer.

Abercrombie, N. and Warde, A. *et al.* (1994) *Contemporary British Society*, 2nd edn, Cambridge: Polity Press.

Acheson, Sir D. (1998) *Independent Inquiry into Inequalities in Health: A Report*, London: Stationery Office. Available at: http://www.archive.official-documents.co.uk/document/doh/ih/ih.htm (accessed 4 July 2008).

Ackernecht, E. W. (1947) 'The role of medical history in medical education', *Bulletin of the History of Medicine*, 21.

Ahmad, W. and Bradby, H. (2008) 'Ethnicity and health', *Current Sociology*, 56, 1: 47–56.

Alanen, L. (1998) 'Children and the family order: constraints and competences', in I. Hutchby and J. Moran-Ellis (eds) *Children and Social Comptence: Arenas of Action*, London: Falmer Press.

Aldridge, J. and Becker, S. (1993a) 'Children as carers', *Archives of Disease in Childhood*, 69: 459–62.

Aldridge, J. and Becker, S. (1993b) 'Punishing children for caring: the hidden cost of young carers', *Children and Society*, 7, 4: 376–87.

Ali, R., Greer, J., Matthews, D., Murray, C., Robinson, S. and Sattar, G. (2006) *General Household Survey 2006: Overview Report*, Newport: Office for National Statistics. Available at: http://www.statistics.gov.uk/downloads/theme_compendia/GHS06/GHS2006overview.pdf (accessed 1 July 2008).

Allan, G. (1985) *Family Life*, Oxford: Basil Blackwell.

Allan, G. and Crow, G. (2001) *Families, Households and Society*, Basingstoke: Palgrave Macmillan.

Allsop, J. (1998) 'Health care', in P. Alcock, A. Erskine and M. May (eds) *The Student's Companion to Social Policy*, Oxford: Blackwell.

Almagor, R. C. (2009) 'Belgian euthanasia law: a critical analysis', *Journal of Medical Ethics*, 35, 436–39.

Alonzo, A. A. and Reynolds, N. R. (1995) 'Stigma, HIV and AIDS: an exploration and elaboration of a stigma trajectory', *Social Science & Medicine*, 41, 3: 303–15.

Anderson, C. (2004) 'An update on the effects of playing violent video games', *Journal of Adolescence*, 27: 113–22.

Anderson, M. (1971) *Family Structure in Nineteenth Century Lancashire*, Cambridge: Cambridge University Press.

Aneshensel, C. S. and Phelan, J. C. (2006) 'The study of mental health: surveying the field', in C. S. Aneshensel, C. S. and J. C. Phelan (eds) *Handbook of the Sociology of Mental Health*, New York: Springer.

Annandale, E. (1998) *The Sociology of Health and Medicine: A Critical Introduction*, Cambridge: Polity Press.

Anspach, R. R. (1979) 'From stigma to identity politics: political activism among the physically disabled and former mental patients', *Social Science & Medicine*, 13A: 765–73.

Arber, S. (1987) 'Social class, non-employment and chronic illness: continuing the inequalities in health debate', *British Medical Journal*, 294: 1069–73.

Arber, S. (1990a) 'Opening the "black box": inequalities in women's health', in P. Abbott and G. Payne (eds) *New Directions in the Sociology of Health*, London: Falmer Press.

Arber, S. (1990b) 'Revealing women's health: re-analysing the General Household Survey', in H. Roberts (ed.) *Women's Health Counts*, London: Routledge.

Arber, S., Gilbert, G. N. and Dale, A. (1985) 'Paid employment and women's health: a benefit or a source of role strain?', *Sociology of Health & Illness*, 7, 3: 375–400.

Arber, S. and Ginn, J. (1991a) *Gender and Later Life: A Sociological Analysis of Resources and Constraints*, London: Sage.

Arber, S. and Ginn, J. (1991b) 'The invisibility of age: gender and class in later life', *Sociological Review*, 39, 2: 260–91.

Arber, S. and Evandrou, M. (1993) 'Mapping the territory: ageing, independence and the life course', in S. Arber and M. Evandrou (eds) *Ageing, Independence and the Life Course*, London: Jessica Kingsley in association with the British Society of Gerontology.

Arber, S. and Ginn, J. (1993) 'Gender and inequalities in later life', *Social Science and Medicine*, 36, 1: 33–46.

Ariès, P. (1962) *Centuries of Childhood*, Jonathan Cape.

Ariès, P. (1974) *Western Attitudes Toward Death: From the Middle Ages to the Present*, London: Marion Boyars.

Ariès, P. (1981) *The Hour of Our Death*, London: Allen Lane.

Armitage, S. (1980) 'Non-compliant recipients of health care', *Nursing Times*, 76: 1–3.

Armstrong, D. (1983a) 'The fabrication of nurse–patient relationships', *Social Science and Medicine*, 17, 8: 457–60.

Armstrong, D. (1983b) *The Political Anatomy of the Body*, Cambridge: Cambridge University Press.

Armstrong, D. (1984) 'The patient's view', *Social Science & Medicine*, 18, 9: 737–44.

Armstrong, D. (1987) 'Silence and truth in death and dying', *Social Science & Medicine*, 24: 651–7.

Arney, W. R. (1982) *Power and the Profession of Obstetrics*, Chicago: University of Chicago Press.

Asmussen, K., Corlyon, J., Hauari, H. and La Placa, V. (2007) *Supporting Parents of Teenagers*, Research Report 830, London: Department for Education and Skills.

Asthana, S., Gibson, A., Moon, G., Brigham, P. and Dicker, J. (2004) 'The demographic and social class basis of inequality in self reported morbidity: an exploration using the Health Survey for England', *Journal of Epidemiology and Community Health*, 58, 4: 303–7.

Atchley, R. (1972) *The Social Forces in Later Life: An Introduction to Social Gerontology*, Belmont: Wadsworth.

Atchley, R. (1976) 'Selected social and psychological differences between men and women in later life', *Journal of Gerontology*, 31: 204–11.

Atkinson, J. M. (1978) *Discovering Suicide: Studies in the Social Organization of Sudden Death*, London: Macmillan.

Atkinson, J. M. and Drew, P. (1979) *Order in Court: The Organisation of Verbal Interaction in Judicial Settings*, London: Macmillan.

Atkinson, P. (1981) *The Clinical Experience: The Construction and Reconstruction of Medical Reality*, Aldershot: Gower.

Audit Commission (1986) *Making a Reality of Community Care*, London: HMSO.

Bajekal, M. (2005) 'Healthy life expectancy by area deprivation: magnitude and trends in England, 1994–1999', *Health Statistics Quarterly*, 25, Spring: 18–27.

Bajekal, M., Blane, D., Grewal, I., Karlsen, S. and Nazroo, J. (2004) 'Ethnic differences in influences on quality of life at older ages: a quantitative analysis', *Ageing & Society*, 24: 709–28.

Baldwin, S., Godfrey, C. and Propper, C. (eds) (1994) *Quality of Life: Perspectives and Policies*, London: Routledge.

Banks, M. H., Beresford, S. A. A., Morrell, D. C., Waller, J. J. and Watkins. C. J. (1975) 'Factors influencing the demand for primary medical care in women aged 20–44 years: a preliminary report', *International Journal of Epidemiology*, 4, 3: 189–95.

Barber, B. (1963) 'Some problems in the sociology of professions', *Daedalus*, 92: 669–88.

Barbigian, H. (1985) 'Schizophrenia epidemiology', in H. Kaplan and E. Saddock (eds) *Comprehensive Textbook of Psychiatry: IV*, Baltimore: Williams and Wilkins.

Barefoot, J. C., Maynard, K. E., Beckham, J. C., Brummett, B. H., Hooker, K. and Siegler, I. C. (1998) 'Trust, health, and longevity', *Journal of Behavioral Medicine*, 21, 6: 517–26.

Barham, P. and Hayward, R. (1996) 'The lives of "users"', in T. Heller, J. Reynolds, R. Gomm, R. Muston and S. Pattison (eds) *Mental Health Matters: A Reader*, Basingstoke: Macmillan in association with Open University Press.

Barnes, H. and Parry, J. (2004) 'Renegotiating identity and relationships: men and women's adjustments to retirement', *Ageing & Society*, 24: 213–33.

Barnes, M. and Morris, K. (2007) 'Networks, connectedness and resilience: learning from the children's fund in context', *Social Policy and Society*, 6: 193–7.

Barrow, S. and Harrison, R. A. (2005) 'Unsung heroes who put their lives at risk? Informal caring, health and neighbourhood attachment', *Journal of Public Health*, 27, 3: 292–7.

Bartley, M. (1987) 'Unemployment and health: selection or causation – a false antithesis', *Sociology of Health & Illness*, 10, 1: 41–67.

Bartley, M. (1994) 'Unemployment and ill health: understanding the relationship', *Journal of Epidemiology and Community Health*, 48: 333–7.

Bartley, M. (2004) *Health Inequality: An introduction to theory, concepts and methods*, Cambridge: Polity.

Barton, R. (1965) *Institutional Neurosis*, 2nd edn, Bristol: Wright.

Bauman, Z. (2001) *Community: Seeking Safety in an Insecure World*, Cambridge: Polity.

Bayley, M. (1973) *Mental Handicap and Community Care: A Study of Mentally Handicapped People in Sheffield*, London: Routledge and Kegan Paul.

Beattie, A. (1991) 'Knowledge and control in health promotion: a test case for social policy and social theory', in J. Gabe, M. Calnan and M. Bury (eds) *The Sociology of the Health Service*, London: Routledge.

Beaumont, J. G. and Kenealy, P. M. (2004) 'Quality of life perceptions and social comparisons in healthy old age', *Ageing and Society*, 24: 755–69.

Bebbington, P. E. (1987) 'Marital status and depression: a study of English national admission statistics', *Acta Psychiatrica Scandinavia*, 75: 640–50.

Beck, U. (1992) *Risk Society: Towards a New Modernity*, London: Sage.

Beck, U. and E. Beck-Gernsheim (2002) *Individualisation*, London: Sage.

Becker, E. (1973) *The Denial of Death*, New York: Collier-Macmillan.

Becker, H. S. (1963) *Outsiders*, New York: Free Press.

Bell, C. and Newby, H. (1971) *Community Studies*, London: Allen and Unwin.

Belle, D. (1990) 'Poverty and women's health', *American Psychologist*, 45, 3: 385–9.

Bender, T. (1978) *Community and Social Change in America*, New Brunswick, NJ: Rutgers University Press.

Bengtson, V. L., Silverstein, M., Putney, N. M. and Gans, D. (eds) (2009) *Handbook of Theories of Aging*, New York: Springer Publishing Company.

Bengtson, V. L., Gans, D., Putney, N. M. and Silverstein, M. (2009) 'Theories about age and aging', in V. L. Bengtson *et al.* (eds) *ibid.*, pp. 3–24.

Benzeval, M., Judge, K. and Whitehead, M. (eds) (1995) *Tackling Inequalities in Health: An Agenda for Action*, London: King's Fund.

Beral, V. (1987) 'Have the changes in women's employment affected their health?', in H. Graheme (ed.) *Women, Health and Work*, London: Women's Medical Federation.

Berger, B. and Berger, P. (1983) *The War Over the Family: Capturing the Middle Ground*, London: Hutchinson.

Berger, P. L. and Berger, B. (1976) *Sociology: A Biographical Approach*, Harmondsworth: Penguin.

Bergner, M., Bobbit, R. A., Kressel, S., Pollard, W. E., Gilson, B. S. and Morris, J. R. (1976) 'The sickness impact profile: conceptual formulation and methodology for the development of a health status measure', *International Journal of Health Services*, 6: 393–415.

Berk, R. A. and Rossi, P. H. (1990) *Thinking About Program Evaluation*, Newbury Park, CA: Sage.

Bernard, J. (1976) *The Future of Marriage*, Harmondsworth: Penguin.

Bernard, M. and Meade, K. (eds) (1993) *Women Come of Age: Perspectives on the Lives of Older Women*, London: Edward Arnold.

Berthoud, R. (1986) *Selective Social Security*, London: Policy Studies Institute.

Berthoud, R. and Nazroo, J. (1997) 'The mental health of ethnic minorities', *New Community*, 23, 3: 309–24.

Bethune, A., Harding, S., Scott, A. and Ffilakti, H. (1995) 'Mortality of longitudinal study 1971 and 1981 census cohorts', in F. Drever (ed.) *Occupational Health – Decennial Supplement*, London: HMSO.

Bhopal, R. S. (2007) *Ethnicity, Race and Health in Multicultural Societies: Foundations for better epidemiology, public health, and health care*, Oxford: Oxford University Press.

Bhopal, R. and White, M. (1993) 'Health promotion for ethnic minorities: past, present and future', in W. I. U. Ahmad (ed.) *'Race' and Health in Contemporary Britain*, Buckingham: Open University Press.

Bhui, K. (1999) 'Common mental disorders among people with origins in or immigrant from India and Pakistan', *International Review of Psychiatry*, 11: 136–44.

Bhui, K., Abdi, A., Abdi, M., Pereira, S., Dualeh, M., Robertson, D., Sathyamoorthy, G. and Ismail, H. (2003) 'Traumatic events, migration characteristics and psychiatric symptoms among Somali refugees', *Social Psychiatry and Psychiatric Epidemiology*, 38: 35–43.

Biener, L. (1983) 'Perceptions of patients by emergency room staff: substance abusers versus non-substance abusers', *Journal of Health and Social Behavior*, 24: 264–75.

Blackburn, A. M. (1989) 'Problems of terminal care in elderly patients', *Palliative Medicine*, 3: 203–6.

Blackhall, L. J., Murphy, S. T., Frank, G., Michel, V. and Azen, S. (1995) 'Ethnicity and attitudes toward patient autonomy', *Journal of the American Medical Association*, 274, 10: 820–5.

Blakely, T. A., Collings, S. C. D. and Atkinson, J. (2003) 'Unemployment and suicide: evidence for a causal association', *Journal of Epidemiology and Community Health*, 57: 594–600.

Blakemore, K. (1989) 'Does age matter? The case of old age in minority ethnic groups', in B. Bytheway, T. Keil, P. Allatt and A. Bryman (eds) *Becoming and Being Old*, London: Sage.

Blane, D. (1985) 'An assessment of the Black Report's "explanations" of health inequalities', *Sociology of Health & Illness*, 7, 3: 423–45.

Blane, D., Smith, G. D. and Bartley, M. (1990) 'Social class differences in years of potential life lost: size, trends and principal causes', *British Medical Journal*, 301: 429–32.

Blane, D. (1991) 'Inequality and social class', in G. Scambler (ed.) *Sociology as Applied to Medicine*, London: Bailliere Tindall.

Blauner, R. (1966) 'Death and social structure', *Psychiatry*, 29: 378–94.

Blaxter, M. and Paterson, E. (1982) *Mothers and Daughters: A Three Generational Study of Health Attitudes and Behaviour*, London: Heinemann Educational Books.

Blaxter, M. (1983) 'The cause of disease: women talking', *Social Science & Medicine*, 17: 59–69.

Blaxter, M. (1985) 'Self-definition of health status and consulting rate in primary care', *Quarterly Journal of Social Affairs*, 1: 131–71.

Blaxter, M. (1987) 'Self-reported health' in B. D. Cox, M. Blaxter, A. L. J. Buckle, N. P. Fenner, J. F. Golding, M. Gore, F. A. Huppert, J. Nickson, Sir M. Roth, J. Stark, M. E. J. Wadsworth and M. Whichelow, *The Health and Lifestyle Survey: preliminary report*, London: The Health Promotion Research Trust.

Blaxter, M. (1989) 'A comparison of measures of morbidity', in A. J. Fox (ed.) *Health Inequalities in European Countries*, Aldershot: Gower.

Blaxter, M. (1990) *Health and Lifestyle*, London: Routledge.

Blennerhassett, S., Farrant, W. and Jones, J. (1989) 'Support for community health projects in the UK: a role for the NHS', *Health Promotion*, 4, 3: 199–206.

Bloor, M. and Horobin, G. (1975) 'Conflict and conflict resolution in doctor/patient interactions', in C. Cox and A. Mead (eds) *A Sociology of Medical Practice*, London: CollierMacmillan.

Bloor, M., Samphier, M. and Prior, L. (1987) 'Artefact explanations of inequalities in health: an assessment of the evidence', *Sociology of Health & Illness*, 9, 3: 231–64.

Blumer, H. (1969) *Symbolic Interactionism: Perspective and Method*, Englewood Cliffs, NJ: Prentice-Hall.

BMA (1999) *Growing up in Britain: Ensuring a Healthy Future for Our Children: A Study of 0–5 Year Olds*, London: British Medical Association.

BMA (2003) *Housing and Health: Building for the Future*, London: British Medical Association.

BMA (2006) *Child and Adolescent Mental Health: A Guide for Healthcare Professionals*, London: British Medical Association. Available at: http://www.bma.jorg.uk?images/ChildAdolescentMental Health_tcm41–20748.pdf (accessed 20 March 2009).

Boardman, A. P., Hodgson, R. E., Lewis, M. and Allen, K. (1997) 'Social indicators and the prediction of psychiatric admission in different diagnostic groups', *British Journal of Psychiatry*, 171: 457–62.

Boase, T. S. R. (1972) *Death in the Middle Ages*, London: Thames & Hudson.

Boeije, H. R., Duijnstee, M. S. H. and Grypdonck, M. H. F. (2003) 'Continuation of caregiving among partners who give total care to spouses with multiple sclerosis', *Health and Social Care in the Community*, 11, 3: 242–52.

Bond, J. and Coleman, P. (eds) (1990) *Ageing and Society: An Introduction to Social Gerontology*, London: Sage.

Bone, M. *et al.* (1995) *Health Expectancy and its Uses*, London: HMSO.

Boneham, M. and Sixsmith, J. (2006) 'The voices of older women in a deprived Community: issues of health and social capital', *Social Science and Medicine*, 62: 269–79.

Bornat, J., Phillipson, C. and Ward, S. (1985) *A Manifesto for Old Age*, London: Pluto Press.

Bottorff, J. L. (2005) 'Nurse–patient interaction', in J. J. Fitzpatrick and M. Wallace (eds) *Encyclopedia of Nursing Research*, 2nd edn, New York: Springer Publishing, pp. 381–2.

Bourdieu, P. (1984) *Distinction: A Social Critique of the Judgment of Taste*, London: Routledge.

Bourke, J. (1994) *Working-Class Cultures in Britain, 1890–1960*, London: Routledge.

Bowling, A. (2005*) Measuring Health: A review of quality of life measurement scales*, 3rd edn, Maidenhead: Open University Press.

Bowling, A. and Gabriel, Z. (2007) 'Lay theories of quality of life in older age', *Ageing & Society*, 27: 827–48.

Bowling, A. and Windsor, J. (2001) 'Towards the good life: a population survey of dimensions of quality of life', *Journal of Happiness Studies*, 2, 1: 55–81.

Boyle, R. and Hibberd, M. (2005) *Review of Research on the Impact of Violent Computer Games on Young People*, Stirling: Stirling Media Research Institute.

Bradbury, M. (1999) *Representations of Death: A Social and Psychological Perspective*, London: Routledge.

Bradbury, M. (2000) 'The "good death"?', in D. Dickenson, M. Johnson and J. S. Katz (eds) *Death, Dying and Bereavement*, London: Open University Press/Sage, pp. 59–63.

Bradford, M. and Winn, S. (1993) 'Practice nursing and health promotion: a case study', in J. Wilson-Barnett and J. Macleod Clark (eds) *Research in Health Promotion and Nursing*, London: Macmillan.

Bradley, C. P., Crowley, M., Barry, C., Stevenson, F. A., Britten, N. and Barber, N. (2000) 'Patient-centredness and outcomes in primary care', *British Journal of General Practice*, 50, 451: 149.

Bradshaw, J. (1988) 'Financing private care for the elderly', in S. Baldwin *et al.* (eds) *Social Security and Community Care*, Aldershot: Avebury.

Braithwaite, V. A. and Gibson, D. M. (1987) 'Adjustment to retirement: what we know and what we need to know', *Ageing & Society*, 7: 1–18.

Bramston, P., Pretty, G. and Chipuer, H. (2002) Unravelling subjective quality of life: an investigation of individual and community determinants', *Social Indicators Research*, 59, 3: 261–74.

Brannen, J., Dodd, K., Oakley, A. and Storey, P. (1994) *Young People, Health and Family Life*, Buckingham: Open University Press.

Bray, H. (2008) '2006-based national population projections for the UK and constituent countries', *Population Trends*, 131: 8–18.

Brayshaw, A. J. (1980) *Public Policy and Family Life*, London: Policy Studies Institute.

Breslow, L. (1995) 'A health promotion primer for the 1990s', in B. Davey, A. Gray and C. Seale (eds) *Health and Disease: A Reader*, 2nd edn, Buckingham: Open University Press.

Britton, M. (1990) *Mortality and Geography: A Review in the Mid-1980s England and Wales*, Series DS, No. 9, London: HMSO.

Bromley, D. B. (1974) *The Psychology of Human Ageing*, Harmondsworth: Penguin.

Brown, G. W. (1981) 'Life events, psychiatric disorder and physical illness', *Journal of Psychosomatic Research*, 25: 461–73.

Brown, G. W. (1989) 'Life events and measurement', in G. W. Brown and T. O. Harris (eds) *Life Events and Illness*, London: The Guilford Press.

Brown, G. W. (1996) 'Life events, loss and depressive disorders', in T. J. Heller *et al.* (eds), op. cit.

Brown, G. W. and Harris, T. O. (1978) *Social Origins of Depression: A Study of Psychiatric Disorder in Women*, London: Tavistock.

Brown, G. W., Bhrolchain, M. N. and Harris, T. (1981) 'Social class and psychiatric disturbance among women in an urban population', in O. Grusky and M. Pollner (eds) *The Sociology of Mental Illness: Basic Studies*, New York: Holt, Rinehart and Winston.

Brown, G. W., Andrews, B., Harris, T. O., Adler, Z. and Bridge, L. (1986) 'Social support, self-esteem and depression', *Psychological Medicine*, 16: 813–31.

Brown, G. W. and Harris, T. O. (1989) 'Interlude: the origins of life events and difficulties', in G. W. Brown and T. O. Harris (eds) *Life Events and Illness*, London: The Guilford Press.

Buckingham, D. with Whiteman, N., Willett, R. and Burn, A. (2007) *The impact of the media on children and young people with a particular focus on computer games and the internet*, a report prepared for the Byron Review on Children and New Technology, Commissioned by the Department for Children, Schools and Families. Available at: http://www.dcsf.gov.uk/byronreview/pdfs/Buckingham%20Impact%20of%20Media%20Literature%20Review%20for%20the%20Byron%20Review.pdf (accessed 14 March 2009).

Buckman, R. (1992) *How to Break Bad News: A Guide for Healthcare Professionals*, London: Pan Books.

Buckman, R. (1998) 'Communication in palliative care: a practical guide', in D. Doyle, G. W. C. Hanks, N. MacDonald (eds) *Oxford Textbook of Palliative Medicine*, 2nd edn, Oxford: Oxford University Press, pp. 141–56.

Bulmer, M. (1987) *The Social Basis of Community Care*, London: Allen and Unwin.

Bungay, H. (2005) 'Cancer and health policy: the postcode lottery of care', *Social Policy and Administration*, 39, 1: 35–48.

Bunton, R., Nettleton, S. and Burrows, R. (eds) (1995) *The Sociology of Health Promotion: Critical Analyses of Consumption, Lifestyle and Risk*, London: Routledge.

Burgess, E. W. (ed.) (1960) *Aging in Western Societies*, Chicago: University of Chicago Press.

Burgess, R. G. (ed.) (1986) *Key Variables in Social Investigation*, London: Routledge and Kegan Paul.

Burgoyne, J. (1987) 'Change, gender and the life course', in G. Cohen (ed.) *Social Change and the Life Course*, London: Tavistock.

Burr, V. (1995) *An Introduction to Social Constructionism*, London: Routledge.

Burrows, R., Nettleton, S. and Bunton, R. (1995) 'Sociology and health promotion: health, risk and consumption under late modernity', in R. Bunton, S. Nettleton and R. Burrows (eds), op. cit.

Bury, M. R. (1986) 'Social constructionism and the development of medical sociology', *Sociology of Health & Illness*, 8: 137–71.

Bury, M. (1997) *Health and Illness in a Changing Society*, London: Routledge.

Busfield, J. (1988) 'Mental illness as social product or social construct: a contradiction in feminists' arguments?', *Sociology of Health & Illness*, 10, 4: 521–42.

Busfield, J. (2001) 'Introduction: rethinking the sociology of mental health', in J. Busfield (ed.) *Rethinking the Sociology of Mental Health*, Oxford: Blackwell, pp. 1–16.

Butterworth, E. and Weir, D. (1984) *The New Sociology of Modern Britain*, Aylesbury: Fontana.

Bytheway, B. (1995) *Ageism*, Buckingham: Open University Press.

Byrne, P. and Long, B. (1976) *Doctors Talking to Patients*, London: HMSO.

Byrne, D., Harrisson, S., Keithly, J. *et al.* (1986) *Housing and Health: The Relationship between Housing Conditions and the Health of Council Tenants*, Aldershot: Gower.

Calnan, M. (1984) 'The functions of the hospital emergency department: a study of patient demand', *Journal of Emergency Medicine*, 2: 57–63.

Calnan, M. (1986) 'Maintaining health and preventing illness: a comparison of the perceptions of women from different social classes', *Health Promotion*, 1, 2: 167–77.

Calnan, M. (1987) *Health and Illness: The Lay Perspective*, London: Tavistock.

Caplan, R. L. (1989) 'The commodification of American health care', *Social Science and Medicine*, 28, 11: 1139–49.

Carpenter, L. and Brockington, I. F. (1980) 'The study of mental illness in Asians, West Indians and Africans living in Manchester', *British Journal of Psychiatry*, 137: 201–5.

Carpenter, M. (1993) 'The subordination of nurses in health care: towards a social divisions approach', in E. Riska and K. Weger (eds) *Gender, Work and Medicine: Women and the Medical Division of Labour*, London: Sage.

Carr, D. (2007) 'Death and dying', in G. Ritzer (ed.) *Blackwell Encyclopedia of Sociology*, Blackwell Publishing, Blackwell Reference Online: http://www.blackwellreference.com/public/tocnode?id=g9781405124331_chunk_g978140512433110_ss1-4 (accessed 22 June 2009).

Carr-Hill, R. (1987) 'The inequalities in health debate: a critical review of the issues', *Journal of Social Policy*, 16, 4: 509–42.

Carr-Hill, R. A. (1991) 'Allocating resources to health care: is the QALY a technical solution to a potential problem?', *International Journal of Health Services*, 21, 2: 351–63.

Carstairs, V. and Morris, R. (1991) *Deprivation and Health in Scotland*, Aberdeen University Press.

Carta, M. G., Bernal, M., Hardoy, M. C., Haro-Abad, J. M. *et al.* (2005) 'Migration and mental health in Europe', *Clinical Practice and Epidemiology in Mental Health*, 1, 13. Also available at: http://www.cpementalhealth.com/content/1/1/13 (accessed 1 April 2009).

Cartwright, A. (1964) *Human Relationships in Hospital Care*, London: Routledge and Kegan Paul.

Cartwright, A. (1967) *Patients and Their Doctors*, London: Routledge and Kegan Paul.

Cartwright, A. and O'Brien, M. (1976) 'Social class variations in health care and in the nature of general practitioner consultations', in Stacey, M. (ed.) *The Sociology of the National Health Service*, University of Keele, Sociological Review Monograph 22.

Cartwright, A. and Anderson, R. (1981) *General Practice Revisited: A Second Study of Patients and Their Doctors*, London: Tavistock Publications.

Central Statistical Office (1993a) *Social Trends 23*, London: HMSO.

Central Statistical Office (1993b) *Monthly Digest of Statistics*, No. 570, London: HMSO.

Central Statistical Office (1994) *Social Trends 24*, London: HMSO.

Chan, W. S. C., Yip, P. S. F., Wong, P. W. C. and Chen, E. Y. H. (2007) 'Suicide and unemployment: what are the missing links?', *Archives of Suicide Research*, 11, 4: 327–35.

Charles, N. and Davies, C. (2005) 'Studying the particular, illuminating the general: community studies and community in Wales', *Sociological Review*, 56: 672–90.

Charmaz, K. (1980) *The Social Reality of Death: Death in Contemporary America*, Reading, MA: Addison-Wesley.

Chesler, P. (1972) *Women and Madness*, New York: Doubleday.

Children's Society (2006) *Good Childhood? A question for our times*, launch report of the Good Childhood Inquiry, London: The Children's Society. Available at: http://www.childrenssociety.org.uk. (accessed 12 March 2009).

ChildWise (2008) *The Monitor Trends Report*, Norwich: ChildWise.

Cho, C-H. and Cheon, H. (2005) 'Children's exposure to negative internet content: Effects of family context', *Journal of Broadcasting and Electronic Media*, 49, 4: 488–509.

Chrisman, N. J. (1977) 'The health-seeking process: an approach to the natural history of illness', *Culture, Medicine and Psychiatry*, 1: 351–77.

Christen, R. N., Alder, J. and Bitzer, J. (2008) 'Gender differences in physicians' communicative skills and their influence on patient satisfaction in gynaecological outpatient consultations', *Social Science & Medicine*, 66: 1474–83.

Christensen, P. H. (1998) 'Differences and similarity: how children's competence is constituted in illness and its treatment', in I. Hutchby and J. Moran-Ellis (eds) op. cit.

Clancy, K. and Gove, W. (1974) 'Sex differences in mental illness: an analysis of response bias in self-reports', *American Journal of Sociology*, 80: 205–15.

Clare, A. (1980) *Psychiatry in Dissent: Controversial Issues in Thought and Practice*, 2nd edn, London: Routledge.

Clark, D. (1993) 'Wither the hospices?' in D. Clark (ed.) *The Future of Palliative Care*, Buckingham: Open University Press.

Clark, D. (1998) 'Originating a movement: Cicely Saunders and the development of St Christopher's Hospice', *Mortality*, 3, 1: 43–63.

Clark, D. (1999a) ' "Total pain": disciplinary power and the body in the work of Cicely Saunders, 1958–1967', *Social Science & Medicine*, 49: 727–36.

Clark, D. (1999b) 'Cradled to the grave? Preconditions for the hospice movement in the UK, 1948–1967', *Mortality*, 4: 225–47.

Clark, D. (2002) 'Between hope and acceptance: the medicalisation of dying', *British Medical Journal*, 324, 905–7, 13 April.

Clark, J. (2003) 'Patient centred death', *British Medical Journal*, 327: 174–5, 26 July.

Clark, J. A. and Mishler, E. G. (1992) 'Attending to patients' stories: reframing the clinical task', *Sociology of Health & Illness*, 14, 3: 344–72.

Clements, L. (2004) *Community Care and the Law*, London: Legal Action Group.

Cochrane, A. L. (1972) *Effectiveness and Efficiency*, London: Nuffield Provincial Hospitals Trust.

Cochrane, R. and Bal, S. S. (1989) 'Mental hospital admission rates of immigrants to England: a comparison of 1971 and 1981', *Social Psychiatry and Psychiatric Epidemiology*, 24: 2–11.

Cockerham, W. C. (1981) *Sociology of Mental Disorder*, Englewood Cliffs, NJ: Prentice-Hall.

Cockerham, W. (2000) *Medical Sociology*, Upper Saddler River, NJ: Prentice-Hall.

Coffield, F. (1987) 'From the celebration to the marginalisation of youth', in G. Cohen (ed.) *Social Change and the Life Course*, London: Tavistock.

Cohen, G. (ed.) (1987) *Social Change and the Life Course*, London: Tavistock.

Cohen, J., Marcoux, I., Bilsen, J., Deboosere, P., van der Wal, G. and Deliens, L. (2006) 'European public acceptance of euthanasia: socio-demographic and cultural factors associated with the acceptance of euthanasia in 33 European countries', *Social Science & Medicine*, 63, 3: 743–56.

Cohen, R. and Hart, T. (1988) *Student Psychiatry Today: A Comprehensive Textbook*, Oxford: Butterworth and Heinemann.

Cole-Hamilton, I. and Lang, T. (1986) *Tightening Belts: A Report on the Impact of Poverty on Food*, London: London Food Commission.

Coleman, D. and Salt, J. (1992) *The British Population: Patterns, Trends and Processes*, Oxford: Oxford University Press.

Coleman, J. (1990) *The Nature of Adolescence*, 2nd edn, London: Routledge.

Coleman, J. and Hagnell, A. (2007) 'The nature of risk and resilience in adolescence', in J. Coleman and A. Hagnell (eds) *Adolescence, Risk and Resilience: Against the Odds*, Chichester: John Wiley and Sons Ltd, pp. 1–16.

Coleman, J. and Hagnell, A. (eds) (2007) *Adolescence, Risk and Resilience: Against the Odds*, Chichester: John Wiley and Sons Ltd.

Coleman, J. and Hendry, L. B. (1999) *The Nature of Adolescence*, London: Routledge.

Coleman, J. and Schofield, J. (2007) *Key Data on Adolescence*, Brighton: Trust for Study of Adolescence.

Coleman, J. S. and Husen, T. (1985) *Becoming Adult in a Changing Society*, Paris: Organisation for Economic Co-operation and Development.

Comaroff, J. (1976) 'Communicating information about non-fatal illnesses: the strategies of a group of general practitioners', *Sociological Review*, 24, 2: 269–90.

Connelly, J. and Crown, J. (1994) *Homelessness and Ill Health*, London: Royal College of Physicians.

Cooper, H. (2002) 'Investigating socio-economic explanations of gender and ethnic inequalities in health', *Social Science & Medicine*, 54: 693–706.

Cooper, H., Arber, S. and Fee, L. *et al.* (1999) *The Influence of Social Support and Social Capital on Health*, London: HEA.

Copp, G. (1998) 'A review of current theories of death and dying', *Journal of Advanced Nursing*, 28, 2: 382–90.

Corea, G. (1985) 'The reproductive brothel', in G. Corea and R. Duelli Klein (eds) *Man-Made Women: How New Reproductive Technologies Affect Women*, London: Hutchinson.

Corner, J. L. and Dunlop, R. (1997) 'New approaches to care', in D. Clark, J. Hockley and S. Ahmedzai (eds) *New Themes in Palliative Care*, Buckingham: Open University Press, pp. 288–302.

Cornwell, J. (1984) *Hard Earned Lives: Accounts of Health and Illness from East London*, London: Tavistock Press.

Corr, C. A. (1992) 'A task-based approach to coping with dying', *Omega*, 24, 2: 81–94.

Costello, J. (2000) 'Truth telling and the dying patient: a silent conspiracy', *International Journal of Palliative Nursing*, 6: 152–8.

Costello, J. (2001) 'Nursing older dying patients: findings from an ethnographic study of death and dying in elderly care wards', *Journal of Advanced Nursing*, 35, 1: 59–68.

Costello, J. (2006) 'Dying well: nurses' experiences of "good and bad" deaths', *Journal of Advanced Nursing*, 54, 5: 594–601.

Coulter, A. (1991) 'Evaluating the outcomes of health care', in J. Gabe, M. Calnan and M. Bury (eds) *The Sociology of the Health Service*, London: Routledge.

Cox, B. D., Blaxter, M. *et al.* (1987) *The Health and Lifestyle Survey: preliminary report*, London: The Health Promotion Research Trust.

Craib, I. (1984) *Modern Social Theory: From Parsons to Habermas*, Hemel Hempstead: Harvester Wheatsheaf.

Crawford, R. (1977) 'You are dangerous to your health: the ideology and politics of victim blaming', *International Journal of Health Services*, 7, 4: 663–80.

Creer, C. and Wing, J. K. (1974) *Schizophrenia at Home*, London: National Schizophrenia Fellowship.

Cribb, A. (1993) 'Health promotion – a human science', in J. Wilson-Barnett and J. Macleod Clark (eds) *Research in Health Promotion and Nursing*, London: Macmillan.

Cribier, F. (1981) 'Changing retirement patterns of the seventies: the example of a generation of Parisian salaried workers', *Ageing & Society*, 1: 51–71.

Cuff, E. C., Sharrock, W. W. and Francis, D. W. (1990) *Perspectives in Sociology*, 3rd edn, London: Unwin Hyman.

Cumming, E. and Henry, W. E. (1961) *Growing Old, the Process of Disengagement*, New York: Basic Books.

Cumming, E. (1963) 'Further thoughts on the theory of disengagement', *International Social Science Journal*, XV: 3.

Cunningham, H. (1995) *Children and Childhood in Western Society since 1500*, Harlow: Longman.

Cunningham, H. (2006) *The Invention of Childhood*, London: BBC Books.

Currer, C. (1986) 'Concepts of well- and ill-being: the case of Pathan mothers in Britain', in C. Currer and M. Stacey (eds) *Concepts of Health, Illness and Disease: A Comparative Perspective*, Leamington Spa: Berg.

Currer, C. and Stacey, M. (eds) (1986) *Concepts of Health, Illness and Disease: A Comparative Perspective*, Leamington Spa: Berg.

Curtis, S. and Jones, I. R. (1998) 'Is there a place for geography in the analysis of health inequality?', *Sociology of Health & Illness*, 20, 5: 645–72.

Daatland, S. O. and Biggs, S. (eds) (2006) *Aging and Diversity: Multiple pathways and cultural migrations*, Bristol: Policy Press.

Dahlberg, L., Demack, S. and Bambra, C. (2007) 'Age and gender of informal carers: a population-based study in the UK', *Health and Social Care in the Community*, 15, 5: 439–45.

Dain, N. (1994) 'Reflections on antipsychiatry and stigma in the history of American psychiatry', *Hospital and Community Psychiatry*, 45, 10: 1010–14.

Dalley, G. (1988) *Ideologies of Caring: Rethinking Community and Collectivism*, London: Macmillan.

Daly, J. and McDonald, I. (1992) 'Introduction: the problem as we saw it', in J. Daly, I. McDonald and E. Willis (eds) *Researching Health Care: Designs, Dilemmas, Disciplines*, London: Tavistock/Routledge.

Davey, B. (2000) 'The blue spotted patient: do-not-resuscitate decisions in the acute surgical wards of an English district general hospital', in D. Dickenson, J. Johnson and J. S. Katz (eds) *Death, Dying and Bereavement*, London: Open University Press/Sage, pp. 250–62.

Davies, C. (1977) 'Continuities in the development of hospital nursing in Britain', *Journal of Advanced Nursing*, 2: 479–93.

Davies, C. (1995) *Gender and the Professional Predicament in Nursing*, Buckingham: Open University Press.

Davis, A., Llewellyn, S. P. and Parry, G. (1985) 'Women and mental health: a guide for the approved social worker', in E. Brook and A. Davis (eds) *Women, the Family and Social Work*, London: Tavistock.

Day, R. (2008) 'Local environments and older people's health: Dimensions from a comparative qualitative study in Scotland', *Health & Place*, 14: 299–312.

DeBord, K. (1999) *Parenting Teens*, Raleigh, NC: North Carolina Cooperative Extension Service. Available at: http://www.ces.ncsu.edu/depts/fcs/pdfs/fcs422.pdf (accessed 5 July 2009).

Deakin, N. (1994) *The Politics of Welfare: Continuities and Change*, London: Harvester Wheatsheaf.

Decker, G. M. (2005) 'Complementary and alternative medicine (CAM) therapies', in C. H. Yarbro, M. H. Frogge and M. Goodman (eds) *Cancer Nursing: Principles and Practice*, 6th revised edn, Massachusetts: Jones and Bartlett Publishers Inc., pp. 590–623.

Delphy, C. (1984) *Close to Home: A Materialist Analysis of Women's Oppression*, London: Hutchinson.

Denzin, N. K. (1970) 'Developmental theories of self and childhood: Some conceptions and misconceptions', revised version of a paper presented at the Annual Meeting of the American Sociology Association, quoted in Murcott, A. (1980) 'The social construction of teenage pregnancy: a problem in the ideologies of childhood and reproduction', *Sociology of Health & Illness*, 2, 1: 1–23.

Department for Communities and Local Government (2007) 'Survey of English Housing, Preliminary Results: 2006/07', *Health Statistics Summary*, 027.

Department for Education and Skills (2001) *Promoting Children's Mental Health within Early Years and School Settings*, Nottingham: DfES Publications.

Department for Education and Skills (2004) *Every Child Matters: Change for Children*, Nottingham: DfES Publications. Also available at: http://www.everychild matters.gov.uk/ (accessed 28 March 2009).

Department of Health (1989) *Caring for People, Community Care in the Next Decade and Beyond*, London: HMSO.

Department of Health (1991) *The Health of the Nation: A Consultative Document for Health in England*, London: HMSO.

Department of Health (1992) *The Health of the Nation – A Strategy for Health in England*, London: HMSO.

Department of Health (1998) *Modernising Social Services*, London: The Stationery Office.

Department of Health (1999a) *Saving Lives: Our Healthier Nation*, London: The Stationery Office.

Department of Health (1999b) *Caring About Carers: A National Strategy for Carers*, London: Department of Health.

Department of Health (2000) *The NHS Plan: A Plan for Investment: A Plan for Reform*, London: Department of Health.

Department of Health (2002) *Tackling Health Inequalities: Summary of the 2002 Cross-Cutting Review*, London: The Stationery Office.

Department of Health (2003a) *Tackling Health Inequalities: A Programme for Action*, London: The Stationery Office. Also available at: http://www.dh.gov.uk/prod_consum_dh/groups/dh_digitalassets/@dh/@en/documents/digitalasset/dh4019362.pdf (accessed 30 July 2008).

Department of Health (2003b) *Building on the Best: Choice, Responsiveness and Equity in the NHS*, London: Department of Health.

Department of Health (2004a) *Choosing Health*, London: The Stationery Office.

Department of Health (2004b) *Departmental Report 2004*, London: The Stationery Office.

Department of Health (2006a) *Fact Sheet on Health Inequalities*, http://www.dh.gov.uk/en/Publicationsandstatistics/Publications/PublicationsPolicyAndGuidance/DH_4139513 (accessed 14 July 2008).

Department of Health (2006b) *Our Health, Our Care, Our Say: A New Direction for Community Services*, London: The Stationery Office. Also available at: http://www.dh.gov.uk/en/Publicationsandstatistics/Publications/PublicationsPolicyAndGuidance/DH_4127453 (accessed 10 May 2009).

Department of Health (2008a) *Carers at the Heart of 21st-century Families and Communities*, London: Department of Health. Also available at: http://www.dh.gov.uk/en/Publicationsandstatistics/Publications/PublicationsPolicyAndGuidance/DH_085345 (accessed 9 May 2009).

Department of Health (2008b) *The Case for Change – Why England Needs a New Care and Support System*, London: Department of Health. Available at: http://careandsupport.direct.gov.uk/wp-content/uploads/2009/03/the-case-for-change-e28093-why-england-needs-a-new-care-and-support-system.pdf (accessed 10 May 2009).

Department of Health, Department for Children, Schools and Families (2009) *Healthy Lives, Brighter Futures: The Strategy for Children and Young People's Health*, London. Also available at: http://www.dh.gov.uk/en/Publicationsandstatistics/Publications/PublicationsPolicyAndGuidance/DH_094400 (accessed 28 March 2009).

Deuchar, N. (1984) 'AIDS in New York City with particular reference to the psycho-social aspects', *British Journal of Psychiatry*, 145: 612–19.

Dex, S. (1985) *The Sexual Division of Work: Conceptual Revolutions in the Social Sciences*, Brighton: Wheatsheaf.

d'Houtaud, A. and Field, M. (1984) 'The image of health: variations in perception by social class in a French population', *Sociology of Health & Illness*, 6, 1: 30–60.

d'Houtaud, A. and Field, M. (1986) 'New research on the image of health', in C. Currer and M. Stacey (eds), op. cit.

DHSS (1976) *Prevention and Health: Everybody's Business*, London: HMSO.

DHSS (1980) *Inequalities in Health*, (The Black Report) London: HMSO.

DHSS (1981a) *Growing Older*, London: HMSO.

DHSS (1981b) *Care in the Community*, London: HMSO.

DHSS (1986) *On the State of Public Health: 1985*, London: HMSO.

DHSS (1987) *Promoting Better Health: The Government's Programme for Improving Primary Health Care*, London: HMSO.

Diener, E., Emmons, R. A., Larson, R. J. and Griffin, S. (1985) 'The satisfaction with life scale', *Journal of Personality Assessment*, 49, 1: 71–5.

Dingwall, R. (1976) *Aspects of Illness*, London: Martin Robertson.

Dingwall, R. and McIntosh, J. (eds) (1978) *Readings in the Sociology of Nursing*, Edinburgh: Churchill Livingstone.

Dingwall, R. and Murray, T. (1983) 'Categorization in accident departments: "good" patients, "bad" patients and children', *Sociology of Health & Illness*, 5, 2: 127–48.

Dini, E. and Goldring, S. (2008) 'Estimating the changing population of the "oldest old"', *Population Trends*, 132: 8–16.

Dohrenwend, B. P. (1975) 'Sociocultural and social-psychological factors in the genesis of mental disorders', *Journal of Health and Social Behavior*, 16: 365–92.

Donabedian, A. (1980) *Explorations in Quality Assessment and Monitoring, Volume I: The Definition of Quality and Approaches to its Assessment*, Ann Arbor, Mich.: Health Administration Press.

Donnison, J. (1977) *Midwives and Medical Men*, London: Heinemann.

Donovan, J. (1986) *We Don't Buy Sickness, It Just Comes*, Aldershot: Gower.

Doran, T. and Whitehead, M. (2003) 'Health of young and elderly informal carers: analysis of UK census data', *British Medical Journal*, 13 December, 327, 7428: 1388.

Douglas, J. D. (1967) *The Social Meanings of Suicide*, Princeton: Princeton University Press.

Dowd, J. J. and Bengston, V. L. (1978) 'Aging in minority populations – an examination of the double jeopardy hypothesis', *Journal of Gerontology*, 33: 427–36.

Doyal, L. and Pennell, I. (1979) *The Political Economy of Health*, London: Pluto Press.

Draper, P. (1983) 'Tackling the disease of ignorance', *Self-Health*, 1: 23–5.

Dreitzel, H. P. (ed.) (1973) *Childhood and Socialization*, London: Macmillan.

Drever, F. and Whitehead, M. (1995) 'Mortality in regions and local authority districts in the 1990s: exploring the relationship with deprivation', *Population Trends*, No. 82, Winter: 19–25.

Drever, F., Whitehead, M. and Roden, M. (1996) 'Current patterns and trends in male mortality by social class (based on occupation)', *Population Trends*, No. 86, Winter: 15–20.

Drever, F. and Whitehead, M. (eds) (1997) *Health Inequalities, Decennial Supplement*, Series DS No. 15, London: The Stationery Office.

Dubos, R. (1995) 'Mirage of health', in B. Davey, A. Gray and C. Seale (eds) *Health and Disease: A Reader*, 2nd edn, Milton Keynes: Open University Press, pp. 4–10.

Duncan, O. D. and Parmelee, L. F. (2006) 'Trends in public approval of euthanasia and suicide in the US, 1947–2003', *Journal of Medical Ethics*, 32, 5: 266–72.

Dunham, H. W. (1977) 'Schizophrenia: the impact of sociocultural factors', *Hospital Practice*, 12: 61–8.

Dunlop, R. J., Davies, R. J. and Hockley, J. M. (1989) 'Preferred versus actual place of death: a hospital palliative care support team experience', *Palliative Medicine*, 3: 197–201.

Dunnell, K. (1995) 'Population review: (2) are we healthier?', *Population Trends*, 82: 12–18.

Dunnell, K. and Cartwright, A. (1972) *Medicine Takers, Prescribers and Hoarders*, London: Routledge and Kegan Paul.

Durkin, K. and Barber, B. (2002) 'Not so doomed: computer game play and positive adolescent development' *Applied Developmental Psychology*, 23: 373–92.

Eaton, W. W. (1985) 'Epidemiology of schizophrenia', *Epidemiologic Review*, 7: 105–26.

Eisenberg, L. (1977) 'Disease and illness: distinctions between professional and popular ideas of sickness', *Culture, Medicine and Psychiatry*, 1: 9–23.

Elias, N. (1985) *The Loneliness of the Dying*, Oxford: Basil Blackwell.

Ell, K. (1996) 'Social networks, social support and coping with serious illness: the family connection', *Social Science & Medicine*, 42, 2: 173–83.

Elliot, J. (1991) 'Demographic trends in domestic life, 1945–1987', in D. Clark (ed.) *Marriage, Domestic Life and Social Change*, London: Routledge.

Elliott, J. A. and Olver, I. N. (2008) 'Dying cancer patients talk about euthanasia', *Social Science & Medicine*, 67: 647–56.

Ellis, J. R. and Hartley, C. L. (1992) *Nursing in Today's World – Challenges, Issues and Trends*, 4th edn, Philadelphia: J. B. Lippincott.

Ellis, R. and Whittington, D. (1993) *Quality Assurance in Health Care: A Handbook*, London: Edward Arnold.

Elston, M. A. (1991) 'The politics of professional power: medicine in a changing health service', in J. Gabe, M. Calnan and M. Bury (eds) *The Sociology of the Health Service*, London: Routledge, pp. 58–88.

Elston, M. A. (1993) 'Women doctors in a changing profession: the case of Britain', in E. Riska and K. Weger (eds) *Gender, Work and Medicine: Women and the Medical Division of Labour*, London: Sage.

Elston, M. A. (2009) *Women and Medicine: The Future*, London: Royal College of Physicians.

Emanuel, E. J. (1994) 'The history of the euthanasia debates in the United States and Britain', *Annals of Internal Medicine*, 121: 793–802.

Engel, G. L. (1977) 'The need for a new medical model: a challenge for biomedicine', *Science*, 196, 4286, 8 April.

Epsom, J. E. (1969) 'The mobile health clinic: a report on the first year's work', in D. Tuckett and J. M. Kaufert (eds) (1978) *Basic Readings in Medical Sociology*, London: Tavistock Publications.

Epstein, R. M., Franks, P., Fiscella, K., Shields, C. G., Meldrum, S. C., Kravitz, R. L. *et al.* (2005) 'Measuring patient-centred communication in patient–physician consultations: Theoretical and practical issues', *Social Science & Medicine*, 61, 7: 1516–28.

Equal Opportunities Commission (1982a) *Caring for the Elderly and Handicapped: Community Care Policies and Women's Lives*, Manchester: Equal Opportunities Commission.

Equal Opportunities Commission (1982b) *Who Cares for the Carers*, Manchester: Equal Opportunities Commission.

Erens, B., Primatesta, P. and Prior, G. (eds) (2001) *Health Survey for England: The Health of Minority Ethnic Groups '99*, London: The Stationery Office. Also available at: http://www.archive.official-documents.co.uk/document/doh/survey99/hse99.htm (accessed 25 July 2008).

Erikson, K. T. (1962) 'Notes on the sociology of deviance', *Social Problems*: 307–14.

Estes, C. L., Swan, J. S. and Gerard, E. (1982) 'Dominant and competing paradigms in gerontology: towards a political economy of ageing', *Ageing & Society*, 2: 151–64.

Etzioni, A. (ed.) (1969) *The Semi-Professions and their Organization*, New York: Free Press.

Evandrou, M. and Glaser, K. (2003) 'Combining work and family life: the pension penalty of caring', *Ageing & Society*, 23: 583–601.

Eve, A., Smith, A. M. and Tebbit, P. (1997) 'Hospice and palliative care services in the UK 1994–5, including a summary of trends 1990–5', *Palliative Medicine*, 11: 31–43.

Exley, C. (2004) 'Review article: the sociology of dying, death and bereavement', *Sociology of Health & Illness*, 26, 1: 110–22.

Exworthy, M., Stuart, M., Blane, D. and Marmot, M. (2003) *Tackling Health Inequalities since the Acheson Inquiry*, Bristol: Policy Press in association with the Joseph Rowntree Foundation. Also available at: http://www.jrf.org.uk/knowledge/findings/socialpolicy/363.asp (accessed 30 July 2008).

Fabrega, H. (1975) 'The need for an ethnomedical science', *Science*, 189: 969–75.

Fadden, G., Bebbington, P. and Knipers, L. (1987) 'The burden of care – the impact of functional psychiatric illness on the patient's family', *British Journal of Psychiatry*, 150: 285–92.

Fagin, L. (1981) *Unemployment and Health in Families*, London: DHSS.

Fagin, L. and Little, M. (1984) *The Forsaken Families*, Harmondsworth: Penguin.

Falkingham, J. (1989) 'Dependency and ageing in Britain: a re-examination of the evidence', *Journal of Social Policy*, 18, 2: 211–33.

Fanshel, S. and Bush, J. W. (1970) 'A health-status index and its application to health-services outcomes', *Operations Research*, 18: 1021–33.

Faris, R. E. L. and Dunham, H. W. (1939) *Mental Disorders in Urban Areas: An Ecological Study of Schizophrenia and Other Psychoses*, Chicago: Chicago University Press.

Farquhar, M. (1995) 'Elderly people's definitions of quality of life', *Social Science & Medicine*, 41, 10: 1439–46.

Faunce, W. A. and Fulton, R. L. (1958) 'The sociology of death: a neglected area of research', *Social Forces*, 36: 205–9.

Featherstone, M. (1991) 'The body in consumer culture', in M. Featherstone, M. Hepworth and B. S. Turner (eds) *The Body: Social Process and Cultural Theory*, London: Sage.

Featherstone, M. and Hepworth, M. (1989) 'Ageing and old age: reflections on the postmodern life course', in B. Bytheway *et al.* (eds), op. cit.

Fennell, G., Phillipson, C. and Evers, H. (1988) *The Sociology of Old Age*, Milton Keynes: Open University Press.

Fernando, S. (1988) *Race and Culture in Psychiatry*, London: Tavistock/Routledge.

Fernando, S. (1991) *Mental Health, Race and Culture*, Basingstoke: Macmillan.

Field, D. (1976) 'The social definition of illness', in D. Tuckett (ed.) *Introduction to Medical Sociology*, London: Tavistock Publications.

Field, D. (1995) 'Terminal illness: views of patients and their lay carers', *Palliative Medicine*, 9: 44–54.

Field, D. (1996) 'Awareness and modern dying', *Mortality*, 1, 3: 255–65.

Field, D. (1998) 'Special not different: general practitioners' accounts of their care of dying people', *Social Science & Medicine*, 46, 9: 1111–20.

Field, D. and Copp, G. (1999) 'Communication and awareness about dying in the 1990s', *Palliative Medicine*, 13, 6: 459–68.

Finch, J. (1989) *Family Obligations and Social Change*, Oxford: Polity Press.

Finch, J. and Wallis, L. (1993) 'Death, inheritance and the life course', in D. Clark (ed.) *The Sociology of Death*, Oxford: Blackwell, pp. 50–68.

Fine, M. and Glendinning, C. (2005) 'Dependence, independence or inter-dependence? Revisiting the concepts of "care" and "dependency"', *Ageing & Society*, 25: 601–21.

Firestone, S. (1974) *The Dialectic of Sex: The Case for Feminist Revolution*, New York: Morrow.

Fisher, S. (1973) *Motionless Body, Body Consciousness*, London: Calder & Boyars.

Fisher, S. (1984) 'Doctor–patient communication: a social and micro-political performance', *Journal of Health and Illness*, 6: 3.

Fisher, S. and Groce, S. B. (1985) 'Doctor–patient negotiation of cultural assumptions', *Sociology of Health & Illness*, 7, 3: 342–74.

Fitton, F. and Acheson, H. W. K. (1979) *Doctor/Patient Relationship: A Study in General Practice*, London: HMSO.

Fitzpatrick, J., Jacobson, B. and Aspinall, P. (2005) *Indications of Public Health in the English Regions: Ethnicity and Health*, Association of Public Health Observatories. Available at: http://www.apho.org.uk/resource/item.aspx?RID=39367 (accessed 26 July 2008).

Fitzpatrick, R., Hinton, J., Newman, S., Scambler, G. and Thompson, J. (eds) (1984) *The Experience of Illness*, London: Tavistock Publications.

Fletcher, R. (1988) *The Shaking of the Foundations: Family and Society*, London: Routledge.

Flint, C. (1986) 'A radical blueprint', *Nursing Times*, 82, 1, 1–7 January: 14.

Forbes, A., While, A. and Mathes, L. (2007) 'Informal carer activities, carer burden and health status in multiple sclerosis', *Clinical Rehabilitation*, 21: 563–75.

Foucault, M. (1965) *Madness and Civilization: The History of Insanity in the Age of Reason*, New York: Random House.

Foucault, M. (1976) *The Birth of the Clinic: An Archaeology of Medical Perception*, London: Tavistock.

Foucault, M. (1980a) 'The politics of health in the eighteenth century', in C. Gordon (ed.) *Power/Knowledge: Selected Interviews and Other Writings, 1972–1977*, Brighton: The Harvester Press.

Foucault, M. (1980b) 'Truth and power', in C. Gordon (ed.), *Power/Knowledge: Selected Interviews and Other Writings, 1972–1977*, Brighton: Harvester.

Fox, A. J. and Goldblatt, P. O. (1982) 'Socio-demographic differences in mortality', *Population Trends*, 27: 8–13.

Fox, A. J., Jones, D. R. and Goldblatt, P. O. (1984) 'Approaches to studying the effects of socio-economic circumstances on geographic differences in mortality in England and Wales', *British Medical Bulletin*, 40, 4: 309–14.

Fox, A. J., Goldblatt, P. O. and Jones, D. R. (1986) 'Social class mortality differentials: artefact, selection or life chances', in Wilkinson, R. G. (ed.) *Class and Health: Research and Longitudinal Data*, London: Tavistock.

Fox, A. J., Goldblatt, P. and Jones, D. (1990) 'Social class mortality differentials: artefact, selection or life circumstances?', in P. Goldblatt (ed.) *Longitudinal Study: Mortality and Social Organisation*, LS no. 6, London: HMSO.

Fraser, N. and Gordon, L. (1994) 'A genealogy of dependency: tracing a keyword of the US welfare state', *Signs*, 19, 2: 309–34.

Freedman, J. (2002) *Media Violence and its Effect on Aggression: Assessing the Scientific Evidence*, Toronto: University of Toronto Press.

Freeman, A. (1984) *Mental Health and the Environment*, Singapore: Longman.

Freidson, E. (1970a) *The Profession of Medicine: A Study of the Sociology of Applied Knowledge*, New York: Dodd, Mead and Company.

Freidson, E. (1970b) *Professional Dominance*, Chicago: Aldine.

Freidson, E. (1975) 'Dilemmas in the doctor/patient relationship', in C. Cox and A. Mead (eds), op. cit.

Freidson, E. (1983) 'The theory of professions – state of the art', in R. Dingwall and P. Lewis (eds) *The Sociology of Professions*, London: Macmillan.

Freidson, E. (1986) *Professional Powers: A Study of the Institutionalisation of Formal Knowledge*, London: University of Chicago Press.

French, J. and Adams, L. (1986) 'From analysis to synthesis: theories of health education', *Health Education Journal*, 45, 2: 71–4.

Freud, S. (1940) *An Outline of Psychoanalysis*, New York: W. W. Norton.

Freund, P. E. S. and McGuire, M. B. (1991) *Health, Illness and the Social Body: A Critical Sociology*, Englewood Cliffs, New Jersey: Prentice Hall.

Frost, H., Klaber Moffett, J. A., Moser, J. S. and Fairbank, J. C. T. (1995) 'Randomized controlled trial for evaluation of a fitness programme for patients with chronic low back pain', *British Medical Journal*, 310: 151–4.

Gabe, J. and Williams, P. (1986) 'Is space bad for your health? The relationship between crowding in the home and the emotional distress in women', *Sociology of Health & Illness*, 8, 4: 351–71.

Gabriel, Z. and Bowling, A. (2004) 'Quality of life from the perspectives of older people', *Ageing & Society*, 24: 675–91.

Gallagher, B. J. (1980) *The Sociology of Mental Illness*, Englewood Cliffs, NJ: Prentice-Hall Inc.

Gallagher, S. K. and Mechanic, D. (1996) 'Living with the mentally ill: effects on the health and functioning of other household members', *Social Science and Medicine*, 42, 12: 1691–701.

Gamarnikow, E. (1978) 'Sexual division of labour: the case of nursing', in A. Kuhn and A. Wolfe (eds) *Feminism and Materialism*, London: Routledge and Kegan Paul.

Garfinkel, H. (1967) *Studies in Ethnomethodology*, Englewood Cliffs, NJ: Prentice-Hall.

Gentile, D. A., Lynch, P., Linder, J. and Walsh, D. (2004) 'The effects of violent video game habits on adolescent hostility, aggressive behaviors, and school performance', *Journal of Adolescence*, 27: 5–22.

Germain, C. (1980) 'Nursing the dying: implications of Kübler-Ross' staging theory', *Annals of the American Academy of Political and Social Science*, 447: 46–58.

Giddens, A. (1989) *Sociology*, Cambridge: Polity Press.

Giddens, A. (1998) *Conversations with Anthony Giddens: Making Sense of Modernity*, Stanford, Calif.: Stanford University Press.

Giddens, A. (2006) *Sociology*, 5th edn, Cambridge: Polity Press.

Gilleard, C. and Higgs, P. (2000) *Cultures of Ageing: Self, Citizen and the Body*, London: Prentice Hall.

Gilleard, C. and Higgs, P. (2002) 'The third age: class cohort or generation?', *Ageing & Society*, 22: 369–82.

Ginn, J. and Arber, S. (2001) 'Pension prospects of minority groups: inequalities by gender and ethnicity', *British Journal of Sociology*, 52: 519–39.

Ginzburg, I. and Link, B. (1993) 'Psycho-social consequences of rejection and stigma feelings in psoriasis patients', *International Journal of Dermatology*, 32: 587–91.

Glaser, B. G. and Strauss, A. L. (1965) *Awareness of Dying*, New York: Aldine.

Glaser, B. G. and Strauss, A. L. (1968) *Time for Dying*, Chicago: Aldine.

Glendinning, C. (1992) *The Costs of Informal Care: Looking Inside the Household*, London: Social Policy Research Unit, HMSO.

Glendinning, A., Hendry, L. and Shucksmith, J. (1995) 'Lifestyle, health and social class in adolescence', *Social Science & Medicine*, 41, 2: 235–48.

Goddard, E. (2006) *General Household Survey 2005: Smoking and drinking among adults, 2005*, London: Office for National Statistics.

Goffman, E. (1961) *Asylums*, Garden City, New York: Doubleday.

Goffman. E. (1968) *Stigma: Notes on the Management of Spoiled Identity*, Harmondsworth: Penguin.

Goffman, E. (1974) *Frame Analysis. An Essay on the Organization of Experience*, New York: Harper.

Goldberg, E. M. and Morrison, S. L. (1963) 'Schizophrenia and social class', *British Journal of Psychiatry*, 109: 785–802.

Goldblatt, P. O. (1989) 'Mortality by social class 1971–1985: an analysis of social class differences in recent mortality data from the OPCS longitudinal study', *Population Trends*, 56, Summer: 6–15.

Goldblatt, P. (ed.) (1990) *Longitudinal Study: Mortality and Organisation*, Series LS No. 1, London: HMSO.

Goldthorpe, J. H., Lockwood, D., Bechhofer, F. and Platt, J. (1969) *The Affluent Worker in the Class Structure*, Cambridge: Cambridge University Press.

Gomm, R. (1996) 'Mental health and inequality', in T. Heller *et al.* (eds), op. cit.

Goode, W. J. (1960) 'Encroachment, charlatanism and the emerging profession: psychology, medicine and sociology', *American Sociological Review*, XXV: 902–14.

Goodinson, S. and Singleton, J. (1989) 'Quality of life: a critical review of current concepts, measures and their clinical implications', *International Journal of Nursing Studies*, 26, 4: 327–41.

Goodman, L. A., Koss, M. P. and Russo, N. F. (1993) 'Violence against women: physical and mental health effects', *Applied and Preventative Psychology*, 2: 79–89.

Gorer, G. (1955) 'The pornography of death', *Encounter*, October.

Gorer, G. (1965) *Death, Grief and Mourning in Contemporary Britain*, London: The Cresecent Press.

Gove, W. R. (1970) 'Societal reaction as an explanation of mental illness: an evaluation', *American Sociological Review*, 35: 873–84.

Gove, W. R. (1972) 'The relationship between sex roles, marital status and mental illness', *Social Forces*, 5: 34–44.

Gove, W. R. (1975) 'Labelling and mental illness', in W. Gove (ed.) *The Labelling of Deviance: Evaluating a Perspective*, New York: Halsted, pp. 35–81.

Gove, W. R. (1980) 'Labelling and mental illness: a critique', in W. R. Gove (ed.) *Labelling Deviant Behavior*, Beverly Hills, CA: Sage.

Gove, W. R. (1982) 'The current status of the labelling theory of mental illness', in W. R. Gove (ed.) *Deviance and Mental Illness*, Beverly Hills, CA: Sage.

Gove, W. R. (1984) 'Gender differences in mental and physical illness: the effects of fixed roles and nurturant roles', *Social Science & Medicine*, 19, 2: 77–91.

Gove, W. R. and Tudor, F. (1973) 'Adult sex roles and mental illness', *American Journal of Sociology*, 78: 812–35.

Grace, V. M. (1991) 'The marketing of empowerment and the construction of the health consumer: a critique of health promotion', *International Journal of Health Services*, 21, 2: 329–43.

Graham, H. (1979) 'Prevention and health: every mother's business: a comment on child health policy in the seventies', in C. Harris (ed.) *The Sociology of the Family: New Directions for Britain*, Sociological Review Monograph 28, University of Keele.

Graham, H. (1983) 'Caring: A Labour of Love', in J. Finch and D. Groves (eds) *A Labour of Love – Women, Work and Caring*, London: Routledge and Keegan Paul.

Graham, H. (1984) *Women, Health and the Family*, London: Tavistock.

Graham. H. (1985) 'Providers, negotiators and mediators: women as the hidden carers', in E. Lewin and V. Oleson (eds) *Women, Health and Healing: Toward a New Perspective*, New York: Tavistock Publications.

Graham, H. (1987) 'Women's smoking and family health', *Social Science & Medicine*, 25: 47–56.

Graham, H. (1990) 'Behaving well: women's health behaviour in context', in H. Roberts (ed.) *Women's Health Counts*, London: Routledge.

Graham, H. and Oakley, A. (1986) 'Competing ideologies of reproduction: medical and maternal perspectives on pregnancy', in C. Currer and M. Stacey (eds), op. cit.

Graham, P. (2004) *The End of Adolescence*, Oxford: Oxford University Press.

Grainger, S. and Robinson, A. (2004) *Housing and Health in Scotland: Analysis of the 2002 Scottish House Conditions Survey*, SHCS Working Paper No. 2, Edinburgh: Communities Scotland Investment and Performance Division. Also available at: http://www.scotland.gov.uk/Resource/Doc/933/0039909.pdf (accessed 15 July 2008).

Gray, J. A. M. (1997) *Evidence Based Health Care: How to Make Health Policy and Management Decisions*, London: Churchill Livingstone.

Green, H., McGinnity, A., Meltzer, H., Ford, T. and Goodman, R. (2005) *Mental Health of Children and Young People in Great Britain, 2004*, Norwich: Palgrave Macmillan/HMSO.

Grewal, I., Nazroo, J., Bajekal, M., Blane, D. and Lewis, J. (2004) 'Influences on the quality of life: a qualitative investigation of ethnic differences among older people in England', *Journal of Ethnic and Migration Studies*, 3: 737–61.

Griffiths, C. and Fitzpatrick, J. (eds) (2001) *Geographic Variations in Health*, Series DS No. 16, London: The Stationery Office.

Griffiths, Sir R. (1988) *Community Care Agenda for Action*, London: HMSO.

Guillemard, A.-M. (1982) 'Old age, retirement and the social class structure: toward an analysis of the structural dynmaics of the later stage of life', in T. K. Hareven and K. J. Adams (eds) *Ageing and Life Course Transitions: An Interdisciplinary Perspective*, London: Tavistock.

Gunaratnam, Y. (1997) 'Culture is not enough: a critique of multi-culturalism in palliative care', in D. Field, J. Hockey and N. Small (eds) *Death, Gender and Ethnicity*, London: Routledge.

Gunnell, D., Middleton, N., Whitley, E., Dorling, D. and Frankel, S. (2003) 'Why are suicide rates rising in young men but falling in the elderly? – a time-series analysis of trends in England and Wales, 1950–1998', *Social Science & Medicine*, 57: 595–611.

Gusfield, J. R. (1975) *Community: A Critical Response*, Oxford: Basil Blackwell.

Gussow, Z. and Tracy, G. S. (1968) 'Status, ideology and adaption to stigmatized illness: a study of leprosy', *Human Organizations*, 27: 316.

Haley, W. E., Levin, E. G., Brown, S. L., Berry, J. W. and Hughes, G. H. (1987) 'Psychological, social and health consequences of caring for a relative with dementia', *Journal of the American Geriatric Society*, 35: 405.

Hall, G. S. (1904) *Adolescence: Its psychology and its relations to physiology, anthropology, sociology, sex, crime, religion and education*, Volumes 1 and 2, New York: Appleton-Century-Crofts.

Hall, P., Brockington, I., Levings, J. and Murphy, C. (1993) 'Comparison of responses to the mentally ill in two communities', *British Journal of Psychiatry*, 162: 99–108.

Hallenbeck, J. L. (2003) *Palliative Care Perspectives*, Oxford: Oxford University Press.

Hamilton, P. M. (1992) *Realities of Contemporary Nursing*, New York: Addison-Wesley Nursing.

Hannay, D., Usherwood, T. and Platts, M. (1992) 'Workload of general practitioners before and after the new contract', *British Medical Journal*, 304: 615–18.

Hannay, D. R. (1979) *The Symptom Iceberg: A Study of Community Health*, London: Routledge and Kegan Paul.

Hansard, (1959) *House of Commons Debates*, 26 January, London: HMSO.

Hanson, D. and Emlet, C. (2006) 'Assessing a community's elder friendliness: a case example of the advantage initiative', *Family and Community Health*, 29: 266–78.

Hanson, L. C., Danis, M. and Garrett, J. (1997) 'What is wrong with end-of-life care? Opinions of bereaved family members', *Journal of the American Gerontological Society*, 45: 1339–44.

Hardey, M. (1999) 'Doctor in the house: the internet as a source of lay health knowledge and the challenge to expertise', *Sociology of Health & Illness*, 21, 6: 820–35.

Harding, S. (1995) 'Social class differences in mortality of men: recent evidence from the OPCS Longitudinal Study, *Population Trends*, No. 80, Summer: 31–7.

Hare, E. H., Price, J. S. and Slater, E. (1972) 'Parental social class in psychiatric patients', *British Journal of Psychiatry*, 121: 515–24.

Harper, S. (2006) *Ageing Societies*, New York: Hodder Arnold.

Harris, J. (2001) *The effects of computer games on young children: a review of the research*, RDS Occasional Paper No. 72, London: Home Office. http://www.homeoffice.gov.uk/rds/pdfs/occ72-compgames.pdf (accessed 14 March 2009).

Harris, N. (1988) 'Social security and the transition to adulthood', *Journal of Social Policy*, 17: 501–23.

Harrison, P. (1973) 'Living with old age', *New Society*, 1 November: 265–8.

Harrison, S. and Hunter, D. J. (1994) *Rationing Health Care*, London: Institute for Public Policy Research.

Hart, B., Sainsbury, P. and Short, S. (1998) 'Whose dying? A sociological critique of the "good death" ', *Mortality*, 3, 1: 65–77.

Hart, N. (1977) 'Parenthood and patienthood: a dialectical autobiography', in A. Davis and G. Horobin (eds) *Medical Encounters: The Experience of Illness and Treatment*, London: Croom Helm.

Hart, N. (1985) 'The sociology of health and medicine', in M. Haralambos (ed.) *Sociology: NewDirections*, Ormskirk: Causeway.

Hart, N. (1989) 'Sex differentials in mortality in Europe', in J. A. Fox (ed.), op. cit.

Hart, T. (1971) 'Inverse care law', *The Lancet*, 27 February: 405–12.

Haug, M. (1973) 'Deprofessionalization: an alternative hypothesis for the future', *Sociological Review Monograph*, 20: 195–211.

Havighurst, R. J. (1963) 'Successful ageing', in R. H. Williams, C. Tibbitts and W. Donahue (eds) *Process of Ageing*, Volume 1, New York: Atherton.

Hawe, P. and Shiell, A. (2000) 'Social capital and health promotion: a review', *Social Science & Medicine*, 51: 871–85.

Hayes, J. and Nutman, P. (1981) *Understanding the Unemployed: The Psychological Effects of Unemployment*, London: Tavistock.

Hearn, J. (1982) 'Notes on patriarchy, professionalization and the semi-professions', *Sociology*, 16: 184–202.

Hearn, J. (1987) *The Gender of Oppression: Men, Masculinity and the Critique of Marxism*, Brighton: Wheatsheaf.

Heath, C. (1981) 'The opening sequence in doctor–patient interaction', in P. Atkinson and C. Heath (eds) *Medical Work: Realities and Routines*, Farnborough: Gower.

Heath, C. (1984) 'Participation in the medical consultation: the co-ordination of verbal and non-verbal behaviour between the doctor and patient', *Sociology of Health & Illness*, 6, 3: 311–38.

Heath, C. (1986) *Body Movement and Speech in Medical Interaction*, Cambridge: Cambridge University Press.

Heginbotham, C. (1993) 'User empowerment in welfare services', in N. Thomas, N. Deakin and J. Doling (eds) *Learning From Innovation; Social Housing and Social Services in the 1990s*, Birmingham: Birmingham Academic Press.

Heller, T., Reynolds, J., Gomm, R., Muston, R. and Pattison, S. (eds) (1996) *Mental Health Matters: A Reader*, Basingstoke: Palgrave Macmillan in association with Open University Press.

Helman, C. (1981) 'Disease versus illness in general practice', *Journal of the Royal College of General Practitioners*, 31: 548–52.

Helman, C. G. (1986) 'Feed a cold, starve a fever: folk models of infection in an English suburban community, and their relation to medical treatment', in C. Currer and M. Stacey (eds), op. cit.

Helman, C. G. (1990) *Culture, Health and Illness: An Introduction for Health Professionals*, 2nd edn, London: Wright.

Henderson, A. S. (1988) *An Introduction to Social Psychiatry*, Oxford: Oxford University Press.

Hendrick, H. (1990) 'Constructions and reconstructions of British childhood: an interpretative survey 1800 to the present', in A. James and A. Prout (eds) *Constructing and Reconstructing Childhood: Contemporary Issues in the Sociological Study of Childhood*, London: Falmer Press.

Heritage, J. (1984) *Garfinkel and Ethnomethodology*, Cambridge: Polity Press.

Herman, N. J. (1993) 'Return to sender: reintegrative stigma-management strategies of ex-psychiatric patients', *Journal of Contemporary Ethnography*, 22, 3: 295–330.

Herzlich, C. (1973) *Health and Illness*, London: Academic Press.

Herzlich, C. and Pierret, J. (1986) 'Illness: from causes to meaning', in C. Currer and M. Stacey (eds), op. cit.

Hess, L. E., Petersen, A. C. and Mortimer, J. T. (2006) 'Youth, unemployment and marginality: the problem and the solution', in A. C. Petersen and J. T. Mortimer (eds) *Youth, Unemployment and Society*, Cambridge: Cambridge University Press.

Hickman, S. E. (2002) 'Improving communication near the end of life', *American Behavioral Scientist*, 46, 2: 252–67.

Hicks, J. and Allen, G. (1999) *A Century of Change: Trends in UK Statistics since 1900*, Research Paper 99/11, 21 December, London: House of Commons Library.

Higgins, P. C. (1981) *Outsiders in a Hearing World: A Sociology of Deafness*, London: Sage.

Hillery, G. A. (1955) 'Definitions of community: areas of agreement', *Rural Sociology*, 20, 2: 111–23.

Hirst, M. (2002) 'Transitions to informal care in Great Britain during the 1990s', *Journal of Epidemiology and Community Health*, 56: 579–87.

Hirst, M. (2003) 'Caring-related inequalities in psychological distress in Britain during the 1990s', *Journal of Public Health and Medicine*, 25: 336–43.

Hockey, J. (1990) *Experiences of Death: An Anthropological Account*, Edinburgh: Edinburgh University Press.

Hockey, J. and James, A. (1993) *Growing Up and Growing Old: Ageing Dependency and the Life Course*, London: Sage.

Hollingshead, A. B. and Redlich, F. C. (1958) *Social Class and Mental Illness: A Community Study*, New York: John Wiley & Sons, Inc.

Holmes, S. (1995) 'Ideology underpinning the issue of community care', *British Journal of Therapy and Rehabilitation*, 2: 246–50.

Holmes, T. H. and Rahe, R. H. (1967) 'The social readjustment rating scale', *Journal of Psychosomatic Research*, 11: 213–18.

Homans, H. (1985) 'Discomforts in pregnancy: traditional remedies and medical prescriptions', in H. Homans (ed.) *The Sexual Politics of Reproduction*, Aldershot: Gower.

Hood-Williams, J. (1990) 'Patriarchy for children: On the stability of power relations in Children's lives', in L. Chisholm, P. Buchner, H-H. Kruger and P. Brown (eds) *Childhood, Youth and Social Change*, London: Falmer Press, pp. 155–71.

hooks, b. (1984) *Feminist Theory: from Margin to Centre*, Boston, MA: South End Press.

Hopkinson, J. B., Hallett, C. E. and Luker, K. A. (2003) 'Caring for dying people in hospital', *Journal of Advanced Nursing*, 44, 5: 525–33.

Hopper, S. (1981) 'Diabetes as a stigmatized condition: the case of low-income clinic patients in the United States', *Social Science & Medicine*, 15, b: 11–19.

Horwitz, A. (1977) 'The pathways into psychiatric treatment: some differences between men and women', *Journal of Health and Social Behaviour*, 18: 169–80.

House of Commons (2001) *Select Committee on Health, Second Report*, London: The Stationery Office.

Howard, S., Dryden, J. and Johnson, B. (1999) 'Childhood resilience: review and critique of literature', *Oxford Review of Education*, 25: 307–23.

Howarth, G. (2007) *Death and Dying: A Sociological Introduction*, Cambridge: Polity.

Hughes, E. C. (1945) 'Dilemmas and contradictions of status', *American Journal of Sociology*, 50: 353–59.

Hughes, E. (1963) 'Professions', *Daedalus*, reprinted in G. Esland, G. Salaman and M. A. Speakman (1975) (eds) *People and Work*, Edinburgh: Holmes McDougall.

Hughes, D. (1980) 'Lay Assessment of Clinical Seriousness: practical decision-making by non-medical staff in a hospital casualty department', unpublished PhD thesis: University of Wales, Swansea.

Hughes, D. (1988) 'When nurse knows best: some aspects of nurse/doctor interaction in a casualty department', *Sociology of Health & Illness*, 10, 1: 1–22.

Hugman, R. (1991) *Power in the Caring Professions*, London: Macmillan.

Humm, M. (ed.) (1992) *Feminisms: A Reader*, Hemel Hempstead: Harvester Wheatsheaf.

Humphreys, L. (1972) *Out of the Closets: The Sociology of Homosexual Liberation*, Englewood Cliffs, NJ: Prentice Hall.

Hunt, K. and Annandale, E. (1999) 'Relocating gender and morbidity: examining men's and women's health in contemporary Western societies', *Social Science & Medicine*, 48, 1: 1–5.

Hunt, S., McEwen, J. and McKenna, S. P. (1985) 'Social inequalities in perceived health', *Effective Health Care*, 2, 4: 151–60.

Hunt, S., McEwen, J. and McKenna, S. (1986) *Measuring Health Status*, London: Croom Helm.

Hunter, R. and MacAlpine, I. (1974) *Three Hundred Years of Psychiatry*, Oxford: Oxford University Press.

Hurrelmann, K. (1988) *Social Structure and Personality Development*, Cambridge: Cambridge University Press.

Hurrelmann, K. (1989) 'The social world of adolescents: a sociological perspective', in K. Hurrelmann and U. Engel (eds) *The Social World of Adolescents: International Perspectives*, Berlin: de Grupter.

Huxley, P. (1993) 'Location and stigma: a survey of community attitudes to mental illness. Part 1: enlightenment and stigma', *Journal of Mental Health*, 2: 73–80.

Hyde, M., Ferrie, J., Higgs, P., Mein, G. and Nazroo, J. (2004) 'The effects of pre-retirement factors and retirement route on circumstances in retirement: findings from the Whitehall II study', *Ageing & Society*, 24: 279–96.

Iley, K. and Nazroo, J. (2001) 'Ethnic inequalities in mental health: a critical examination of the evidence', in L. Culley and S. Dyson (eds) *Sociology, Ethnicity and Nursing Practice*, Basingstoke: Palgrave, pp. 67–89.

Illich, I. (1977) *Limits to Medicine: Medical Nemesis: The Expropriation of Health*, Harmondsworth: Penguin.

Ineichen, B. (1979) *Mental Illness*, London: Longman.

Information Centre (2006) *Drug use, smoking and drinking among young people in England in 2005*, London: The Information Centre, NHS. Available at: http://www.ic.nhs.uk/pubs/youngpeopledruguse-smoking-drinking2005 (accessed 19 March 2009).

James, A. and Prout, A. (eds) (1990) *Constructing and Reconstructing Childhood: Contemporary Issues in the Sociological Study of Childhood*, London: Falmer Press.

James, N. and Field, D. (1992) 'The routinization of hospice: charisma and bureaucratization', *Social Science & Medicine*, 34, 12: 1363–75.

Jeffery, R. (1979) 'Normal rubbish: deviant patients in casualty departments', *Sociology of Health and Illness*, 1, 1: 90–107.

Jefferys, M. and Sachs, H. (1982) *Rethinking General Practice*, London: Tavistock.

Jenkinson, C. (ed.) (1997) *Assessment and Evaluation of Health and Medical Care: A Methods Text*, Buckingham: Open University Press.

Jenkinson, C. and McGee, H. (1997) 'Patient assessed outcomes: measuring health status and quality of life', in C. Jenkinson (ed.), op. cit.

Jenkinson, C. (1998) *Health Status Measurement: A brief but critical introduction*, Oxford: Radcliffe Medical Press.

Jenks, C. (1996) *Childhood*, London: Routledge.

Jenks, C. (2004) 'Editorial: Many Childhoods?', *Childhood*, 11: 5–8.

Jobling, R. (1977) 'Learning to live with it: an account of a career of chronic dermatological illness and patienthood', in A. Davis and G. Horobin (eds) *Medical Encounters: The Experience of Illness and Treatment*, London: Croom Helm.

Johansen, S., Hole, J. C., Kaasa, S., Loge, H. J. and Materstvedt, L. J. (2005) 'Attitudes towards, and wishes for, euthanasia in advanced cancer patients at a palliative care unit', *Palliative Medicine*, 19, 6: 454–60.

Johnson, M. (1976) 'That was your life: a biographical approach to later life', in J. M. A. Munnichs, W. J. A. Van Den Heuval (eds) *Dependency or Interdependency in Old Age*, The Hague: Martinus Nijhoff.

Johnson, M. (1990) 'Dependency and Interdependency', in J. Bond and P. Coleman (eds), op. cit.

Johnson, M. M. and Martin, H. W. (1965) 'A sociological analysis of the nurse role', in J. K. Skipper and R. C. KLeonard (eds) *Social Interaction and Patient Care*, Philadelphia: J. B. Lippincott.

Jones, C., Woods, K. and Taylor, G. O. (1997) 'Social deprivation and tooth decay in Scottish schoolchildren', *Health Bulletin*, 55: 11–5.

Jones, D. E. and Vetter, N. J. (1984) 'A survey of those who care for the elderly at home: their problems and their needs', *Social Science & Medicine*, 19: 511.

Jones, D. W. (1996) 'Families and the experience of mental distress', in T. Heller *et al.* (eds), op. cit.

Jones, E., Farina, A., Hastorf, A., Markus, H., Miller, D. T. and Scott, R. (1984) *Social Stigma: The Psychology of Marked Relationships*, New York: Freeman and Company.

Jones, G. and Wallace, C. (1992) *Youth, Family and Citizenship*, Milton Keynes: Open University Press.

Jones, I. G. and Cameron, D. (1984) 'Social class: an embarrassment to epidemiology?', *Community Medicine*, 6: 37–46.

Jones, K. (1988) *Experience in Mental Health: Community Care and Social Policy*, London: Sage.

Jones, K., Gould, M. I. and Duncan, C. (2000) 'Death and deprivation: an exploratory analysis of deaths in the Health and Lifestyle Survey', *Social Science & Medicine*, 50: 1059–79.

Jordanova, L. J. (1990) 'New worlds for children in the eighteenth century: problems of historical interpretation', *History of Human Sciences*, 3: 71–83.

Karlsen, S. and Nazroo, J. Y. (2002) 'Relation between racial discrimination, social class and health among ethnic minority groups', *American Journal of Public Health*, 92, 4: 624–31.

Kart, G. (1987) 'Review essay: the end of conventional gerontology?', *Sociology of Health & Illness*, 9: 76–88.

Kastenbaum, R. (1985) 'Do we die in stages?', in S. Wilcox and M. Sutton (eds) *Understanding Death and Dying: An Interdisciplinary Approach*, 3rd edn, Palo Alto: Mayfield Publishing Company.

Katz, J. S. (1989) *Context and Care: Nurses' Accounts of Stress and Support on a Cancer Ward*, unpublished PhD thesis, University of Warwick.

Katz, J. S. with Komaromy, C. (2004) *Death & Dying: Workbook 2: Caring for Dying People*, 3rd edn, Milton Keynes: Open University.

Kawachi, I., Kennedy, B. P. and Glass, R. (1999) 'Social capital and self-rated health: A contextual analysis', *American Journal of Public Health*, 89, 8: 1187–93.

Kawachi, I., Kennedy, B. P., Lochner, K. and Prothrow-Stith, D. (1997) 'Social capital, social inequality, and mortality', *American Journal of Public Health*, 87, 9: 1491–98.

Kelaher, M., Paul, S., Lambert, H., Ahmad, W., Paradies, Y. and Smith, G. D. (2008) 'Discrimination and health in an English study', *Social Science & Medicine*, 66: 1627–36.

Kellehear, A. (1984) 'Are we a death-denying society? A sociological review', *Social Science & Medicine*, 18: 713–23.

Kellehear, A. (1990) *Dying of Cancer: The final year of life*, Melbourne: Harwood Academic Publishers.

Kelly, A. E., Schochet, T. and Landry, C. F. (2004) 'Risk taking and novelty seeking in adolescence', *The Annals of the New York Academy of Sciences,* 1021: 27–32.

Kelly, M. P. and May, D. (1982) 'Good patients and bad patients: a review of the literature and a theoretical critique', *Journal of Advanced Nursing*, 7: 147–56.

Kelner, M. J. and Bourgeault, I. L. (1993) 'Patient control over dying: responses from health care professionals', *Social Science & Medicine*, 36: 757–65.

Keniston, K. (1970) 'Youth – A "new" stage of life', *The American Scholar*, 39, 4: 631–54.

Keogh, J. (1997) 'Professionalization of nursing: development, difficulties and solutions', *Journal of Advanced Nursing*, 25: 302–8.

Keown, J. (2002) *Euthanasia, Ethics and Public Policy: An Argument Against Legalisation*, Cambridge: Cambridge University Press.

Kerr, M. (1958) *The People of Ship Street*, London: Routledge and Kegan Paul.

Kickbush, I. (1981) 'Involvement in health: a social concept of health education', *International Journal of Health Education*, 24: 3–15.

Kiernan, K. and Wicks, M. (1990) *Family Change and Future Policy*, London: Family Policy Study Centre.

Kincey, J., Bradshaw, P. and Ley, P. (1975) 'Patients' satisfaction and reported acceptance of advice in general practice', *Journal of the Royal College of General Practitioners*, 25: 558–62.

Kind, P., Rosser, R. and Williams, A. (1982) 'Validation of quality of life: some psychometric evidence', in M. W. Jones-Lee (ed.) *The Value of Life and Safety*, Leiden: North Holland.

Kind, P., Gudex, C. and Godfrey, G. (1994) 'Introduction: What are QALYS?', in S. Baldwin, C. Godfrey and C. Propper (eds) *Quality of Life: Perspectives and Policies*, London: Routledge.

Kirke, P. N. (1980) 'Mothers' views of obstetric care', *British Journal of Obstetrics and Gynaecology*, 87: 1029–33.

Kirkham, M. J. (1983) 'Labouring in the dark: limitations on the giving of information to enable patients to orientate themselves to the likely events and timescale of labour', in J. Wilson-Barnet (ed.) *Nursing Research: Ten Studies in Patient Care*, Chichester: Wiley.

Kitsuse, J. I. (1962) 'Social reaction to deviant behaviour', *Social Problems*, 9: 247–56.

Klee, G. D., Spiro, E., Bahn, A. K. and Gorwitz, K. (1967) 'An ecological analysis of diagnosed mental illness in Baltimore', in R. R. Monroe, G. D. Klee and E. B. Brody (eds) *Psychiatric Epidemiology and Mental Health Planning*, Psychiatric Research Report No. 22, Washington: American Psychiatric Association.

Kleinman, A. (1980) *Patients and Healers in the Context of Culture*, Berkeley: University of California Press.

Kleinman, A. (1987) 'Anthropology and psychiatry: The role of culture in cross-cultural research on illness', *British Journal of Psychiatry*, 151: 447–54.

Kleinman, A., Eisenberg, L. and Good, B. (1978) 'Culture, illness and care: clinical lessons from anthropological and cross-cultural research', *Annals of International Medicine*, 88: 251.

Knight, I. (1984) *The Height and Weight of Adults in Great Britain*, London: OPCS/HMSO.

Knowles, R. (1987) 'Who's a pretty girl then?', *Nursing Times*, 83, 27: 58–9.

Kratz, C. R. (1979) (ed.) *The Nursing Process*, London: Balliere Tindall.

Kübler-Ross, E. (1969) *On Death and Dying*, New York: Macmillan.

La Fontaine, J. S. (1979) *Sex and Age as Principles of Social Differentiation*, London: Academic Press.

Laing, R. D. (1967) *The Politics of Experience*, Harmondsworth: Penguin.

Lakey, J. (2001) *Youth Unemployment, Labour Market Programmes and Health: A review of the literature*, London: Policy Studies Institute/Central Books.

Lakey, J. (2002) *Health Impacts of New Deal for Young People*, London: Policy Studies Institute/Central Books.

Lang, T., Andrews, C., Hunt, J. *et al.* (1984) *Jam Tomorrow?*, Food Policy Unit, Hollings Faculty, Manchester Polytechnic.

Langwell, K. M. (1982) 'Differences by sex in economic returns with physician specialization', *Journal of Health Politics, Policy and Law*, 6: 752–61.

Lareau, A. (2008) 'Introduction: Taking stock of class', in A. Lareau and D. Conley (eds) *Social Class: How Does it Work?*, New York: Russell Sage Foundation, pp. 3–24.

Laslett, P. (1987) 'The emergence of the third age', *Ageing & Society*, 7: 133–60.

Laslett, P. (1996) *A Fresh Map of Life*, London: Macmillan.

Laslett, P. and Wall, R. (1974) *Household and Family in Past Time*, Cambridge: Cambridge University Press.

Last, J. (1963) 'The iceberg: completing the clinical picture in general practice', *Lancet* 2: 28–31.

Lawless, S., Kippax, S. and Crawford, J. (1996) 'Dirty, diseased and undeserving: the positioning of HIV positive women', *Social Science & Medicine*, 43, 9: 1371–77.

Lawrence, B. (1987) 'The fifth dimension – gender and general practice', in A. Spenser and D. Podmore (eds) *In a Man's World: Essays on Women in Male-dominated Professions*, London: Tavistock.

Lawton, J. (2000) *The Dying Process*, London: Routledge.

Layard, R. and Dunn, J. (2009) *A Good Childhood: Searching for Values in a Competitive Age*, London: The Children's Society.

Leach, E. (1968) 'Ritual', in *International Encyclopaedia of the Social Sciences*, New York: Free Press/Macmillan.

Lee, D. and Newby, H. (1983) *The Problem of Sociology*, London: Hutchinson.

Leeson, J. and Gray, J. (1978) *Women and Medicine*, London: Tavistock.

Lemert, E. M. (1967) *Human Deviance, Social Problems and Social Control*, Englewood Cliffs, NJ: Prentice-Hall.

Leonard, D. (1990) 'Persons in their own right: children and sociology in the UK', in L. Chisholm *et al.* (eds), op. cit.

Lerner, R. M. and Galambos, N. L. (1998) 'Adolescent development: challenges and opportunities for research, programmes and policies', *Annual Review of Psychology*, 49: 413–46.

L'Esperance, J. (1977) 'Doctors, women and nineteenth century society: sexuality and role', in J. Woodwards and D. Richards (eds) *Health Care and Popular Medicine in Nineteenth Century England*, London: Croom Helm.

LeTouze, D. and Watters, C. (2003) 'Good practices in mental health and social care provision for refugees and asylum seekers. Report on the United Kingdom', in C. Watters and D. Ingleby (eds) *Final Report on Good practices in mental health and social care provision for asylum seekers and refugees*, Bruxelles: European Commission (European Refugee Fund).

Levin, E., Sinclair, I. and Gorbach, P. (1989) *Families, Services and Confusion in Old Age*, Aldershot: Gower.

Levy, S. M. (1979) 'Temporal experience in the aged: body integrity and the social milieu', *International Journal of Ageing and Human Development*: 313–44.

Lewis, J. (1980) *The Politics of Motherhood: Child and Maternal Welfare in England, 1900–1939*, London: Croom Helm.

Li, L., Manor, O. and Power, C. (2004) 'Are inequalities in height narrowing? Comparing effects of social class on height in two generations', *Archives of Disease in Childhood*, 89: 1018–23.

Li, L. and Power, C. (2004) 'Influences on childhood height: comparing two generations in the 1958 British birth cohort', *International Journal of Epidemiology*, 33, 6: 1320–8.

Link, B. G. and Cullen, F. T. (1983) 'Reconsidering the social rejection of ex-mental patients: levels of attitudinal response', *American Journal of Community Psychology*, 11: 261–73.

Link, B. G. and Cullen, F. (1986) 'Contact with the mentally ill and perceptions of how dangerous they are', *Journal of Health and Social Behaviour*, 27: 289–303.

Link, B. G., Cullen, F. T., Struening, E., Shrout, P. and Dohrenwend, B. P. (1989) 'A modified labeling theory approach in the area of the mental disorders: an empirical assessment', *American Sociological Review*, 54: 400–23.

Link, B. G., Struening, E. L., Rahav, M., Phelan, J. C. and Nuttbrock, L. (1997) 'On stigma and its consequences: evidence from a longitudinal study of men with dual diagnoses of mental illness and substance abuse', *Journal of Health and Social Behaviour*, 38: 177–90.

Litman, T. J. (1974) 'The family as a basic unit in health and medical care: a social-behavioural overview', *Social Science & Medicine*, 8: 495–519.

Livingstone, S. and Bober, M. (2003) *UK Children Go Online: Listening to Young People's Experience*, LSE: LSE Research Online: http://eprints.lse.ac.uk/archive/0000388 (accessed 15 March 2008).

Livingstone, S. and Bober, M. (2005) *UK Children Go Online: Final Report of Key Project Findings*, London: London School of Economics.

Locker, D. (1979) *Symptoms and Illness*, London: Tavistock Publications.

Lorber, J. (1975) 'Good patients and problem patients: conformity and deviance in a general hospital', *Journal of Health and Social Behaviour*, 16: 213–25.

Lowry, S. (1991a) *Housing and Health*, London: British Medical Journal.

Luthar, S. and Zelazo, L. B. (2003) 'Research on resilience: an integrative review', in S. Luthar, *Resilience and Vulnerability: Adaptation in the Context of Childhood Adversities*, Cambridge/New York: Cambridge University Press, pp. 510–49.

Lynch, J. W., Kaplan, G. A. and Shema, S. J. (1997) 'Cumulative impact of sustained economic hardship on physical, cognitive, psychological and social functioning', *New England Journal of Medicine*, 337: 1889–95.

Lynch, J. W., Smith, G. D., Kaplan, G. A. and House, J. S. (2000) 'Income inequality and mortality: importance to health of individual income, psychosocial environment, or material conditions', *British Medical Journal*, 320: 1200–4.

Macdonald, E. (2004) 'The doctor's perspective', in E. Macdonald (ed.) *Difficult Conversations in Medicine*, Oxford: Oxford University Press, pp. 46–76.

Macfarlane, A. and Mugford, M. (1984) *Birth Counts: Statistics of Pregnancy and Childbirth*, National Perinatal Epidemiology Unit/OPCS, London: HMSO.

Macfarlane, A. and Cole, T. (1985) 'From depression to recession – evidence about the effects of unemployment on mothers' and babies' health 1930s–1980s' in *Born Unequal: Perspectives on Pregnancy and Childbearing in Unemployed Families*, London: Maternity Alliance.

Macfarlane, A. and Mugford, M. (2000) *Birth Counts; statistics of pregnancy and childbirth: Volume 1*, 2nd edn, London: The Stationery Office.

Macfarlane, A., Mugford, M., Henderson, J., Furtado, A., Stevens, J. and Dunn, A. (2000) *Birth Counts: Statistics of pregnancy and childbirth, Volume 2*, London: Stationery Office.

Macintrye, S. (1977) *Single and Pregnant*, London: Croom Helm.

Macintyre, S. (1986) 'The patterning of health by social position in contemporary Britain: directions for sociological research', *Social Science & Medicine*, 23, 4: 393–415.

Macintyre, S. (1997) 'The Black Report and beyond: what are the issues?', *Social Science & Medicine*, 44, 6: 723–45.

Macintyre, S., Hunt, K. and Sweeting, H. (1996) 'Gender differences in health: are things as simple as they seem?', *Social Science & Medicine*, 42, 4: 617–24.

Macintyre, S., McKay, L. and Ellaway, A. (2005) 'Who is more likely to experience common disorders: men, women, or both equally? Lay perceptions in the West of Scotland', *International Journal of Epidemiology*, 34, 2: 461–6.

Mackay, L. (1990) 'Nursing: just another job?' in P. Abbott and C. Wallace (eds), op. cit.

MacLeod, R. D. (2001) 'On reflection: doctors learning to care for people who are dying', *Social Science & Medicine*, 52: 1719–27.

MacLeod, R. D. and Nash, A. (1991) 'Teaching palliative care in general practice: a survey of educational needs and preferences', *Journal of Palliative Care*, 7, 4: 9–12.

Macleod Clark, J. (1993) 'From sick nursing to health nursing: evolution or revolution', in J. Wilson-Barnett and J. Macleod Clark (eds) *Research in Health Promotion and Nursing*, London: Macmillan.

Maddox, G. (1966) 'Retirement as a social event', in J. C. McKinney and F. T. de Vyer (eds) *Aging and Social Policy*, New York: Appleton-Century-Croft.

MAFF (1985) *Household Food Consumption and Expenditure*, Report of the National Food Survey Committee, London: HMSO.

Maher, J. and Green, H. (2002) *Carers 2000*, London: The Stationery Office. Also available at: http://www.statistics.gov.uk/downloads/theme_health/carers2000.pdf (accessed 7 May 2009).

Maher, J. and Macfarlane, A. (2004) 'Inequalities in infant mortality: trends by social class, registration status, mother's age and birthweight, England and Wales, 1976–2000', *Health Statistics Quarterly*, 24, Winter: 14–22.

Marmot, M. (2002) 'The influence of income on health: views of an epidemiologist. Does money really matter? Or is it a marker for something else?', *Health Affairs*, 21, 2: 31–46.

Marmot, M. (2004) *Status Syndrome: how your social standing directly affects your health and life expectancy*, London: Bloomsbury.

Marmot, M. G. *et al.* (1981) 'Changes in heart disease mortality in England and Wales and other countries', *Health Trends*, 13: 33–8.

Marmot, M. G., Shipley, M. J. and Rose, G. (1984) 'Inequalities in death: specific explanations of a general pattern', *Lancet*, i: 1003–6.

Marmot, M. G. (1986) 'Social inequalities in mortality: the social environment', in Wilkinson, R. G. (ed.) (1986) op. cit.

Marmot, M., Banks, J., Blundell, R., Lessof, C. and Nazroo, J. (2002) *Health, Wealth and Lifestyles of the Older Population in England: The 2002 English Longitudinal Study of Ageing*, London: Institute of Fiscal Studies. Also see http://www.ifs.org.uk/elsa/ (accessed 2 April 2008).

Marmot, M. G. and McDowall, M. E. (1986) 'Mortality decline and widening social inequalities', *Lancet*, ii: 274–76.

Martin, J. P. (1984) *Hospitals in Trouble*, Oxford: Basil Blackwell.

Martin, J. and Roberts, C. (1984) *Women and Employment: A Lifetime Perspective*, London: HMSO.

Maughan, B., Iervolino, A. C. and Collishaw, S. (2005) 'Time trends in child and adolescent mental disorders', *Current Opinion in Psychiatry*, 18: 381–5.

Mayall, B. (1993) 'Keeping healthy at home and school: "it's my body, so it's my job" ', *Sociology of Health & Illness*, 15, 4: 464–87.

Mayall, B. (1994a) *Children's Childhoods: Observed and Experienced*, London: Falmer Press.

Mayall, B. (1994b) *Negotiating Health: Children at Home and Primary School*, London: Cassell.

Mayall, B. (1998a) 'Towards a sociology of child health', *Sociology of Health & Illness*, 20, 3: 269–88.

Mayall, B. (1998b) 'Children, emotions and daily life', in G. Bendelow and S. Williams (eds) *Emotions in Social Life*, London: Routledge.

Mayall, B. and Foster, M.-C. (1989) *Child Health Care: Living with Children, Working for Children*, Oxford: Heinemann Professional Publications.

Maynard, M. (1990) 'The reshaping of sociology? Trends in the study of gender', *Sociology*, 24, 2: 269–90.

McCarthy, M. (1985) 'Taking Control', *Nursing Times*, 81, 15: 52.

McConnell, H. and Wilson, B. (2007) 'Families', in S. Smallwood and B. Wilson (eds) *Focus on Families*, Office for National Statistics, Basingstoke: Palgrave Macmillan, pp. 2–18.

McCreadie, R., Wiles, D. H., Moore, J. W. *et al.* (1987) 'The Scottish first episode schizophrenia study, IV: psychiatric and social impact on relatives', *British Journal of Psychiatry*, 150: 340.

McDowell, I. (2006) *Measuring Health: A Guide to Rating Scales and Questionnaires*, 3rd edn, New York: Oxford University Press.

McGlone, F., Park, A. and Smith, K. (1998) *Families and Kinship*, London: Family Policy Studies Centre.

McHoul, A. (1978) 'The organisation of turns at formal talk in the classroom', *Language in Society*, 7: 183–213.

McInerney, F. (2006) 'Heroic frames: discursive constructions around the requested death movement in Australia in the late 1990s', *Social Science & Medicine*, 62: 654–67.

McIntosh, J. (1981) 'Communicating with patients in their own homes', in W. Bridge and J. Clark (eds) *Communication in Nursing Care*, London: HM and M.

McKay, R. (1973) 'Conceptions of children and models of socialization', in H. P. Dreitzel (ed.) *Childhood and Socialization*, Recent Sociology, No. 5, Collier-Macmillan.

McKeown, L. P., Porter-Armstrong, A. and Baxter, G. (2003) 'The needs and experiences of caregivers of individuals with multiple sclerosis: a systematic review', *Clinical Rehabilitation*, 17: 234–48.

McKeown, T. (1976) *The Role of Medicine: Dream, Mirage or Nemesis*, London: Nuffield Provincial Hospitals Trust.

McKie, J., Richardson, J., Singer, P. and Kuhse, H. (1998) *The Allocation of Health Care Resources: An Ethical Evaluation of the 'QALY' Approach*, Aldershot: Dartmouth Ashgate.

McKinlay, J. B. and McKinlay, S. B. (1977) 'Questionable contribution of medical measures to the decline of mortality in the United States in the twentieth century', *Milbank Memorial Fund Quarterly (Health and Society)*, 55: 405–28.

McKinlay, J. (1973) 'Social networks, lay consultation and help-seeking behavior', *Social Forces*, 51: 275–81.

McKinlay, J. and Arches, J. (1985) 'Towards the proletarianization of physicians', *International Journal of Health Services*, 15: 161–95.

McKinley, J. (1977) 'The business of good doctoring or doctoring as good business: reflections on Freidson's view of the medical game', *International Journal of Health Services*, 7, 3: 459–83.

McMahon, C. and Ford, T. (1955) 'Surviving the first five years of retirement', *Journal of Gerontology*, 10: 212–15.

McNamara, B., Waddell, C. and Colvin, M. (1994) 'The institutionalization of the good death', *Social Science & Medicine*, 39: 1501–8.

McNamara, B., Waddell, C. and Colvin, M. (1995) 'Threats to the good death: the cultural context of stress and coping among hospice nurses', *Sociology of Health & Illness*, 17: 222–44.

McWhinney, I. R. (1995) 'Why we need a new clinical method', in M. Stewart, J. B. Brown, W. W. Weston, I. R. McWhinney, C. L. McWilliam and T. R. Freeman (eds) *Patient-Centred Medicine: Transforming the Clinical Method*, Thousand Oaks, CA: Sage, pp. 1–18.

Mead, G. H. (1934) *Mind, Self and Society*, Chicago: Chicago University Press.

Mechanic, D. and Volkart, E. H. (1961) 'Stress, illness behaviour and the sick role', *American Sociological Review*, 26: 51–8.

Meehl, P. E. (1962) 'Schizotaxia, schizotypy, schizophrenia', *American Psychologist*, 17: 827–38.

Mellor, P. A. (1993) 'Death in high modernity: the contemporary presence and absence of death', in D. Clark (ed.) *The Sociology of Death*, Oxford: Basil Blackwell, pp. 11–30.

Meltzer, H. (2007) 'Childhood mental disorder in Great Britain: An epidemiological perspective', *Child Care in Practice*, 13, 4: 313–26.

Meltzer, H., Gatward, R., Ford, T. and Goodman, R. (2000) *The Mental Health of Children and Adolescents in Great Britain*, London: The Stationery Office.

Meltzer, H., Gill, B., Pettigrew, M. and Hinds, K. (1995) 'The prevalence of psychiatric morbidity among adults living in private households', *OPCS Surveys of Psychiatric Morbidity in Great Britain, Report 1*, London: HMSO.

Mercer, J. R. (1968) 'Labeling the mentally retarded' in E. Rubington and M. S. Weinberg (eds) *Deviance: The Interactionist Perspective*, New York: Macmillan.

Meredith, H. (1991) 'Young carers: the unacceptable face of community care', *Social Work and Social Services Review*, 3: 47–51.

Midgley, J. (1991) 'The radical right, politics and society' in H. Glennerster and J. Midgley (eds) *The Radical Right and the Welfare State: An International Assessment*, London: Harvester Wheatsheaf.

Miles, A. (1981) *The Mentally Ill in Contemporary Society*, Oxford: Martin Robertson.

Miles, A. (1988) *Women and Mental Illness*, Brighton: Wheatsheaf.

Miles, A. (1991) *Women, Health and Medicine*, Milton Keynes: Open University Press.

Millerson, G. L. (1964) *The Qualifying Association*, London: Routledge and Kegan Paul.

Millett, K. (1970) *Sexual Politics*, London: Abacus.

Millwood Hargrave, A. and Livingstone, S. (2007) *Harm and Offence in Media Content: Updating the 2005 Review*, London: Ofcom.

Ministry of Health (1962) *A Hospital Plan for England and Wales*, London: HMSO.

Ministry of Health (1968*) Findings and Recommendations Following Enquiries into Allegations Concerning the Care of Elderly Patients in Certain Hospitals*, 1973, London: HMSO.

Minkler, M. and Estes, C. L. (eds) (1984) *Readings in the Political Economy of Aging*, Farmingdale, New York: Baywood Publishing.

Mitchell, K. J., Finkelhor, D. and Wolak, J. (2003) 'The Exposure of Youth to Unwanted Sexual Material on the Internet: A national survey of risk, impact, and prevention', *Youth & Society*, 34, 3: 330–58.

Mohaupt, S. (2008) 'Review Article: Resilience and social exclusion', *Social Policy & Society*, 8, 1: 63–71.

Morgan, D. H. J. (1975) *Social Theory and the Family*, London: Routledge & Kegan Paul.

Morgan, D. (1994) 'The family', in M. Haralambos (ed.) *Developments in Sociology*, vol. 10, Ormskirk: Causeway.

Morgan, M., Calnan, M. and Manning, N. (1985) *Sociological Approaches to Health and Medicine*, London: Croom Helm.

Morgan, O. and Baker, A. (2006) 'Measuring deprivation in England and Wales using 2001 Carstairs scores', *Health Statistics Quarterly*, 31, Autumn: 28–33.

Moriarty, J. and Butt, J. (2004) 'Inequalities in quality of life among older people from different ethnic groups', *Ageing & Society*, 24, 5: 729–53.

Morrison, M. F. (1998) 'Obstacles to doctor–patient communication at the end of life', in M. D. Steinberg and S. J. Youngner (eds) *End-of-Life Decisions: A Psychosocial Perspective*, Washington, DC: American Psychiatric Press, pp. 109–36.

Morse, J. M. (1991) 'Negotiating commitment and involvement in the nurse–patient relationship', *Journal of Advanced Nursing*, 16: 455–68.

Moser, K. A., Fox, A. J. and Jones, D. R. (1984) 'Unemployment and mortality in the OPCS longitudinal study', *Lancet*, ii: 1324–8.

Moser, K. A., Goldblatt, P. O., Fox, A. J. *et al.* (1987) 'Unemployment and mortality: a comparison of the 1971 and 1981 longitudinal study census samples', *British Medical Journal*, 294: 86–90.

Mulkay, M., Ashmore, M. and Pinch, T. (1987) 'Measuring the quality of life: a sociological invention concerning the application of economics to health care', *Sociology*, 21, 4: 541–64.

Munday, D., Dale, J. and Murray, S. (2007) 'Choice and place of death: individual preferences, uncertainty and the availability of care', *Journal of the Royal Society of Medicine*, May, 100: 211–15.

Murcott, A. (1981) 'On the typification of "bad patients"', in P. Atkinson and C. Heath (eds) *Medical Work: Realities and Routines*, Aldershot: Gower.

Murphy, E. (2007) 'Images of childhood in mothers' accounts of contemporary childrearing', *Childhood*, 14: 105–27.

Mynors-Wallis, L. M., Gath, D. H., Lloyd-Thomas, A. R. and Tomlinson, D. (1995) 'Randomized controlled trial comparing problem solving treatment with amitriptyline and placebo for major depression in primary care', *British Medical Journal*, 310: 441–5.

Nathanson, C. (1980) 'Social roles and health status among women: the significance of employment', *Social Science & Medicine*, 14a: 463–71.

National Association of Health Authorities (1988) *Action Not Words*, Birmingham: NAHA.

National Cancer Alliance (1996) *'Patient-Centred Services?' What Patients Say*, London: National Cancer Alliance.

National Statistics Online (2008) Standardised Mortality Ratios for Wards in England and Wales, 1999–2003, http://www.statistics.gov.uk/statbase/Product.asp?vlnk=14359 (accessed 3 July 2008).

Navaie-Waliser, M., Feldman, P. H., Gould, D. A., Levine, C., Kuerbis, A. N. and Donelan, K. (2001) 'The experiences and challenges of informal caregivers: Common themes and differences among Whites, Blacks and Hispanics', *The Gerontologist*, 41: 733–41.

Navarro, V. (1976) *Medicine Under Capitalism*, London: Croom Helm.

Navarro, V. (1980) 'Work, ideology and science', *International Journal of Health Services*, 10, 4: 523–50.

Nazroo, J. Y. (1997) *The Health of Britain's Ethnic Minorities*, London: Policy Studies Institute.

Nazroo, J. and King, M. (2002) 'Psychosis – symptoms and estimated rates', in K. Sproston and J. Nazroo, *Ethnic Minority Illness Rates in the Community (EMPIRIC) – Quantitative Report*, London: The Stationery Office, pp. 47–62.

Nazroo, J. and Sproston, K. (2002) 'Introduction', in K. Sproston and J. Nazroo, *Ethnic Minority Illness Rates in the Community (EMPIRIC) – Quantitative Report*, London: The Stationery Office, pp. 9–24.

Nettleton, S. (1995) *The Sociology of Health & Illness*, Cambridge: Polity Press.

Nettleton, S. and Bunton, R. (1995) 'Sociological critiques of health promotion', in R. Bunton, S. Nettleton and R. Burrows (eds), op. cit., pp. 41–58.

New, B. (ed.) (1997) *Rationing: Talk and Action in Health Care*, London: King's Fund and BMJ Publishing Group.

Newby, H. (1980) *Green and Pleasant Land? Social Change in Rural England*, Harmondsworth: Penguin.

Niebrój, L. T. (2006) 'Defining health/illness: societal and/or clinical medicine?', *Journal of Physiology and Pharmacology*, 57, 4: 251–62.

Nilchaikovit, T., Hill, J. M. and Holland, J. C. (1993) 'The effects of culture on illness behaviour and medical care: Asian and American differences', *General Hospital Psychiatry*, 15, 1: 41–50.

Nissel, M. and Bonnerjea, L. (1982) *Family Care of the Handicapped Elderly: Who Pays?*, London: Policy Studies Institute.

Norman, A. (1985) *Triple Jeopardy: Growing Old in a Second Homeland*, London: Centre for Policy on Ageing.

Oakley, A. (1972) *Sex, Gender and Society*, London: Temple Smith.

Oakley, A. (1974) *Housewife*, London: Allen Lane.

Oakley, A. (1979) *Becoming a Mother*, Oxford: Martin Robertson.

Oakley, A. (1980) *Women Confined: Towards a Sociology of Childbirth*, Oxford: Martin Robertson.

Oakley, A. (1982) *Subject Women*, London: Fontana.

Oakley, A. (1984) *The Captured Womb: A History of the Medical Care of Pregnant Women*, Oxford: Blackwell.

Oakley, A. (1990) 'Who's afraid of the randomized controlled trial? Some dilemmas of the scientific method and "good" research practice', in H. Roberts (ed.) *Women's Health Counts*, London: Routledge.

Obama, B. (2008) *Dreams from My Father: A Story of Race and Inheritance*, Edinburgh: Canongate Books Ltd.

O'Boyle, C. A. (1997) 'Measuring the quality of later life', *Philosophy Transactions of the Royal Society of London*, 352: 1871–9.

O'Brien, M. (1981) *The Politics of Reproduction*, London: Routledge and Kegan Paul.

Ofcom (2009) 'What is media literacy?', http://www.ofcom.org.uk/advice/media_literacy/of_med_lit/whatis/ (accessed 19 March 2009).

Office for National Statistics (1997) *Social Focus on Families*, London: The Stationery Office.

Office for National Statistics (1998a) *Social Trends 28*, London: The Stationery Office.

Office for National Statistics (1998b) *Informal Carers*, London: The Stationery Office.

Office for National Statistics (1998c) *Living in Britain: Results from the 1996 General Household Survey*, London: Stationery Office.

Office for National Statistics (2000) *Social Trends 30*, London: The Stationery Office.

Office for National Statistics (2004) *Living in Britain: Results from the 2002 General Household Survey*, Palgrave, Macmillan. Also see http://www.statistics.gov.uk/cci/nugget.asp?id=826 (accessed 1 July 2008).

Office for National Statistics (2006) http://www.statistics.gov.uk/cci/nugget.asp?id=1657 (ccessed 27 July 2008).

Office for National Statistics (2007a) 'Infant and perinatal mortality 2006: Health areas, England and Wales', *Health Statistics Quarterly*, 35, web supplement, http://www.statistics.gov.uk/downloads/theme_health/Infant_and_perinatal_report_HSQ35.pdf (accessed 25 June 2008).

Office for National Statistics (2007b) *Social Trends, No. 37*, Basingstoke, Hants: Palgrave Macmillan.

Office for National Statistics (2007c) 'UK population set to increase to 65 million over the next ten years', News Release, 23 October 2007. Available at: http://www.statistics.gov.uk/pdfdir/pproj1007.pdf (accessed 18 August 2008).

Office for National Statistics (2007d) 'Variations persist in life expectancy by social class, 2002–2005 data released', News release, 24 October 2007. Available at http://www.statistics.gov.uk/pdfdir/le1007.pdf (accessed 18 July 2009).

Office for National Statistics (2008a) http://www.statistics.gov.uk/CCI/nugget.asp?ID=332&Pos=&ColRank=1&Rank=374 (accessed 15 July 2008).

Office for National Statistics (2008b) 'Large differences in infant mortality by ethnic group', New Release, News Release, 24 June 2008. Available at: http://www.statistics.gov.uk/pdfdir/imeth0608.pdf (accessed 23 July 2008).

Office for National Statistics (2008c) 'Life expectancy continues to rise', News release, 22 February 2008. Available at: http://www.statistics.gov.uk/cci/nugget.asp?ID=168 (accessed 15 August 2008).

Office for National Statistics (2008d) *Social Trends, No. 38*, Basingstoke, Hants: Palgrave Macmillan. Also available at: http://www.statistics.gov.uk/socialtrends38/ (accessed 1 March 2009).

Office for National Statistics (2008e) 'Divorce rate lowest for 26 years', News Release, 29 August 2008. Available at: http://www.statistics.gov.uk/pdfdir/div0808.pdf (accessed 7 May 2009).

Office for National Statistics (2009) *Social Trends, No. 39*, Basingstoke, Hants: Palgrave Macmillan. Also available at: http://www.statistics.gov.uk/socialtrends39/ (accessed 1 May 2009).

Ong, L. M. L., de Haes, J. C. J. M., Hoos, A. M. and Lammes, F. B. (1995) 'Doctor–patient communication: a review of the literature', *Social Science & Medicine*, 40, 7: 903–18.

OPCS (1986) *Registrar General's Dicennial Supplement on Occupational Mortality 1979–83*, London: HMSO.

OPCS (1988) *Occupational Mortality: Childhood Supplement 1979–80, 1982–83*, London: HMSO.

OPCS (1991) *General Household Survey 1989*, London: HMSO.

OPCS (1992) *General Household Survey 1990*, London: HMSO.

OPCS (1993) *Population Trends*, 71, Spring: 5.

Osborn, A. F., Butler, N. R. and Morris (1984) *The Social Life of Britain's Five-Year Olds: A Report of the Child Health and Education Study*, London: Routledge & Kegan Paul.

Pahl, R. (1984) *Divisions of Labour*, Oxford: Basil Blackwell.

Palmore, E. G., Burchett, B., Fillenbaum, G., George, L. and Wallman, L. (1985) *Retirement: Causes and Consequences*, New York: Springer.

Parker, G. (1990) *With Due Care and Attention: A Review of Research on Informal Health Care*, 2nd edn, London: Family Policy Studies Centre.

Parker, G. (1993) *With This Body: Caring and Disability in Marriage*, Buckingham: Open University Press.

Parker, R. (1981) 'Tending and social policy', in E. M. Goldberg and S. Hatch (eds), *A New Look at the Personal Social Services*, London: Policy Studies Institute.

Parker, S. (1980) *Older Workers and Retirement*, OPCS, London: HMSO.

Parkin, F. (1979) *Marxism and Class Theory: A Bourgeois Critique*, London: Tavistock.

Parliamentary Office of Science and Technology (2006) *Healthy Life Expectancy*, Postnote, February, No. 257. Also available at: http://www.parliament.uk/documents/upload/postpn257.pdf. (accessed 10 March 2008).

Parliamentary Office of Science and Technology (2007) *Ethnicity and Health*, Postnote, January, No. 276. Also available at: http://www.parliament.uk/documents/upload/postpn276.pdf (accessed 25 July 2008).

Parry, N. and Parry, J. (1976) *The Rise of the Medical Profession*, London: Croom Helm.

Parsons, T. (1942) 'Age and sex in the social structure of the United States', *American Sociological Review*, 7: 604–16.

Parsons, T. (1951) *The Social System*, Glencoe, IL: The Free Press.

Parsons, T. (1956) *Family, Socialisation and Interaction Process*, London: Routledge and Kegan Paul.

Parsons, T. (1972) 'Definitions of health and illness in the light of American values and social structure', in E. G. Jaco (ed.) *Patients, Physicians and Illness*, New York: Macmillan, pp. 107–27.

Parsons, T. (1975) 'The sick role and the role of the physician reconsidered', *Millbank Memorial Fund Quarterly: Health and Society*, 53: 257–78.

Parsons, T. (1978) 'Death in the Western world', in T. Parsons, *Action Theory and the Human Condition*, New York: Free Press, pp. 331–51.

Parsons, T. and Fox, R. C. (1953) 'Illness, therapy and the modern urban American family', *Journal of Social Issues*, 8: 31–44.

Parsons, T. and Lidz, V. (1967) 'Death in American society', in E. Schneidman (ed.) *Essays in Self Destruction*, New York: Science House, pp. 133–70.

Patel, S. and Gaw, A. C. (1996) 'Suicide among immigrants from the Indian subcontinent: a review', *Psychiatry Services*, 47: 517–21.

Patrick, D. and Peach, H. (1989) *Disablement in the Community*, Oxford: Oxford University Press.

Payne, S. (1991) *Women, Health and Poverty: An Introduction*, Hemel Hempstead: Harvester Wheatsheaf.

Peace, S. (1986) 'The forgotten female: social policy and older women', in C. Phillipson and Walker, A. (eds) *Ageing and Social Policy: A Critical Assessment*, Aldershot: Gower.

Pearlin, L., Mullan, J., Semple, S. and Skaff, M. (1990) 'Caregiving and the stress process: an overview of concepts and their measures', *The Gerontologist*, 30, 5: 583–94.

Peberdy, A., Katz, J. S. and Komaromy, C. (2004) *Death & Dying: Workbook 1: Life and Death*, 3rd edn, Milton Keynes: Open University.

Pendleton, D. and Brochner, S. (1980) 'The communication of medical information in general practice consultations as a function of patients' social class', *Social Science and Medicine*, 14A, 6: 669–73.

Penn, D., Guynan, K., Daily, T., Spaulding, W., Garbin, C. and Sullivan, M. (1994) 'Dispelling the stigma of schizophrenia: what sort of information is best?', *Schizophrenia Bulletin*, 20, 3: 567–74.

Perloff, R. M., Bonder, B., Ray, G. B., Ray, E. B. and Siminoff, L. A. (2006) 'Doctor–patient communication, cultural competence and minority health: theoretical and empirical perspectives', *American Behavioural Scientist*, 49: 835–52.

Perry, M. J. (1996) 'The relationship between social class and mental disorder', *Journal of Primary Prevention*, 17, 1: 17–30.

Perry, N. (1974) 'The two cultures and the total institution', *British Journal of Sociology*, 25: 345–55.

Petrou, S., Kupeck, E., Hockley, C. and Goldacre, M. (2006) 'Social class inequalities in childhood mortality and morbidity in an English population', *Paediatric and Perinatal Epidemiology*, 20, 1: 14–23.

Philips Report (1954) *Report of the Committee on the Economic and Financial Problems of the Provision for Old Age*, London: HMSO.

Philimore, P., Beattie, A. and Townsend, P. (1994) 'Widening inequality of health in Northern England, 1981–1991', *British Medical Journal*, 308: 1125–8.

Phillips, D. L. and Segal, B. E. (1969) 'Sexual status and psychiatric symptoms', *American Sociological Review*, 34: 58–72.

Phillips, J. (2007) *Care*, Cambridge: Polity Press.

Phillipson, C. (1981) 'Women in later life: patterns of control and subordination', in B. Hutter and G. Williams (eds) *Controlling Women: The Normal and the Deviant*, London: Croom Helm.

Phillipson, C. (1982) *Capitalism and the Construction of Old Age*, London: Macmillan.

Phillipson, C. (1987) 'The Transition to Retirement', in G. Cohen (ed.), op. cit.

Phillipson, C. (1990) 'The sociology of retirement', in J. Bond and P. Coleman (eds), op. cit.

Phillipson, C. (2007) 'The "elected" and the "excluded": sociological perspectives on the experience of place and community in old age', *Ageing & Society*, 27: 321–42.

Phillipson, C., Bernard, M., Phillips, J. and Ogg, J. (2001) *The Family and Community Life of Older People*, London: Routledge.

Phillipson, C., Bernard, M. and Strang, P. (eds) (1986) *Dependency and Interdependency in Old Age – Theoretical Perspectives and Policy Alternatives*, London: Croom Helm.

Phillipson, C. and Walker, A. (1986) *Ageing and Social Policy: A Critical Assessment*, Aldershot: Gower.

Philo, G., Secker, J., Platt, S., Henderson, L., McLaughlin and Burnside, J. (1996) 'Media images of mental distress', in T. J. Heller *et al.* (eds), op. cit., pp. 163–70.

Pickard, L. (2007) 'Unpaid care and the family', in S. Smallwood and B. Wilson (eds) *Focus on Families*, Office for National Statistics, Basingstoke: Palgrave Macmillan, pp. 20–34.

Pierret, J. (1992) 'Coping with AIDS in everyday life', *Current Sociology*, 40, 3: 66.

Pietroni, P. (1991) *The Greening of Medicine*, London: Victor Gollanaz.

Pilgrim, D. and Rogers, A. (1993) *A Sociology of Mental Health and Illness*, Buckingham: Open University Press.

Pill, R. and Stott, N. C. H. (1986) 'Concepts of illness causation and responsibility: some preliminary data from a sample of working-class mothers' in C. Currer and M. Stacey (eds), op. cit.

Plaja, A. and Cohen, S. (1968) 'Communication between physicians and patients in out-patient clinics: social and cultural factors', *Milbank Memorial Fund Quarterly*, 46: 161–213.

Platt, L. (2007) *Poverty and Ethnicity in the UK*, Bristol: Policy Press in association with the Joseph Rowntree Foundation. Also available at: http://www.jrf.org.uk/bookshop/eBooks/2006-ethnicity-poverty-UK.pdf (accessed 26 July 2008)

Platt, S. D., Martin, C. J., Hunt, S. M. and Lewis, C. W. (1989) 'Damp housing, mould growth and symptomatic health state', *British Medical Journal*, 298: 1673–8.

Platt, S., Martin, C., Hunt, S. and Tantam, D. (1990) 'The mental health of women with children living in deprived areas of Great Britain: the role of living conditions, poverty and unemployment', in D. Goldberg (ed.) *The Public Health Impact of Mental Disorder*, Gottingen, Hogrefe & Huber.

Pollock, A. M., with Leys, C., Price, D., Rowland, D. and Gnani, S. (2004) *NHS plc: The Privatisation of Our Health Care*, London: Verso.

Pollock, K. (1984) *Mind and matter: a study of conceptions of health and illness among three groups of English families with particular reference to multiple sclerosis, schizophrenia and 'nervous breakdown'*, PhD thesis, University of Cambridge.

Pollock, K. (2005) *Concordance in Medical Consultations: A Critical Review*, Oxford: Radcliffe Publishing.

Pollock, L. (1983) *Forgotten Children*, Cambridge: Cambridge University Press.

Polusny, M. A. and Follette, V. M. (1995) 'Long-term correlates of child sexual abuse: theory and review of the empirical literature', *Applied and Preventative Psychology*, 4: 143–66.

Poortinga, W. (2006) 'Social relations of social capital? Individual and community health effects of bonding social capital', *Social Science & Medicine*, 63: 255–70.

Porter, S. (1991) 'A participant observation study of power relations between nurses and doctors in a general hospital', *Journal of Advanced Nursing*, 16: 728–35.

Porter, S. (1992) 'Women in a women's job: the gendered experience of nurses', *Sociology of Health & Illness*, 14, 4: 510–27.

Pratchett, R. (2005) *Gamers in the UK: Digital Play, Digital Lifestyles*, London: BBC.

Preston, B. (1978) 'Further statistics of inequality', *Sociological Review*, 27, 2: 343–50.

Prior, L. (1989) *The Social Organization of Death: Medical Discourses and Social Practices in Belfast*, Basingstoke: Macmillan.

Prior, L., Pang, L. C. and See, B. H. (2000) 'Beliefs and accounts of illness. Views from two Cantonese-speaking communities in England', *Sociology of Health & Illness*, 22, 6: 815–39.

Prout, A. (1979) 'Children and childhood in the sociology of medicine', paper presented at the British Sociological Association Medical Sociology Conference, University of Warwick.

Prout, A. (1986) 'Wet children and little actresses: going sick in primary school', *Sociology of Health and Illness*, 8, 2: 111–36.

Prout, A. (1988) '"Off school sick": mothers' accounts of school sickness', *Sociological Review*, 36, 4: 765–89.

Prout, A. and James, A. (1990) 'A new paradigm for the sociology of childhood? Provenance, promise and problems', in A. James and A. Prout (eds), op. cit.

Ptacek, J. T. and Eberhardt, T. L. (1996) 'Breaking bad news: a review of the literature', *Journal of the American Medical Association*, 276, 6: 496–502.

Ptacek, J. T. and Ptacek, J. J. (2001) 'Patients' perceptions of receiving bad news about cancer', *Journal of Clinical Oncology*, 19: 4160–4.

Qvortrup, J. (1991) *Childhood as a Social Phenomenon*, Eurosocial Report, 36, Hungary: Publicitas.

Rahkonen, O., Arber, S. and Lahelma, E. (1995) 'Health inequalities in early adulthood: a comparison of young men and women in Britain and Finland'. *Social Science and Medicine*, 41: 163–71.

Rainey, L. (1988) 'The experience of dying', in H. Wass, F. Berardo, F. and R. Neimeyer (eds) *Dying: Facing the Facts*, 2nd edn, Washington: Hemisphere, pp. 137–57.

Raleigh, V. S. and Polato, G. M. (2004) *Evidence of Health Inequalities*, London: Healthcare Commission. Also available at: http://www.healthcarecommission.org.uk/db/documents/04017601.pdf (accessed 28 July 2008).

Ramsden, S. and Smee, C. (1981) 'The health of the unemployed: DHSS cohort study', *Employment Gazette*, 89: 397–401.

Ranger, C. (1989) 'Race, culture and "cannabis psychosis": the role of social factors in the construction of a disease category', *New Community*, 15, 3: 357–69.

Rasulo, D., Bajekal, M. and Yar, M. (2007) 'Inequalities in health expectancies in England and Wales: small area analysis from the 2001 census', *Health Statistics Quarterly*, 34, Summer: 35–45.

Reidy, A. (1984) 'Marxist functionalism in medicine: a critique of the work of Vicente Navarro on health and medicine', *Social Science & Medicine*, 19, 9: 897–910.

Renaud, M. (1975) 'On the structural constraints to state intervention in health', *International Journal of Health Services*, 5, 4: 559–72.

Retterstøl, N. (1993) *Suicide: A European Perspective*, Cambridge: Cambridge University Press.

Richard, L., Laforest, S., Dufresne, F. and Sapinski, J. (2005) 'The quality of life of older adults living in an urban environment: professional and lay perspectives', *Canadian Journal of Aging*, 24: 19–30.

Riley, M. W., Johnson, M. and Foner, A. (1972) *Aging and Society (3): A Sociology of Age Stratification*, New York: Russell Sage.

Robb, B. (ed.) (1967) *Sans Everything: A Case to Answer*, London: Nelson.

Robbins, M. A (1998) *Evaluating Palliative Care*, Oxford: Oxford University Press.

Roberts, H., Smith, S. J. and Bryce, C. (1995) *Children at Risk?*, Buckingham: Open University Press.

Roberts, K. (1984) 'Problems and initiatives in youth employment', *Journal of Community and Health Care*, 62: 320–6.

Robinson, D. (1971) *The Process of Becoming Ill*, London: Routledge and Kegan Paul.

Rodberg, L. and Stevenson, G. (1977) 'The health care industry in advanced capitalism', *Review of Radical Political Economics*, 9: 1.

Rodmell, S. and Watt, A. (eds) (1986) *The Politics of Health Education*, London: Routledge and Kegan Paul.

Rogers, A., Karlsen, S. and Addington-Hall, J. (2000) 'All the services were excellent. It is when the human element comes in that things go wrong: dissatisfaction with hospital care in the last year of life', *Journal of Advanced Nursing*, 31, 4: 768–74.

Rogers, A. and Pilgrim, D. (2005) *A Sociology of Mental Health and Illness*, 3rd edn, Maidenhead: Open University Press.

Romeri, E., Baker, A. and Griffiths, C. (2006) 'Mortality by deprivation and cause of death in England and Wales, 1999–2003', *Health Statistics Quarterly*, 32, Winter: 19–34.

Rosenfield, S. (1997) 'Labelling mental illness: the effects of received services and perceived stigma on life satisfaction', *American Sociological Review*, 62, 4: 660–72.

Rosenhan, D. L. (1973) 'On being sane in insane places', *Science*, 179: 250–8.

Rosenthal, C. J., Marshall, V. W. Macpherson, A. S. and French, S. E. (1980) *Nurses, Patients and Families*, London: Croom Helm.

Roslender, R. (1992) *Sociological Perspectives on Modern Accountancy*, London: Routledge.

Rosser, C. and Harris, C. C. (1965) *The Family and Social Change*, London: Routledge & Kegan Paul.

Rosser, R. and Kind, P. (1978) 'A scale of valuations of states of illness. Is there a social consensus?', *International Journal of Epidemiology*, 7: 247–58.

Rossi, P. H. and Freeman, H. E. (1993) *Evaluation: A Systematic Approach*, 5th edn, Newbury Park, CA: Sage.

Roter, D. L. and Hall, J. A. (2004) 'Physician gender and Patient-centred communication: a Critical review of empirical research', *Annual Review of Public Health*, 25: 497–519.

Roter, D. L. and Hall, J. A. (2006) *Doctors Talking with Patients/Patients Talking with Doctors: Improving Communication in Medical Visits*, 2nd revised edn, Westport, CT: Praeger Publishers.

Roter, D. L., Hall, J. A. and Aoki, Y. (2002) 'Physician gender effects in medical communication: a meta-analytic review', *Journal of the American Medical Association*, 288, 6: 756–64.

Roth, J. (1963) *Timetables: Structuring the Passage of Time in Hospital Treatment and Other Careers*, New York: Bobbs-Merrill.

Roth, J. A. (1972) 'Some contingencies of the moral evaluation and control of clientele', *American Journal of Sociology*, 77, 5: 839–86.

Roth, J. A. (1984) 'Staff–inmate bargaining tactics in long-term treatment institutions', *Sociology of Health and Illness*, 6, 2: 111–31.

Roth, M. (1976) 'Schizophrenia and the theories of Thomas Szasz', *British Journal of Psychiatry*, 129: 317–26.

Rowe, J. W. and Kahn, R. L. (1997) 'Successful aging', *The Gerontologist*, 37, 4: 433–41.

Rowles, G. and Chaudhury, H. (eds) (2005) *Home and Identity in Later Life: International Perspectives*, New York: Springer Publishing Company.

Royal Commission on the Law Relating to Mental Illness and Mental Deficiency (The Percy Report) (1957) London: HMSO.

Rutter, M. (1985) 'Resilience in the face of adversity. Protective factors and resistance to psychiatric disorder', *British Journal of Psychiatry*, 47: 598–611.

Rutter, M. (1990) 'Psychosocial resilience and protective mechanism', in J. Rolf, A. Masten, D. Cicchetti, K. Neuchterlein and S. Weintraub (eds) *Risk and Protective Factors in the Development of Psychopathology*, New York: Cambridge University Press.

Salvage, J. (1985) *The Politics of Nursing*, London: Heinemann.

Salvage, J. and Kershaw, B. (1990) *Models for Nursing*, London: Scutari Press.

Salway, S., Platt, L., Chowbey, P., Harriss, K. and Bayliss, E. (2007) *Long-term Ill Health, Poverty and Ethnicity*, Bristol: Policy Press in association with the Joseph Rowntree Foundation. Also available at: http://www.jrf.org.uk/knowledge/findings/socialpolicy/2060.asp (accessed 26 July 2008).

Samson, C. (1995) 'The fracturing of medical dominance in British psychiatry?', *Sociology of Health & Illness*, 17, 2: 245–68.

Saunders, C. (1992) 'Voluntary euthanasia', *Palliative Medicine*, 6: 1–5.

Saunders, C. and Baines, M. (1983) *Living with Dying: The Management of Terminal Disease*, Oxford: Oxford University Press.

Savage, W. (1986) *A Savage Enquiry: Who Controls Childbirth?*, London: Virago.

Scambler, G. (1984) 'Perceiving and coping with stigmatizing illness', in R. Fitzpatrick *et al.* (eds), op. cit.

Scambler, G. (1989) *Epilepsy*, London: Routledge.

Scambler, G., Scambler, A. and Craig, D. (1981) 'Kinship and friendship networks and women's demand for primary care', *Journal of the Royal College of General Practitioners*, 26: 746–50.

Scambler, G. and Scambler, A. (1984) 'The illness iceberg and aspects of consulting behaviour', in R. Fitzpatrick *et al.* (eds), op. cit.

Scambler, G. and Hopkins, A. (1986) 'Being epileptic: coming to terms with stigma', *Sociology of Health and Illness*, 8: 26–43.

Scharf, T., Phillipson, C., Smith, A. E. and Kingston, P. (2002) *Growing Older in Socially Deprived Areas*, London: Help the Aged.

Scheff, T. J. (1966) *Being Mentally Ill: A Sociological Theory*, Chicago: Aldine.

Scheff, T. J. (1975) 'The labeling theory of mental illness', in T. Scheff (ed.) *Labeling Madness*, Englewood Cliffs, NJ: Prentice-Hall.

Schon, D. (1991) *The Reflective Practitioner*, 2nd edn, San Francisco: Jossey Bass.

Schoon, I. (2006) *Risk and Resilience: Adaptations in Changing Times*, Cambridge: Cambridge University Press.

Schrock, R. (1982) 'Is health visiting a profession?', *Health Visitor*, 55: 104–7.

Schulz, R., Noelker, L. S., Rockwood, K. and Sprott, R. L. (2006) (eds) *The Encyclopedia of Aging*, Vol. I, 4th edn, New York: Springer Publishing Co. Inc.

Schuman, J. (1998) 'Childhood, infant and perinatal mortality, 1996; social and biological factors in deaths of children aged under 3', *Population Trends*, Summer, 92: 5–14.

Schutz, A. (1967) 'Concept and theory formation in the social sciences', in M. Natanson (ed.) *Alfred Schutz, Collected Papers*, vol. 1, The Hague: Nijhoff.

Scott, R. (1969) *The Making of Blind Men*, New York: Russell Sage Foundation.

Scull, A. (1983) 'The asylum as community or the community as asylum: paradoxes and contradictions of mental health care', in P. Bean (ed.) *Mental Illness: Changes and Trends*, Chichester: John Wiley and Sons Ltd.

Seale, C. (1989) 'What happens in hospices: a review of research evidence', *Social Science & Medicine*, 28: 551–9.

Seale, C. (1998) *Constructing Death: The Sociology of Dying and Bereavement*, Cambridge: Cambridge University Press.

Seale, C. and Addington-Hall, J. (1995) 'Dying at the best time', *Social Science and Medicine*, 40, 5: 589–95.

Seale, C. F., Addington-Hall, J. and McCarthy, M. (1997) 'Awareness of dying: prevalence, causes and consequences', *Social Science & Medicine*, 45, 3: 477–84.

Seale, C. F. and Cartwright, A. (1994) *The Year Before Death*, Aldershot: Avebury.

Seale, C. and Kelly, M. (1997) 'A comparison of hospice and hospital care for people who die: views of the surviving spouse', *Palliative Medicine*, 11: 93–100.

Seebohm Report (1968) *Report of the Committee on Local Authority and Allied Social Services*, London: HMSO.

Sehnert, K. W. and Eisenberg, H. (1975) *How To Be Your Own Doctor – Sometimes*, New York: Grossett and Dunlap.

Select Committee on Economic Affairs (2003) *Aspects of the Economics of an Ageing Population*, Fourth Report, Volume I, HL Paper 179-I, London: The Stationery Office. Also available at: http://www.publications.parliament.uk/pa/ld200203/ldselect/ldeconaf/179/179.pdf (accessed 15 August 2008).

Senior, P. and Bhopal, R. S. (1994) 'Ethnicity as a variable in epidemiological research', *British Medical Journal*, 309: 327–9.

Seymour, J. E. (1999) 'Revisiting medicalisation and "natural" death', *Social Science & Medicine*, 49: 691–704.

Seymour, J. E., Bellamy, G., Gott, M., Ahmedzai, S. H. and Clark, D. (2002) 'Good deaths, bad deaths: older people's assessments of the risks and benefits of morphine and terminal sedation in end-of-life care', *Health, Risk and Society*, 4, 3: 287–303.

Shanas, E., Townsend, P., Wedderburn, B., Friis, H., Milhoj, P. and Stehouwer, J. (1968) *Old People in Three Industrial Societies*, London: Routledge and Kegan Paul.

Shanas, E. (1970) 'Health and adjustment in retirement', *The Gerontologist*, 10: 19–21.

Sharkey, P. (2007) *Essentials of Community Care*, Basingstoke: Palgrave Macmillan.

Shelter (2006) *Against the Odds*, London: Shelter.

Shepperd, S., Doll, H. and Jenkinson, C. (1997) 'Randomized controlled trials', in C. Jenkinson (ed.), op. cit.

Shetland, M. L. (1965) 'Teaching and learning in nursing', *American Journal of Nursing*, 65, 9, 112–16.

Siegler, V., Langford, A. and Johnson, B. (2008) 'Regional differences in male mortality inequalities using the National Statistics Socio-economic Classification, England and Wales, 2001–03', *Health Statistics Quarterly*, 40, Winter: 6–17.

Simpson, I. H., Back, K., Ingles, T., Kerckhoff, A. and McKinney, J. C., (1979) *From Student to Nurse: A Longitudinal Study of Socialization*, Cambridge: Cambridge University Press.

Singh-Manoux, A. and Marmot, M. (2005) 'Role of socialization in explaining social inequalities in health', *Social Science & Medicine*, 60: 2129–33.

Sixsmith, A. J. (1986) 'Independence and home in later life', in C. Phillipson, M. Bernard and P. Strang (eds), op. cit.

Slevin, M. L., Plant, H., Lynch, D., Drinkwater, J. and Gregory, W. M. (1988) 'Who should measure quality of life, the doctor or the patient?', *British Journal of Cancer*, 57: 109–12.

Smaje, C. (1995) *Health, 'Race' and Ethnicity: Making Sense of the Evidence*, London: King's Fund Institute.

Smallwood, S. and Chamberlain, J. (2005) 'Replacement fertility, what has it been and what does it mean?', *Population Trends*, 119: 16–27.

Smelser, N. J. (1994) *Sociology*, Cambridge, Massachusetts: Basil Blackwell.

Smith, A. (1986) *The Science of Social Medicine*, London: Staples.

Smith, A. and Jacobson, B. (eds) (1988) *The Nation's Health: A Strategy for the 1990s*, London: King's Fund.

Smith, A. E. (2000) 'Quality of life: a review', *Education and Ageing*, 15, 3: 419–35.

Smith, A. E., Sim, J., Scharf, T. and Phillipson, C. (2004) 'Determinants of quality of life amongst older people in deprived neighbourhoods', *Ageing & Society*, 24: 793–814.

Smith, D. E. (1987) *The Everyday World as Problematic: A Feminist Sociology*, Milton Keynes: Open University Press.

Smith, G. D., Bartley, M. and Blane, D. (1990) 'The Black Report on socio-economic inequalities and health ten years on', *British Medical Journal*, 301: 373–7.

Smith, P. and Natalier, K. (2004) *Understanding Criminal Justice: Sociological Perspectives*, London: Sage.

Smith, R. (1985) 'Occupationless health', *British Medical Journal*, 16 November: 1409.

Smith, R. (1987) *Unemployment and Health*, Oxford: Oxford University Press.

Smith, R. (ed.) (1991) *Health of the Nation: The BMJ View*, London: BMJ.

Smith, R. (2000) 'A good death', *British Medical Journal*, 320: 129–30.

Smith-Rosenberg, C. (1984) 'The hysterical woman: sex roles and role conflict in nineteenth century America', in N. Black *et al.* (eds) *Health and Disease: A Reader*, Milton Keynes: Open University Press.

Social Services Inspectorate (1995) *Young Carers: Something to Think About*, London: Department of Health.

Social Services Select Committee (1985) *Community Care*, vol. I, Report HC 13-1, London: HMSO.

Somerville, S. M., Rona, R. J. and Chinn, S. (1988) 'Passive smoking and respiratory conditions in primary school children', *Journal of Epidemiology and Community Health*, 42: 105–10.

Spencer, N. J. (1984) 'Parents' recognition of the ill child', in J. A. Macfarlane (ed.) *Progress in Child Health*, Edinburgh: Churchill-Livingstone.

Spitzer, W. O., Dobson, A. J., Hall, J. *et al.* (1981) 'Measuring the quality of life of cancer patients: a concise QL index for use by physicians', *Journal of Chronic Disease*, 34: 585–99.

Sproston, K. and Nazroo, J. (eds) (2002) *Ethnic Minority Illness Rates in the Community (EMPIRIC) – Quantitative Report*, London: The Stationery Office.

Srole, L., Langer, T. S., Michael, S. T., Opler, M. K. and Rennie, T. A. C. (1962) *Mental Health in the Metropolis: The Midtown Manhattan Study*, New York: McGraw-Hill Inc.

Stacey, J. (1993) 'Untangling feminist theory', in D. Richardson and V. Robinson (eds) *Introducing Women's Studies*, London: Macmillan.

Stacey, M. (1969) 'The myth of community studies', *British Journal of Sociology*, 20, 2: 134–47.

Stacey, M. (1976) 'The health service consumer: a sociological misconception', in *Sociology of the National Health Service*, Sociological Review Monograph 22, Keele: University of Keele.

Stacey, M. (1988) *The Sociology of Health and Healing: A Textbook*, London: Unwin Hyman.

Stacey, M. (1991) 'Medical sociology and health policy: an historical overview', in J. Gabe, M. Calnan and M. Bury (eds) *The Sociology of the Health Service*, London: Routledge.

Starr, P. (1982) *The Social Transformation of American Medicine*, New York: Basic Books.

Steele, D. J., Blackwell, B., Gutmann, M. C. and Jackson, T. C. (1987) 'The activated patient: dogma, dream or desideratum', *Patient Education and Counseling*, 10: 3–23.

Stein, L. (1978) 'The doctor–nurse game', in R. Dingwall and J. McIntosh (eds), op. cit.

Stern, J. (1983) 'Social mobility and the interpretation of social class mortality differentials', *Journal of Social Policy*, 12, 1: 27–49.

Stimson, G. and Webb, B. (1975) *Going to See the Doctor*, London: Routledge and Kegan Paul.

St Leger, A. S., Schnieden, H. and Walsworth-Bell, J. P. (1992) *Evaluating Health Services' Effectiveness*, Milton Keynes: Open University Press.

Stockwell, F. (1972) *The Unpopular Patient*, London: Royal College of Nursing.

Stone, L. (1977) *The Family, Sex and Marriage in England, 1500–1800*, London: Weidenfeld and Nicolson.

Strauss, A. *et al.* (1963) 'The hospital and its negotiated order', in E. Freidson (ed.) *The Hospital in Modern Society*, New York: Free Press of Glencoe.

Strauss, A. (1966) 'The structure and ideology of American nursing: an interpretation' in F. Davis (ed.) *The Nursing Profession: Five Sociological Essays*, New York: Wiley.

Strauss, A. (1978) *Negotiations: Varieties, Contexts, Processes and Social Order*, San Francisco: Jossey Bass.

Strieb, G. F. and Schneider, C. J. (1971) *Retirement in American Society*, Ithaca, N. Y.: Cornell University Press.

Strong, P. M. (1979) *The Ceremonial Order of the Clinic: Patients, Doctors and Medical Bureaucracies*, London: Routledge and Kegan Paul.

Suchman, E. A. (1965) 'Stages of illness and medical care', *Journal of Health and Human Behavior*, 6: 114–28.

Sulkava, R., Wikstrom, J., Aromaa, A., Raitasalo, R., Lehtinen, V., Lahtela, K. and Palo, J. (1985) 'Prevalence of severe dementia in Finland', *Neurology*, 35: 1025–9.

Susman, J. (1994) 'Disability, stigma and deviance', *Social Science & Medicine*, 38, 1: 15–22.

Sutter, G. (2000) '"Nothing New Under the Sun": Old fears and new media', *International Journal of Law and Information*, 8, 3: 338–78.

Szasz, T. (1961) *The Myth of Mental Illness*, New York: Harper.

Szasz, T. (1971) *The Manufacture of Madness*, London: Routledge & Kegan Paul.

Szasz, T. (1974a) *The Second Sin*, London: Routledge & Kegan Paul.

Szasz, T. (1974b) *Ideology and Insanity*, Harmondsworth: Penguin Books.

Szasz, T. S. and Hollender, M. H. (1956) 'A contribution to the philosophy of medicine: the basic models of the doctor–patient relationship', *Archives of Internal Medicine*, 97: 585–92.

Szinovacz, M. (1982) 'Research on women's retirement', in M. Szinovacz (ed.), *Women's Retirement: Policy Implications of Recent Research*, London: Sage.

Talbot-Smith, A. and Pollock, A. M. (2006) *The New NHS: A Guide*, Abingdon: Routledge.

Taske, N., Taylor, L., Mulvihill, C. and Doyle, N. *et al.* (2005) *Housing and public health: a review of reviews of interventions for improving health: evidence briefing*, London: National Institute for Health and Clinical Excellence. Also available at: http://www.nice.org.uk/niceMedia/pdf/housing_MAIN%20FINAL.pdf (accessed 15 July 2008).

Taylor, B. (1993) 'Hospice nurses tell their stories about a good death; the value of storytelling as a qualitative health research method', *Annual Review of Health Social Sciences*, 3: 97–108.

Taylor, L. (2006) 'Positive features of video games', in N. Dowd, D. Singer and R. Wilson (eds) *Handbook of Children, Culture and Violence*, London: Sage pp. 247–65.

Taylor, R. and Ford, G. (1983) 'Inequalities in old age: an examination of age, sex and class differences in a sample of community elderly', *Ageing & Society*, 3: 183–208.

Taylor, S. and Field, D. (1993) *Sociology of Health and Health Care*, Oxford: Blackwell.

Taylor, M. and Quayle, E. (2003) *Child Pornography: An Internet Crime*, London: Brunner-Routledge.

ten Have, H. (2001) 'Suffering and death: introductory comments', in H. ten Have and B. Gordijn (eds) *Bioethics in a European Perspective*, Dordrecht: Kluwer, pp. 407–9.

Thane, P. (1981) 'Childhood in history', in M. King (ed.) *Childhood Welfare Justice*, London: Batsford.

Thane, P. (1989) 'Old age: burden or benefit?', in H. Joshi (ed.) *Changing Population of Britain*, Oxford: Blackwell.

Thomas, R. K. (2003) *Society and Health: Sociology for Health Professionals*, New York: Kluwer Academic/Plenum Publishers.

Thornburgh, D. and Lin, H. (2002) *Youth, Pornography and the Internet*, Washington DC: National Academies Press.

Thorogood, N. (1992) 'What is the relevance of sociology for health promotion', in R. Bunton and G. Macdonald (eds) *Health Promotion: Disciplines and Diversity*, London: Routledge.

Thumma, S. (1991) 'Negotiating a religious identity: the case of the gay evangelical', *Sociological Analysis*, 52, 4: 333–47.

Timmermans, S. (1994) 'Dying of awareness: the theory of awareness contexts revisited', *Sociology of Health and Illness*, 16, 3: 322–39.

Titmuss, R. (1963) 'Community care: fact or fiction', in H. Freeman and J. Farndale (eds) *Trends in the Mental Health Services*, London: Pergamon Press.

Tones, B. K. (1993) 'The theory of health promotion: implications for nursing', in J. Wilson-Barnett and J. Macleod Clark (eds), op. cit.

Tönnies, F. (1957) *Community and Society*, New York: Harper and Row [1887].

Torrey, E. F. (1994) 'Violent behaviour by individuals with serious mental illness', *Hospital and Community Psychiatry*, 45, 7: 653–62.

Townsend, J., Frank, A., Fermont, D., Dyer, S., Karran, O. *et al.* (1990) 'Terminal cancer and patients' preferences for place of death: a prospective study', *British Medical Journal*, 301: 415–17.

Townsend, P. (1957) *The Family Life of Old People: An Inquiry in East London*, London: Routledge and Kegan Paul.

Townsend, P. (1973) *The Social Minority*, London: Allen Lane.

Townsend, P. (1979) *Poverty in the United Kingdom: A Survey of Household Resources and Standards of Living*, Harmondsworth: Penguin.

Townsend, P. (1981) 'The structured dependency of the elderly: creation of social policy in the twentieth century', *Ageing & Society*, 1: 5–28.

Townsend, P. (1986) 'Ageism and social policy', in C. Phillipson and A. Walker (eds), op. cit.

Townsend, P. (1987) 'Poor health', in A. Walker and C. Walker (eds), op. cit.

Townsend, P. (1990) 'Individual or social responsibility for premature death: current controversies in the British deabate about health', *International Journal of Health Studies*, 20: 373–92.

Townsend, P., Corrigan, P. and Kowarzik, O. (1986) *Poverty and the London Labour Market*, London: Low Pay Unit.

Townsend, P. and Davidson, N. (1982) *Inequalities in Health: the Black Report*, Harmondsworth: Penguin.

Townsend, P. and Davidson, N. (eds) (1992) *Inequalities in Health*, Harmondsworth: Penguin.

Townsend, P., Davidson, N. and Whitehead, M. (1992) *Inequalities in Health: The Black Report* and *The Health Divide*, in one volume, 2nd edn, Harmondsworth: Penguin.

Townsend, P., Phillimore, P. and Beattie, A. (1988) *Health and Deprivation: Inequality and the North*, London: Croom Helm.

Tuckett, D., Bolton, M., Olson, C. and Williams, A. (1985) *Meetings Between Experts: An Approach to Sharing Ideas in Medical Consultations*, London: Tavistock.

Tucker, N. (1977) *What is a Child?*, London: Fontana – Open Books.

Tunstall, J. (1962) *The Fisherman*, London: McGibbon and Kee.

Turner, B. S. (1987) *Medical Power and Social Knowledge*, London: Sage.

Twaddle, A. C. (1974) 'The concept of health status', *Social Science & Medicine*, 8, 1: 29–38.

Tweed, P., Molineux, C. and Edwards, M. (2008) 'Ethics', in M. Edwards (ed.) *The Informed Practice Nurse*, 2nd edn, West Sussex: John Wiley & Sons Ltd, pp. 1–30.

Twigg, J. and Atkin, K. (1994) *Carers Perceived: Policy and Practice in Informal Care*, Buckingham: Open University Press.

United Kingdom Central Council for Nursing, Midwifery and Health Visiting (UKCC) (1984) *Code of Professional Conduct for the Nurse, Midwife and Health Visitor*, London: UKCC.

Ungerson, C. (1983) 'Why do women care?', J. Finch and D. Groves (eds) *A Labour of Love: Women, Work and Caring*, London: Routledge & Kegan Paul.

Ungerson, C. (1987) *Policy is Personal: Sex, Gender and Informal Care*, London: Tavistock.

Ungerson, C. (1998) 'The informal sector', in P. Alcock, A. Erskine and M. May (eds) *The Student's Companion to Social Policy*, Oxford: Blackwell.

Ustun, T. B. (1998) 'The primary care setting-relevance, advantages, challenges', in R. Jenkins and T. B. Ustun (eds) *Preventing Mental Illness: Mental Health Promotion in Primary Care*, Chichester: John Wiley and Sons.

Vaillant, G. E. (2002) *Ageing Well: Surprising Guideposts to a Happier Life from the Landmark Study of Adult Development*, Boston, Massachusetts: Little, Brown and Company.

Valentine, G. (2004) *Public Space and the Culture of Childhood*, Basingstoke: Ashgate.

Victor, C. (1987) *Old Age in Modern Society: A Textbook of Social Gerontology*, London: Croom Helm.

Vostanis, P. (2002) 'Mental health of homeless children and their families', *Advances in Psychiatric Treatment*, 8: 463–9.

Wadsworth, M. E. J., Butterfield, W. J. H. and Blaney, R. (1971) *Health and Sickness: The Choice of Treatment*, London: Tavistock Publications.

Wadsworth, M. E. J. (1986) 'Serious illness in childhood and its association with later-life achievement', in Wilkinson, R. G. (ed.), op. cit.

Wagg, S. (1992) ' "I blame the parents": childhood and politics in modern Britain', *Sociology Review*, 1, 4, April: 10–15.

Wahl, H. W. and Lang, F. R. (2004) 'Aging in context across the adult life course: integrating physical and social environmental research perspectives', in H. W. Wahl, R. Scheidt and P. Windley (eds) *Focus on Aging in Context: Socio-Physical Environments: Annual Review of Gerontology and Geriatrics 23*, New York: Springer Publishing Company, pp. 1–33.

Waitzkin, H. B. (1985) 'Information giving in medical care', *Journal of Health and Social Behaviour*, 26: 81–101.

Waitzkin, H. B. (1989) 'A critical theory of medical discourse: ideology, social control and the processing of social context in medical encounters', *Journal of Health and Social Behaviour*, 30: 220–39.

Walby, S. (1990) *Theorizing Patriarchy*, Oxford: Blackwell.

Wald, N., Nanchahal, K., Thompson, S. G. and Cuckle, H. S. (1986) 'Does breathing other people's tobacco smoke cause lung cancer', *British Medical Journal*, 293: 1217–22.

Walker, A. (1980) 'The social creation of poverty and dependency in old age', *Journal of Social Policy*, 9, 1: 45–75.

Walker, A. (1981) 'Towards a political economy of old age', *Ageing & Society*, 1: 73–94.

Walker, A. (1982) 'Dependency and old age', *Social Policy and Administration*, 16: 115–35.

Walker, A. (1986a) 'The politics of ageing in Britain', in C. Phillipson *et al.* (eds), op. cit.

Walker, A. (1986b) 'Pensions and the production of poverty in old age', in C. Phillipson and A. Walker (eds), op. cit.

Walker, A. (1987) 'The poor relation; poverty among old women', in C. Glendinning and J. Millar (eds) *Women and Poverty in Britain*, Brighton: Wheatsheaf.

Walker, A. (1993) 'Community care policy: from consensus to conflict', in J. Bornat *et al.* (eds) *Community Care: A Reader*, London: Macmillan.

Walker, A. (1996) *Young Carers and their Families*, London: The Stationery Office.

Walker, A. and Walker, C. (1987) *The Growing Divide: A Social Audit 1979–1987*, London: Child Poverty Action Group.

Wallen, J., Waitzkin, H. and Stoeckle, J. D. (1979) 'Physician stereotypes about female health and illness', *Women and Health*, 4: 135–46.

Walter, T. (1990) *Funerals and How to Improve Them*, London: Hodder & Stoughton.

Walter, T. (1991) 'Modern death: taboo or not taboo?', *Sociology*, 25: 293–310.

Walter, T. (1996) 'Facing death without tradition', in G. Howarth and P. Jupp (eds) *Contemporary Issues in the Sociology of Death, Dying and Disposal*, Basingstoke: Macmillan.

Walter, T. (2003) 'Historical and cultural variants on the good death', *British Medical Journal*, 327, 7408: 218–20.

Walter, T., Littlewood, J. and Pickering, M. (1995) 'Death in the news: the public invigilation of private emotion' *Sociology*, 29: 579–96.

Walton, J. (1980) 'Urban political economy', *Comparative Urban Research*, 7: 1.

Ware, J. E. (1992) Measures for a new era of health assessment, in A. L. Stewart and J. E. Ware (eds) *Measuring Functioning and Well-Being*, London: Duke University Press.

Ware, J. E., Snow, K. K., Kosinski, M. and Gandek, B. (1993) *The SF36 Health Survey Manual and Interpretation Guide*, Boston, Massachusetts: The Health Institute, New England Medical Center.

Warr, P. (1983) 'Work, jobs and unemployment', *Bulletin of the British Psychological Society*, 36: 305–11.

Warr, P. (1987) *Work, Unemployment and Mental Health*, Oxford: Clarendon Press.

Watson, J. (1988) *Nursing: Human Science and Human Care*, New York: National League for Nursing.

Waxler, N. E. (1975) 'The normality of deviance: an alternate explanation of schizophrenia in the family', *Schizophrenia Bulletin*, 14: 38–47.

Weich, S. and McManus, S. (2002) 'Common mental disorders', in K. Sproston and J. Nazroo (eds) *Ethnic Minority Illness Rates in the Community (EMPIRIC) – Quantitative Report*, London: The Stationery Office, pp. 25–45.

Weiss, R. S. (1974) 'The provisions of social relationships', in Z. Rubin (ed.) *Doing Unto Others*, Englewood Cliffs, NJ: Prentice Hall.

Weisman, A. D. (1992) Commentary on Corr's 'A task-based approach to coping with dying', *Omega*, 24, 2: 95–6.

Weissman, M. M. (1979) 'Environmental factors in affective disorders', *Hospital Practice*, 14: 103–9.

Weissman, M. M. and Klerman, G. L. (1977) 'Sex differences and the epidemiology of depression', *Archives of General Psychiatry*, 34: 98–111.

Weitz, R. (1989) 'Uncertainty and the lives of persons with AIDS', *Journal of Health and Social Behaviour*, 30: 270–81.

West, C. (1983) '"Ask me no questions. . . .": an analysis of queries and replies in physician–patient dialogues', in S. Fisher and A. Todd (eds) *The Social Organization of Doctor–Patient Communication*, Norwood, N. J.: Ablex.

West, P. (1997) 'Health inequalities in the early years: is there equalisation in youth?', *Social Science and Medicine*, 44: 833–58.

West, P., Macintyre, S., Annandale, E. *et al.* (1990) 'Social class and health in youth: findings from the West of Scotland Twenty-07 Study', *Social Science & Medicine*, 30: 665–73.

West, P. and Sweeting, H. (2003) 'Fifteen, female and stressed: changing patterns of psychological distress over time', *Journal of Child Psychology and Psychiatry*, 44: 399–411.

Wheller, L., Baker, A. and Griffiths, C. (2006) 'Trends in premature mortality in England and Wales 1950–2004', *Health Statistics Quarterly*, 31: 34–41.

Wheller, L., Baker, A., Griffiths, C. and Rooney, C. (2007) 'Trends in avoidable mortality in England and Wales, 1993–2005', *Health Statistics Quarterly*, 34, Summer: 6–17.

White, C., van Galen, F. and Chow, Y. H. (2003) 'Trends in social class differences in mortality by cause, 1986 to 2000', *Health Services Quarterly*, 20, Winter: 25–37.

White, C., Glickman, M., Johnson, B. and Corbin, T. (2007) 'Social inequalities in adult male mortality by National Statistics Socio-economic Classification', *Health Statistics Quarterly*, 36, Winter: 6–18.

White, C., Edgar, G. and Siegler, V. (2008) 'Social inequalities in male mortality for selected causes of death by the National Statistics Socio-economic Classification, England and Wales, 2001–2003', *Health Statistics Quarterly*, 38, Summer: 19–32.

White, K. (1991) 'The Sociology of health and illness', *Current Sociology*, 39, 2: 1–115.

Whitehead, M. (1988) *The Health Divide*, Harmondsworth: Penguin.

Wicks, S., Hjern, A., Gunnell, D. *et al.* (2005) 'Social adversity in childhood and the risk of developing psychosis: A national cohort study', *American Journal of Psychiatry*, 162: 1652–7.

Wigley, K. and Clarke, B. (2000) *Kids.net*, London: National Opinion Poll (quoted in Livingstone, S. and M. Bober, 2003, op. cit.).

Wild, S. H., Fischbacher, C., Brock, A., Griffiths, C. and Bhopal, R. (2007) 'Mortality from all causes and circulatory disease by country of birth in England and Wales 2001–2003, *Journal of Public Health*, 29, 2: 191–8.

Wilkinson, G. S. (1975) 'Patient–audience social status and the social construction of psychiatric disorders: toward a differential frame of reference hypothesis', *Journal of Health and Social Behaviour*, 16: 28–38.

Wilkinson, R. G. (1986) 'Income and mortality', in R. G. Wilkinson (ed.) *Class and Health: Research and Longitudinal Data*, London: Tavistock.

Wilkinson, R. and Marmot, M. (eds) (1998) *The Social Determinants of Health: The Solid Facts*, Geneva: World Health Organisation.

Williams, J. and Watson, G. (1996) 'Mental health services that empower women' in T. J. Heller *et al.* (eds), op. cit.

Williams, R. (1976) *Keywords: A Vocabulary of Culture and Society*, London: Fontana.

Williams, R. G. A. (1983) 'Concepts of health: an analysis of lay logic', *Sociology*, 17: 185–204.

Willmott, P. (1984) *Community in Social Policy*, Discussion Paper No. 9, London: Policy Studies Institute.

Willmott, P. (1986) *Social Networks, Informal Care and Public Policy*, London: Policy Studies Institute.

Willmott, P. (1987) 'Community and social structure', *Policy Studies*, 8, 1: 52–63.

Willmott, P. (1989) *Community Initiatives: Patterns and Prospects*, London: Policy Studies Institute.

Wing, J. K. (1973) 'Schizophrenia: medical and social models', unpublished paper quoted in A. Clare (1980), op. cit.

Wing, J. K. (ed.) (1975) *Schizophrenia from Within*, London: National Schizophrenia Fellowship.

Wing, J. K. (ed.) (1982) 'Long-term community care: experience in a London borough', *Psychological Medicine*, 12, Supplement 2: 1–97.

Witz, A. (1990) 'Patriarchy and professions: the gendered politics of occupational closure', *Sociology*, 24, 4: 675–90.

Woods, L. M., Rachet, B., Riga, M., Stone, N., Shah, A. and Coleman, M. P. (2005) 'Geographical variation in life expectancy at birth in England and Wales is largely explained by deprivation', *Journal of Epidemiology and Community Health*, 59: 115–20.

World Health Organisation (WHO) (1959) *Mental Health Problems of Ageing and the Aged*, Technical report, no. 171, WHO.

World Health Organisation (WHO) (1984) *Report of the Working Group on Concepts and Principles of Health Promotion*, WHO.

World Health Organisation (WHO) (1986) *Ottawa Charter for Health Promotion*, Canada: WHO.

World Health Organisation (2001) *Strengthening Mental Health Promotion*, Geneva: WHO, Fact sheet No. 220.

Wrong, D. H. (1961) 'The oversocialised conception of man', *American Sociological Review*, 26: 183–93.

Wyke, S. and Hewison, J. (eds) (1991) *Child Health Matters: Caring for Children in the Community*, Milton Keynes: Open University Press.

Young, J. T. (2004) 'Illness behaviour: a selective review and synthesis', *Sociology of Health & Illness*, 26, 1: 1–31.

Young, M. and Willmott, P. (1957) *Family and Kinship in East London*, London: Routledge and Kegan Paul.

Young, M. and Willmott, P. (1973) *The Symmetrical Family*, London: Routledge and Kegan Paul.

Zandbelt, L. C., Smets, E. M. A., Oort, F. J., Godfried, M. H. and de Haes, H. C. J. M. (2006) 'Determinants of physicians' patient-centred behaviour in the medical specialist encounter', *Social Science & Medicine*, 63: 899–910.

Zborowski, M. (1952) 'Cultural components in response to pain', *Journal of Social Issues*, 8: 16–30.

Zelizer, V. A. (1985) *Pricing the Priceless Child: The Changing Social Value of Children*, New York: Basic Books.

Zimmermann, C. and Rodin, G. (2004) 'The denial of death thesis: sociological critique and implications for palliative care', *Palliative Medicine*, 18: 121–8.

Zola, I. K. (1966) 'Culture and symptoms: an analysis of patients presenting complaints', *American Sociological Review*, 31: 615–30.

Zola, I. K. (1973) 'Pathways to the doctor – from person to patient', *Social Science and Medicine*, 7: 677–89.

Zola, I. K. (1983) *Socio-Medical Inquiries: Recollections, Reflections and Reconsiderations*, Philadelphia: Temple University Press.

Index